A Practical Synopsis Of Cutaneous Diseases: According To The Arrangement Of Dr. Willan

Thomas Bateman, Robert Willan, Anthony Todd Thompson

EIGHT ORDERS
of
Cutaneous Diseases.

1. Pimples.

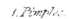
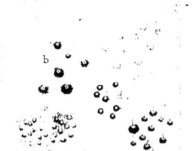

2. Scales.

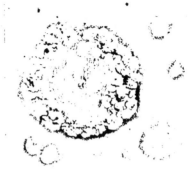

3. Rashes.

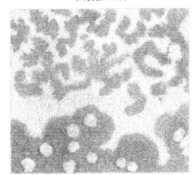

4. Bullæ.

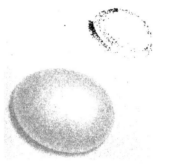

5. Pustules.

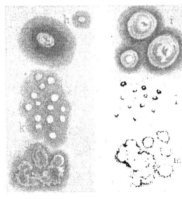

6. Vesicles.

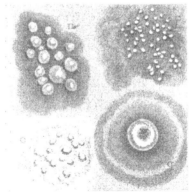

7. Tubercles.

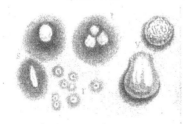

8. Spots.

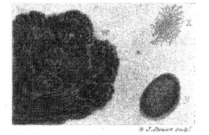

T. B. delin.

J. Stewart Sculp.

Pub.d by Longman & C.o May. 1829.

A

PRACTICAL SYNOPSIS

OF

CUTANEOUS DISEASES,

ACCORDING TO THE ARRANGEMENT OF

DR. WILLAN;

EXHIBITING A CONCISE VIEW OF THE DIAGNOSTIC
SYMPTOMS AND THE METHOD OF TREATMENT.

BY THOMAS BATEMAN, M.D. F.L.S.

PHYSICIAN TO THE PUBLIC DISPENSARY, AND CONSULTING PHYSICIAN
TO THE FEVER INSTITUTION.

THE SEVENTH EDITION.

EDITED BY

ANTHONY TODD THOMSON, M.D. F.L.S.

MEMBER OF THE ROYAL COLLEGE OF PHYSICIANS,
AND PROFESSOR OF MATERIA MEDICA AND PHARMACY IN THE
UNIVERSITY OF LONDON, ETC. ETC.

LONDON:

PRINTED FOR
LONGMAN, REES, ORME, BROWN, AND GREEN,
PATERNOSTER-ROW.
1829.

LONDON:
Printed by A. & R. Spottiswoode,
New-Street-Square.

ADVERTISEMENT.

In putting forth a new edition of this work of the late Dr. Bateman, the Editor has purposely refrained from altering the arrangement of the diseases of which it treats; from a desire that the work should still retain the stamp and impression given to it by its excellent Author. In stating his conviction that no arrangement is free from imperfections, the Editor does not mean to enlist himself with those who affect to despise nosological arrangements: on the contrary, he accords with every sentiment of the Author on this subject*; and believes that it is not by the loose manner of imparting information, which has of late years prevailed in medical writings, that a correct knowledge of the healing art can be communicated to the uninitiated, and the boundaries of the science of medicine extended.

* See the Preface.

A 2

The chief object of the Editor has been to render the work as useful to the student as possible; with this view he has added the synonyms of each genus and species; and, by giving the definitions in a distinct form, has endeavoured to impress on the whole a more definite character. The opportunities which have been afforded to him, from his connection with two extensive medical, charitable institutions, have enabled him to add considerably to the practical part of the work; and he trusts that, in this respect, the present edition will be found not unworthy of the confidence of the practitioner. It is the wish of the Editor still to improve this portion of the volume; and he shall anxiously embrace every opportunity which his brethren may afford him of doing so, conscious that much may be done in improving the treatment of a class of diseases, which have hitherto been regarded more as affording opportunities for empirical experiment, than for the application of those principles which are founded upon an accurate knowledge of physiology and pathology. Another change, from which he hopes the student will derive advantage, is the addition, at the close of each genus, of lists of the works which may be consulted on the diseases that constitute the genera. Much of the difficulty, indeed, which a young man has to encounter in the early pursuit of his profession, arises from his ignorance of the sources whence he can derive information; the Editor, therefore, is assured that this part of his labours will be justly appreciated.

The advantage of plates to aid the descriptions of cutaneous eruptions is undeniable; for without such an appeal to the eye it is almost impossible for the student to form a correct idea of the most accurate description. The delineations of the Author of the Synopsis are admirably calculated to fulfil such an object; but they are executed on a scale of expense which places them far beyond the reach of the student. To supply a remedy for this obstacle in the path of the student, the Atlas of Plates, now appended, as it were, to the Synopsis, has been constructed. It contains almost all that really relates to the diseases delineated in Dr. Bateman's plates, with the addition of several original representations. To give them the character of demonstrations, the different stages of the eruptions, and other peculiarities necessary to be pointed out, are marked upon the plates.

By this plan the troublesome method of examining plates by means of letters and figures of reference is avoided; and without lessening in any degree the beauty of the representation, the utility of the plates is greatly enhanced.

The Editor is perfectly sensible that his part of the volume is not free from defects: he trusts, however, notwithstanding these, that the merit of having endeavoured to improve a most useful work will not be denied to him. He is responsible for all the parts, in the text, contained within inverted commas, and for those notes marked with his initial. Such as this edition is, he commits it to the Public and to the Profession; and is willing to abide by their award, whether it be favourable or adverse.

A. T. T.

3, Hinde-street, Manchester-square,
April, 1829.

THE AUTHOR'S
PREFACE.

To prevent any misapprehension in regard to the nature and object of this volume, it may be necessary to state, that it is not brought forward with any pretensions to supply the deficiencies which have been left in the valuable treatise of Dr. Willan, or to be considered as the completion of that original work. Its sole purpose is to present an abstract of the classification proposed by that respected author, together with a concise view of all the genera and species, which he intended that it should comprehend. The materials for the description of the first four Orders have been obtained principally from Dr. Willan's publication, of which the first part of this Synopsis may be regarded as an abridgment; some additional facts, however, have been supplied from subsequent observation. The remainder

of the matter has been derived partly from
personal experience and research, but principally from a constant intercourse with Dr.
Willan, upon the subject of these diseases,
during a period of ten years, while his colleague
at the Public Dispensary, and from his own
communications in his last illness, before he
departed for Madeira, when he kindly under-
took a cursory perusal of his unfinished MSS.
for my information, during which I made
notes relative to those points with which I
was least acquainted. For it was, in fact, his
wish, that the Profession should possess a
sketch of the whole of his arrangement, even
when the completion of his own treatise,
though distant, was not without hope. Were
I capable of following my learned preceptor
through the literary and historical researches
which enriched his publication, it would be
altogether incompatible with my plan. I
have, however, deemed it advisable to introduce into notes some brief illustrations and
references, which, without interrupting the
practical details, may satisfy the reader that
the principles of the classification and nomenclature were not adopted without the sanction
of reason and authority.

I am far from maintaining that this arrangement of cutaneous diseases is altogether free from material imperfections; (for what artificial arrangement of natural objects has yet been devised, to which imperfections may not be imputed?) but I apprehend, it will be impossible to study it carefully and practically, without deriving benefit from the exercise. I am aware, indeed, that there are many individuals, professing themselves to be practical men, who affect a contempt for all nosological disquisitions, and deem the discussions relating to nomenclature, in particular, very idle and frivolous, or, at the best, a sort of literary amusement, which is not conducive, in the smallest degree, to the improvement of the medical art. But this I conceive to be a mistaken view of the subject, originating perhaps from indolence, or from a want of habitual precision in the use of language. The inferences of slight and superficial observation may, indeed, be detailed without recourse to a very definite vocabulary; for, where little discrimination is exercised, very little nicety can be requisite in regard to the import of the language employed. But it is not by such means that the boundaries of science are extended.

Among the manifest advantages of a copious

and definite nomenclature, may be mentioned, in the first place, the necessity, which it demands, of an accurate investigation of phænomena, or, in other words, the habitual analytic turn which it tends to give to our enquiries, and therefore the general improvement of the talent of observation, which it must ultimately produce. Secondly, it contributes to facilitate the means of discrimination, by multiplying, as it were, the instruments of distinct conception; for from a deficiency of terms we are apt to think and even to observe indistinctly. But, above all, a definite nomenclature supplies us with the means of communicating, with precision, the information which we acquire, and therefore contributes directly to the advancement of knowledge, or at least removes an otherwise insurmountable impediment to its progress.

In this view, such a nomenclature, as far as regards the diseases of the skin, is obviously a great desideratum. For, while the language taught us by the fathers of medicine, relative to all other classes of disease, is clear and intelligible, the names of cutaneous disorders have been used in various acceptations, and without much discrimination, from the days of Hippocrates, and still more vaguely since

the revival of learning in modern times.
From that period, indeed, the diseases of the
skin have been generally designated by some
few terms of universal import, which therefore
carried no import at all. Hence the words
Leprosy, Scurvy, Herpes, Scabies, Dartres,
and some other appellations, have become so
indefinite, as to be merely synonyms of
cutaneous disease. Even the more scientific
enquirers, whose knowledge of diseases was not
always equal to their learning, or whose learning fell short of their pathological skill, have
interpreted the generic and specific appellations of the ancients in various senses. They
have not only differed, for instance, in their
acceptation of general terms, such as of the
words *pustule, phlyctæna, exanthema, erythema,
phyma, phlyzacium*, &c.; but the particular
appellations *Lichen, Psora, Herpes, Impetigo,
Porrigo, Scabies*, and many others, have been
arbitrarily appropriated to very different
genera of disease. The practical errors, which
must necessarily have resulted from such a
confusion in the use of terms, are very numerous, as every one must be satisfied, who
has attempted to study the subject in books.
It may be sufficient to allude to the gross
misapplication of the remedies of the petechial

or sea-scurvy, which have been prescribed for the cure of inflammatory, scaly, and pustular diseases, merely because the epithet *scorbutic* has been vaguely assigned to them all; and to specify the single instance of the administration of tincture of cantharides in the scaly Lepra, on the recommendation of Dr. Mead; who, however, seems to have spoken of the tubercular Elephantiasis, or the non-squamous Leuce; although it would be very difficult to ascertain his meaning.

Most of the writers, who have composed express treatises on cutaneous diseases, in modern times, have implicitly adopted the nomenclature of the ancients, without attempting to render it more definite, or to improve upon the diagnosis which they had pointed out. The essays of Mercurialis, Hafenreffer, Bonacursius, and Turner, were written after this manner; and even Lorry, in his able and elegant work, does not step far out of the ancient path. About the year 1780, however, an elaborate classification of the diseases of the skin was published by Prof. Plenck, of the university of Buda; and subsequently to the commencement of Dr. Willan's publication, a sort of arrangement has been proposed, in the splendid and pompous performance of M. Alibert, which however is altogether destitute of method.

The arrangement of Plenck is founded upon the same principles as that of Dr. Willan, namely, upon the external appearances of the eruptions: but, in filling up the scheme, he has deviated widely from the strict laws of classification which naturalists have established. Nine of his fourteen classes very nearly correspond with the eight orders of Dr. Willan. * These are, 1. Maculæ; 2. Pustulæ; 3. Vesiculæ; 4. Bullæ; 5. Papulæ; 6. Crustæ; 7. Squamæ; 8. Callositates; and 9. Excrescentiæ. But the five remaining classes comprise, 10. Ulcera; 11. Vulnera; 12. Insecta cutanea; 13. Morbi Unguium; and 14. Morbi Capillorum, which are less judiciously devised. But such a classification must fail to answer its end, because it requires the different stages of the same disease to be considered as so many distinct maladies, and to be arranged in several classes. For example, the Crustæ

---

* It seems probable, indeed, that Dr. Willan was indebted to this work of Professor Plenck for the groundwork of his classification; since his definitions, as well as his terms, accord accurately with those of the Hungarian nosologist.

and the Ulcera cutanea are equally the result of Pustules, Vesicles, and Bullæ, and sometimes even of Scales: hence, while Smallpox and Scabies are arranged among the Pustules, and Lepra (by which he understands Elephantiasis) among the Papulæ, the Crusts, which succeed them, are all brought together as species of one genus, in the class of Crustæ. In like manner, particular symptoms are classed as distinct genera: thus the " Rugositas" and the " Rhagades" of the same Elephantiasis are found in the classes of Squamæ and Ulcera respectively. In short, this Elephantiasis is divided into no less than four genera, and its parts arranged under four different classes — an error, which renders the purposes of the classification almost nugatory.

M. Alibert, with loud pretensions to superior skill, and much vaunting of the services which he has rendered this department of medicine, has, in fact, contributed nothing to the elucidation of the obscurity in which it is veiled. The merit of his publication belongs principally to the artists, whom he has had the good fortune to employ: for he has adopted the ancient confusion of terms, without a single definition to fix their acceptation; and he has not scrupled to borrow the nomen-

clature of the vulgar, in its most vague and
indeterminate sense. He has, moreover,
thrown together his genera, without any attention to their affinity or dissimilarity,
making an arbitrary whole of disjointed parts.
Thus his arrangement commences with " Les
Teignes" (Porrigo), which are followed by
" Les Pliques" (Plica or Trichiasis), and by
" Les Dartres" (which seems to be equivalent
to our vulgar and indefinite term *Scurvy*) ; —
and he then passes to the discolorations,
called " Ephélides," to some eruptions, which
he chooses to call " Cancroides," but which
are not intelligibly described, — to the com-
prehensive Lepra, — to Framboesia, — and to
Ichthyosis.

But the total defect of discrimination and
of method is still more obvious in M. Alibert's distribution of the species. The Dartres, for instance, are said to be of seven kinds,
— furfuraceous, scaly, crustaceous, phagedenic, pustular, vesicular, and erythemoid ; so
that, in fact, the appellation has an universal
fitness to almost every form of cutaneous
disease ; it includes at least the Pityriasis,
Psoriasis, Lepra, Impetigo, Ecthyma, Herpes,
Acne, Sycosis, Lupus, and Erythema of this
classification. In like manner, the Lepra in-

cludes some forms of the scaly disease properly so called, together with Leuce or Vitiligo, the tubercular Elephantiasis, and the Barbadoes leg. Thus he unites, under the same generic name, diseases which have no affinity with each other.

From these gross errors the classification of Dr. Willan appears to be entirely free; and the imperfections, which confessedly belong to it, are probably inseparable from the nature of the subject. The truth is, that the various genera of cutaneous disease, as characterized by their external appearances, do not differ in the same essential degree in which the diseases of organs of various structure differ from each other. The same exciting cause will produce different kinds of cutaneous disorder in different individuals: thus, certain substances, which suddenly derange the organs of digestion, sometimes produce Urticaria, sometimes Erythema and Roseola, and sometimes even Lepra and Psoriasis; yet each of these shall retain its specific character, and follow its peculiar course: thus also certain external irritants will, in one case, excite the pustules of Impetigo, and in another the vesicles of Eczema. Again, the diseases which commence with one generic character

are liable occasionally to assume another, in
the course of their progress : — thus, some of
the papular eruptions become scaly, and still
more frequently pustular, if their duration be
long protracted; the Lichen simplex and
circumscriptus, for instance, sometimes pass
into Psoriasis; the Lichen agrius and Prurigo
formicans are occasionally converted into Impetigo; and the Prurigo mitis is changed to
Scabies. Moreover, it frequently happens,
that the characteristic forms of eruptive diseases are not pure and unmixed, but with the
more predominant appearance there is combined a partial eruption of another character;
thus, with the papular Strophulus, with the
rashes of Measles and Scarlet Fever, and with
the pustular Impetigo and Scabies, there is
occasionally an intermixture of lymphatic
vesicles. And, lastly, the natural progress of
many eruptions is to assume a considerable
variety of aspect; so that it is only at some
particular period of their course that their
character is to be unequivocally decided.
Thus in the commencement of Scabies papuliformis and lymphatica, the eruption is of a
vesicular character, although its final tendency
is to the pustular form : and, on the contrary,
in all the varieties of Herpes, the general cha-

racter of the eruption is purely vesicular : yet,
as it advances in its progress, the inclosed
lymph of the vesicles acquires a considerable
degree of opacity, and might be deemed
purulent by cursory observers.   In like manner, the original pustular character of some
of the forms of Porrigo is frequently lost in
the accumulating crusts, the confluent ulcerations, and the furfuraceous exfoliations,
which ensue, and which conceal its true
nature from those who have not seen, and
are unacquainted with, the whole course of
its advancement.

These circumstances constitute a series of
natural impediments to every attempt at a me-
thodical arrangement of cutaneous diseases.
But it is more philosophical, as well as practically useful, to compromise these difficulties,
by retaining in the same station the different
appearances of a disease, in its different stages
and circumstances, when our knowledge of the
causes and remedies, as well as of the natural
progress and termination of it, is sufficient to
establish its identity,—than to separate the
varying symptoms of the same disorder, and to
distribute the *disjecta membra*, not only under
different genera, but into different classes of
the system, after the manner of Prof. Plenck.

Such was the method adopted by Dr. Willan; and although it may sometimes diminish the facility of referring individual appearances to their place in the nosological system, yet it greatly simplifies the classification, as well as the practical indications to which it conducts us.

If, then, the adoption of the arrangement and nomenclature, of which a Synopsis is here given, should lead to more clear and definite views of the various forms of cutaneous disease, and should enable practitioners to write and converse respecting them with perspicuity, by fixing the meaning of the terms which they employ, we may consider this as an important object gained: and it will at length, perhaps, be found, that, for the successful treatment of these diseases, the discovery of new medicines is less necessary than a discriminate appropriation of those which we already possess.

I am fully aware that it is very difficult to convey by words, used in an acceptation that is not familiar, distinct notions of many of the minute changes of appearance in the skin; and that one great deficiency, which Dr. Willan's larger work was calculated to supply, by means of the engravings which accompanied it, will

be left unprovided for by this Synopsis. Perhaps, however, this defect will be partially obviated by the plate prefixed to this volume, in
which I have endeavoured to convey an idea of
the fundamental principles of the classification,
as well as to designate the characters of some
of the more remarkable genera of cutaneous
disease.

T. B.

SKETCH

THE LIFE AND CHARACTER

THOMAS BATEMAN, M. D.*

THOMAS BATEMAN, the learned and ingenious author of this Synopsis, was born at Whitby, in Yorkshire, on the 29th of April 1778. He was of a feeble constitution, and in consequence, perhaps, of that circumstance, naturally diffident and reserved. At four years of age he was placed at a day-school, a step, on the part of his parents, which may be regarded as calculated rather to repress a timid child, than to inspire him with that fearless spirit of enquiry which usually belongs to childhood. This plan was continued until young Bateman was seven years of age, when he was removed from the charge of Mr. Watson, the master of the school, an intimate friend of his father, and a dissenting minister of great learning and talents.

* The materials for this Sketch are furnished by the Life written by his sister.

a 3

It is remarkable, that, during his childhood,
young Bateman discovered no indications of that
reflective and powerful mind which he afterwards
displayed; he showed little pleasure in the acqui-
sition of knowledge, and seldom, voluntarily, sought
the occupation of reading. Thus, in common
with many other great men, his mind resembled a
plant, which, secretly and slowly arriving at maturity, blows with a fresher hue and purer odour
than its companion bud, suddenly and prematurely
disclosed.

It happened that young Bateman was sent into
the country to regain his strength after the measles,
his father, who was an eminent medical practitioner,
remaining at Whitby, and visiting him occasionally
only, when his avocations permitted. At these
times, the anxious and busy parent was grieved to
find that his son had quite abandoned his books
and tasks, and passed the days sitting on the top
of a gate near the house. The remark naturally
was, that " that boy would never be good for any
thing." The fact is, that children who are allowed
to sink into these natural reveries, experience a
relief to their spirits ; and frequently employ such
intervals in digesting the information which they
have attained, or in originating ideas which, at
some future period, are developed and brought
into action.

During this period of apparent inertia, Mr.
Watson had given up his school, and young Bateman was, in consequence, placed with the curate,

who succeeded him. From the tuition of this
gentleman he derived so little advantage, that he
soon became aware, even from his own simple
perception, that he was making little progress; and
on being called up with some other boys, to spell
English, he became so convinced of his master's
deficiency in classical learning, that he earnestly
persuaded his parents to remove him from the
school. He was placed, therefore, under the care
of the Rev. Michael Macheretti, at Thornton, a
village near Whitby; and the most beneficial effects upon his character were soon observable. To
his serious studies he devoted himself with a degree of ardour which was quickly repaid with distinction; his relaxations, music, drawing, and
especially botany, had something above the common
school-boy in them; and he even abstained from
sports, to which, cricket especially, he was partial.

The intellectual powers thus stimulated to activity, his ingenuity was now called into play. His
walks in the fields were enlivened and made salutary,
in two senses, by the collection of a Hortus siccus;
and in this close investigation of nature, materials
for philosophy and religion were created in his
mind. He delighted in Astronomy and Electricity;
and, with wonderful dexterity, contrived to make
a planetarium and an electrical machine from the
drawings in Chambers's Dictionary, cutting the
wheels with his pen-knife; and then transferring
his exertions to the fabrication of an Eolian harp.
It was remarked by his instructors, that the pro-

minent features of his mind were judgment and
energy; in quickness and brilliancy he was deficient. His disposition at this time gave promise
of future eminence in piety and virtue. It is a
beautiful example to the young, that he never required, nor received, punishment when at school.

Dr. Bateman was not deficient in fancy nor in
humour. Some of his early poetic translations from
the Greek and Latin were preserved by his master;
and a few original verses, rallying one of his young
companions upon his want of taste in music. Like
most highly-gifted people when young, he had a
quick perception of what is ludicrous.

At the age of fifteen he lost his father. In consequence of this calamity, young Bateman was
removed from school to the occupation of an apothecary's shop, in order to acquire a knowledge of
Pharmacy. It was wisely thought expedient that he
should continue his general studies, under his old
master. In the plan thus chalked out for him, the
science of mathematics was included : but for this
branch of knowledge Dr. Bateman, at no period of
his life, had any predilection; he was accustomed
to say, that it was the only one which did not give
him pleasure.

At nineteen years of age he was advised to go
to London to pursue his medical education. He
attended the lectures in Windmill-street in 1797
and 1798 ; and, as a physician's pupil, in Guy's
Hospital, he had the advantage of receiving the
instructions of Dr. Baillie, then in the zenith of

his reputation. For this great, and justly-honoured physician, Dr. Bateman always entertained a profound respect, enhanced, probably, by the congeniality of their moral sentiments. Looking at his profession, not merely as a means of acquiring money, but as a mode of practising benevolence and charity, the assiduity of the young student was stimulated by the pure example of similar motives which the conduct of Dr. Baillie presented.

From 1798 until 1801 Mr. Bateman resided at Edinburgh, where he acted as clinical clerk of the elder Professor Duncan, at the Infirmary, and entered with full spirit into all the institutions of the University. In the Medical Society, in particular, Mr. Bateman distinguished himself; for, although his speeches had little rhetorical ornament to attract the attention of the indifferent listener, yet they were always fraught with good sense, and displayed such a masterly acquaintance with the details of his subject, that they carried conviction with them in favour of the side which he espoused. The great importance of such societies in a university is undeniable. In the Medical Society of Edinburgh, some of the leading doctrines which have governed, at different periods, both the practice and the opinions of the medical world, were first submitted to the test of criticism : and some of the greatest men that have adorned the profession essayed their talents in that society. It is a curious fact, that few of those students who have taken the lead in the discussions of the Medical Society of Edin-

sent to him through his ambassador : at the same time a ring, of a hundred guineas value, was pre- sented to Dr. Bateman as a testimony of imperial approbation.

While honours and success thus rewarded his exertions, his health, which had never been strong, was irremediably injured by incessant application. Periodical head-aches, loss of sight in the right eye, and danger of total blindness, impeded his labours in the cause of Science. Occasional resi- dence at the sea-side mitigated indeed these symp- toms; but the digestive organs being much impaired, his health was never restored. From this circum- stance he was obliged to absent himself frequently from London, and in his visits to the romantic parts of our island, he now experienced the happy effects of an early and long-cherished love of Nature, and of her hand-maiden, Poetry. His en- joyment of our English classics was genuine, and it proves how easily even the most refined cultivation of general knowledge may be combined with scien- tific pursuits. But all his various attainments, both in knowledge and virtue, were destined to be sur- rendered, at an early period of life, to the Heavenly Being who had implanted the seeds of goodness. It was consistent with the tenour of his life that the very sacrifice of it was in the exercise of bene- volence. An epidemic fever at this time raged in London ; and seven hundred of the sufferers were received into the Fever Hospital under Dr. Bate- man's charge. The medical officers and attendants

of the hospital suffered from the contagion, and
Dr. Da Costa, who was studying the practice of
medicine in fevers there, died of it.   Dr. Bateman
had the disease slightly, but experienced the worst
effects from the fatigue and anxiety incident to his
unremitting attention to his patients.   From this
time his decline was perceptible; and in 1819 an
attack of his complaints, more severe than usual,
seized him on his road from London to Middleton,
in Durham, whither he was going for the benefit
of the sulphureous springs.   With difficulty he
reached the village of Bishop Burton, near Bever-
ley.   He had already resigned his situation at the
Fever Institution, which he had held fourteen years,
and which was exchanged for that of consulting
physician.   He now determined not to return to the
metropolis, regarding it as too exciting a scene for
one in his shattered state; and on this account he
prepared to relinquish also his arduous duties at the
Public Dispensary.   He was immediately appointed
a life-governor by the committee of that Institution,
and a piece of plate voted to him.   The first of these
testimonies to his merit was declined with reluct-
ance, although originating from Dr. Laird, the
beloved and justly-valued friend of Dr. Bateman,
with whom an intercourse of twenty years' duration
had cemented early prepossessions into mutual
and unalienable regard.

And now the close of an active and useful life
became, to all human observation, inevitable. Frequent indications of some fatal disease, from the

state of languor into which he relapsed, again and again prevented his taking up his abode at Whitby with his sister, and a temporary habitation at Bishop Burton was therefore provided for him. Of his own disease he had the most decided apprehensions, and was at one time persuaded that some organic affection of the heart threatened every hour of his existence, producing, as it were, a fearful vibration of that thread upon which his feeble being hung. It appears, however, that the digestive organs were chiefly affected.

The natural enquiry, upon reviewing the last days of any gifted individual, is, " How did such a man die?" " What were the fears, or recollections, or expectations, by which his moments of solitude and of sickness were disturbed, or cheered?"

To the mere man of the world such questions as these may appear to partake of what is unfairly termed *cant*, or what is superficially deemed hypocrisy. To the rational enquirer, however, the death of no fellow-mortal can be imparted without awakening such feelings as suggest the queries that have just been hinted. This digression must be pardoned as a necessary introduction to the affecting and singular termination of Dr. Bateman's life.

In common with many men mixing in the busy world, Dr. Bateman had cherished and practised a code of morality founded upon those principles of expediency and propriety which constitute what is commonly called " honour." He went farther, too, than many mere superficial characters would have been in danger of doing : he leaned towards materialism; and even doubted the truth of Divine Revelation. It was for sickness and hopelessness of this world's prolonged enjoyments to bring his chastened heart to truth. The narrative of what may be termed his conversion has been succinctly, and we believe accurately, related by the friend who was, under Providence, the instrument of effecting this great change in the mind of Dr. Bateman; but, whilst every sincere believer must rejoice at the good work, it is to be lamented, for the sake of Christianity, that the zeal of the pious agent in this good cause has couched the narrative in terms neither likely to convince the sceptical, nor to reclaim the depraved portion of society. Unless we can minutely follow the workings of the heart, confidentially imparted, as in the case of Lord Rochester; and unless those emotions are imparted in simple language, free from the infusion of any prevailing doctrines; we are apt to wonder at the suddenness of the conversion, and to doubt whether anxiety to illustrate particular modes of faith does not add vivacity to the description.

Such are the impressions incident to the first perusal of the account of Dr. Bateman's change, published in the Christian Observer. Upon a more deliberate revision of the statement, it appears, however, not extraordinary that a strong mind, indifferent, if not averse, to religious enquiry, should, on bending its great force to the overwhelming subject of Revelation, be suddenly in a

state of conviction to which weaker understand-
ings would be slower in arriving. One leading
truth once admitted, the great fabric of religious
belief would soon be reared. Still there are many
drawbacks to the certainty of a satisfactory
conviction; and the variations of his persuasion
and of his hopes kept the mind of Dr. Bateman
in a state of great anxiety for a considerable time.
Sometimes, security and peace, he longed to
depart before this happy confidence could subside. Then, in an agony of doubt concerning
the miracles of our Saviour, he dreaded lest the
hour of dissolution should find him in this dismal
and heart-rending uncertainty. Unhappily, his
well-intentioned but ill-judging friends directed his
attention too much to points of doctrine, which
have been stumbling-blocks even to the pious, and
of which the great God of Nature has given us only
intimations, not proofs. Perplexed by dread, and
agitated by spiritual conflicts, the situation of Dr.
Bateman presents an awful lesson to those who put
by the work of religious reflection till the shadow
of death approaches, and a weakened and trembling
mind can offer but an imperfect tribute of belief
and praise to its Creator. At last, however, the
" fitful" fever of Dr. Bateman's agitated spirit
subsided. A temporary gleam of restored health
mercifully lent its aid. His hopes became settled;
his belief firm; and he was enabled even to bless
the bodily afflictions which had brought him to a
proper sense of religion. Patience, resignation,

and charity, were the happy fruits of this "living" faith. He would not permit his maladies to be called sufferings, nor allow them to be any thing but inconveniences. Once, to his afflicted mother, who was watching his bed-side in the night, he said, " Surely you are not in tears. Mine is a case that calls for rejoicing, not for sorrow. Only think what it will be to drop this poor, frail, perishing body, and go to the glories which are set before me!" At length the struggle ceased; and, with a full conviction of the truth, he expired, calmly, and without convulsions, on the 9th of April, the very day twelvemonths on which he had first been aroused from his state of infidelity.

Such was Dr. Bateman as a man: as a physician, few whose labours have terminated at so early a period of life deserve a higher eulogium. Dr. Bateman's mind was not of a character to be satisfied with a superficial knowledge of any subject whatsoever, which attracted his attention. He carried his enquiries into the minutest details, and was dissatisfied until he felt assured that he understood every point of his investigation, in all its bearings. As we have had occasion already to remark, his reading was most extensive, and he was unwearied in his researches into every part of any subject that could be elucidated by observation. His mode of investigating disease was extremely happy; the questions he put had always some bearing upon the obscure points of the case; and

b

his mode of putting them was such as to convince his patient that his utmost attention was given to the subject; and, consequently, his manner was admirably calculated to secure the confidence of both the patient and his friends.

Dr. Bateman's Medical writings speak for themselves. His *Synopsis* and *Delineations*, whatever differences of opinion may exist respecting the arrangement and classification of the diseases, have done more to advance the knowledge of cutaneous affections than any works which have preceded them. His Account of the *Typhus or Contagious Fever*, exemplified in the Epidemic which prevailed in the metropolis in 1817 and 1818, displays a talent for observation, a correct discrimination of symptoms, a decision in the application of remedies, and a simplification of treatment, which would be honourable to a physician of any standing; and afforded to his medical friends an anticipation of the high rank which its author, had he lived, was destined to hold as a practical physician. Besides these works, and the articles in the medical department of *Rees's Encyclopædia*, which our author avowed as the productions of his pen, Dr. Bateman furnished the excellent reports of the Carey-street Dispensary, and much of the valuable information connected with the practice of the metropolis, which, for many years, enriched the pages of the Edinburgh Medical and Surgical Journal. He also, in conjunction with others, his medical friends, contributed largely to the *Annual Medical Register*, a work that was published in 1809-10; and which, like many other productions intended to advance solely the science of the profession, did not meet with patronage sufficient to justify its continuance.

Upon the whole, it may be truly said of the Author of the Synopsis, that few men have achieved so much in so short a course of years; that he sacrificed his life to the love of his profession; and that he has deservedly merited a place among the honoured few, whose exertions have contributed to dispel the clouds which so long obscured the light of Science from the paths of Practical Medicine.

April 6th, 1829.

EXPLANATION OF THE PLATE.

THE eight compartments of the plate exhibit the eight forms of cutaneous eruptions.

Fig. 1. represents five varieties of *Papulæ*, as they are seen in (a) Strophulus confertus, (b) Lichen simplex, (c) Lichen pilaris, (d) Lichen lividus, and (e) Prurigo mitis.

Fig. 2. shows the *Scales* and circular patches of Lepra vulgaris.

Fig. 3. exhibits two forms of *Exanthemata* or *Rashes*, viz. (f) the Measles, and (g) the febrile Nettle-rash.

Fig. 4. shows the *Bullæ* of Pompholyx diutinus, in different stages of their progress.

Fig. 5. illustrates the four forms of *Pustules*, namely, the *Phlyzacia*, as they appear in (h) Ecthyma vulgare, and in (i) Scabies purulenta upon the hands; — the *Psydracia*, as they arise in (k) Impetigo, and afterwards form a scab; — the *Achores* (l), of Porrigo scutulata, on the scalp; — and the *Favi* (m), as they appear on the scalp and other parts.

Fig. 6. contains three genera of *Vesicles;* namely, patches of (n) Herpes zoster, and (o) Herpes phlyctænodes; (p) Miliary vesicles; and (q) the Vaccine vesicle.

Fig. 7. exhibits different forms of *Tubercles;* as in (r) Acne punctata, and (s) Acne indurata; in (t) Sycosis; and in (v) Molluscum.

Fig. 8. contains specimens of *Maculæ;* viz. (w) a Nævus compared to the stain of red wine; (x) a spider Nævus; and (y) a mole.

The Diseases of the Skin were arranged by Dr. WILLAN in eight Orders, according to their external forms, as in the following Table.

Recently were published by Longman, Rees, Orme, Brown, and Green, London.

1. DELINEATIONS of the CUTANEOUS DISEASES comprised in the Classification of the late Dr. Willan; including the greater part of the Engravings of that Author, in an improved State, and completing the Series as intended to have been finished by him.

By the late T. BATEMAN, M.D. F.L.S., &c.

In one volume, 4to. with upwards of 70 coloured plates, price 12*l.* 12*s.* boards.

The Series of New Engravings, representing those Diseases which should have been figured in the subsequent Parts of Dr. Willan's unfinished Work, may be had by the possessors of that Work, separate, price 7*l.* boards.

2. A SUCCINCT ACCOUNT of the CONTAGIOUS FEVER of this COUNTRY, as exemplified in the Epidemic now prevailing in London; with the appropriate Method of Treatment as practised in the House of Recovery.

To which are added,

OBSERVATIONS on the NATURE and PROPERTIES of CONTAGION, tending to correct the popular Notions on this Subject, and pointing out the Means of Prevention.

By the late THOMAS BATEMAN, M.D. F.L.S., &c.

3. REPORTS on the DISEASES of LONDON, and the State of the Weather, from 1804 to 1816, including practical Remarks on the Causes and Treatment of the former.

By the late THOMAS BATEMAN, M.D. In 8vo. 9*s.* bds.

A

PRACTICAL SYNOPSIS

OF

CUTANEOUS DISEASES.

Order I.

·PAPULÆ.

SYN. Ἐξόρμια (*G.*): Exormia (*Good*): Papula (*Sauv. Lin.*): Bouton, Elevure, Papule (*F.*): die Finne, Knoten (*Ger.*): Sheri (*Arab.*): *Pimples.*

Def. PAPULA (*Pimple*); A SMALL AND ACUMI-NATED ELEVATION OF THE CUTICLE, WITH AN INFLAMED BASE, VERY SELDOM CONTAINING A FLUID, OR SUPPURATING, AND COMMONLY TERMI-NATING IN SCURF. *

---

* The term Papula has been used in various acceptations by the older writers, but the nosologists have nearly agreed in restricting it to the sense here adopted. Sauvages defines it, " Phyma parvulum, desquamari solitum." (Nosol. Meth. class i. Synops. ord. ii. 6.) The definition of Linnæus is " Tuberculum faretum, coloratum, inflam-matum, vix suppurandum." (Linnæi Gen. Morbor. class xi. ord. 4.) In this sense also Celsus seems to have understood the term, although he uses it generally : for when he calls it a disease, in which " the skin is made *rough* and *red* by very minute pustules," he means obviously dry papulæ; as by the word pustula he understands every *elevation* of the skin, even wheals. (De Med. lib. v. cap. 28. §§ 15. and 18.)

B

PAPULÆ, or Pimples, are generally supposed to originate in an inflammation of the papillæ of the skin, by which these are enlarged, elevated, and indurated, and made to assume more or less of a red colour. It is, however, equally probable that the minute elevation which constitutes a pimple, is the consequence of inflammation in a capillary vessel ; and as Mr. Plumbe has suggested, " a minute escapement of lymph" from it.* We even perceive, sometimes, that a slight effusion of lymph has taken place, which gives a vesicular appearance to several of the papulæ ; but the fluid is re-absorbed without breaking the cuticle ; and papulæ terminate for the most part in scurf.

The varieties of papulous eruptions are comprehended in this arrangement under three genera ; namely,

    1. STROPHULUS,
    2. LICHEN †,
    3. PRURIGO.

Dr. Mason Good derives the term Papula from πωππος, the sprouting of down or buds ; and regards the radical sense to be " production, or putting forth." He derives the terminating diminutive from the Greek ὕλη, " materia, materies," thus, Papula, " of the matter or nature of Pappus." (Nosology, p. 460.) T.

* Prac. Treatise on Diseases of the Skin. 1st ed. p. 187.

† Rayer regards Strophulus merely as a modification of Lichen in young infants ; and there is much probability in his remark. See *Traité Théorique et Pratique des Maladies de la Peau*, 8vo. Paris, 1826. vol. i. p. 360. T.

Genus I. STROPHULUS.

Syn. Licheniasis Strophulus (*Young*) : Exanthema Strophulus (*Parr*): Bouton, Efflorescence cutanée, Ebullition, Feux de Dents, Strophulus (*F.*): Carpang (*Tamool*): *Gum Rash.*

Def. An eruption of pimples in early infancy, chiefly on the face, neck, arms, and loins; generally in clusters, surrounded with a reddish halo.

This genus comprises several papular affections, peculiar to infants, which are known by the common appellations of *red gum, tooth-eruption,* &c. They arise, in consequence of the extreme vascularity and irritability of the skin at that period of life, when the constitution is accidentally disturbed by irritations, either in the alimentary canal or other parts of the habit; or in the gums. Much of the irritation in the alimentary canal is connected with irregularities in the diet of the mother; and from overfeeding the infant even when it is nourished entirely upon the breast. As these eruptions are not, however, very important objects of medical practice, but interesting only from their occasional resemblance to some of the exanthemata, I shall not dwell upon them at any length. " It is necessary, however, to guard the infant from sudden exposure to cold during the continuance of these eruptions; for, when repelled, the system generally suffers, and sometimes convulsions supervene."

There are five species of Strophulus :

1. S. *intertinctus.*   4. S. *volaticus.*
2. S. *albidus.*   5. S. *candidus.*
3. S. *confertus.*

SPECIES 1.   STROPHULUS *intertinctus,* RED GUM
or GOWN.

Syn. Taches de Lait, Efflorescence benigne (*F.*):
Rothe (*Ger.*): Cheng Carapang (*Tamool*): Kurpān
(*Duk.*): Cārāpānie (*Tel.*): Rooshitum (*Sans.*): *Red
Gum.*

This species of Strophulus (Plate I. of BATEMAN;
Pl. 1. of THE ATLAS,) is characterized by papulæ
of a vivid red colour, situated most commonly on
the cheeks, fore-arms, and back of the hands, but
sometimes universally diffused. They are usually
distinct from one another; but are intermixed with
red dots, or stigmata, and often with large red
patches, which have no elevation. Occasionally a
few small vesicles appear on the hands and feet;
but these soon desiccate, without breaking. " It
generally terminates in scurf."

This eruption is often obviously connected in
young infants with a weak, irritable state of the
alimentary canal, and consequent indigestion * ;
whence it is frequently preceded by sickness of
stomach, and sometimes by diarrhœa. But in its
ordinary mild form it is not inconsistent with good
health, and requires little medical treatment. Daily
ablutions with tepid water, which remove sordes,

---

* Dr. Underwood, with much truth, remarks, that every species of
Strophulus is the effect of a predominant acid. Treat. on the Diseases
of Children, 8vo. 8th edition, p. 167. T.

and promote an equal perspiration, are beneficial; and a proper attention should be enforced both to the kind and quantity of the aliment, and to the regularity of exercise afforded to the child. The cold bath, or even exposure to a stream of cold air, should be avoided during the occurrence of this eruption; and if, in consequence of want of caution in this respect, the eruption shall have disappeared, and sickness, purging, or any other internal disorder have ensued, a warm bath affords the most speedy relief: — " mild aperients, as Rhubarb and Magnesia, combined with a few drops of the Spiritus Ammoniæ compositus internally, or some other slight cordial, and the stimulus of a blister externally, have been found beneficial under these circumstances." *

SPĒCIES 2. STROPHULUS *albidus*, WHITE GUM.

This species (Plate II. of BATEMAN; Pl. 1. of THE ATLAS,) is rather a variety of the preceding than a distinct species; and is occasionally intermixed with it; the papulæ consisting of minute, hard, whitish specks, a little elevated, and sometimes surrounded by a slight redness, and appearing chiefly on the face, neck, and breast.

---

* See Underwood on the Diseases of Children, vol. i. p. 79. 5th edit., and Armstrong on the same subject, p. 84. These alternations of internal and superficial disorder, though not so frequently seen under modern management as under that of the older physicians, take place occasionally in Strophulus, as well as in the measles, and some other exanthemata. In such cases, diarrhœa, tormina, sickness, and sometimes a tendency to syncope or convulsions, ensue.

SPECIES 3. STROPHULUS *confertus*, RANK RED GUM, the TOOTH-RASH.

Strophulus *confertus* (Plate III. fig. 1. of BATE-MAN; Pl. 1. of THE ATLAS,) is distinguished principally by the more extensive crop of papulæ which appears, " and the degree of feverish excitement with which it is generally attended." The patches of papulæ are chiefly seated on the cheeks and forehead, when they occur about the fourth or fifth month, and are smaller, more crowded, and less vivid in their colour, than in the first species. But in children seven or eight months old, they appear in large irregular patches, on the outside of the hands, arms, shoulders, and loins, and are hard and close set, so as to give to the whole surface a high red colour. In about a fortnight they begin to fade and exfoliate, and gradually disappear.

Sometimes, though rarely, a variety of the S. confertus appears on the legs, spreading upwards even to the loins and navel, producing a general redness of the cuticle (not unlike Intertrigo*), which cracks and separates in large pieces, occasioning much distress to the child. " The patches on the lower extremities are always accompanied with troublesome itching." This form of the disease is liable to recur at short intervals, for the space of two or three months.

The S. confertus requires no specific medical treatment, as it appears to be one of the numerous

---

* In Intertrigo the surface is free from papulæ; is shining and uniformly red; and is generally confined to the nates and thighs. T.

symptoms of irritation arising from dentition, and recedes soon after the cutting of the first teeth.* It can only be alleviated " by scarifying the gums, so as to assist the protrusion of the teeth; by the administration of mild aperients, such as Hydrargyrus cum creta;" and by the general treatment proper for the state of teething, with great attention to cleanliness, and frequent tepid ablution with milk and water. In India, the native physicians touch the excoriated parts with a little pure castor oil.

SPECIES 4. STROPHULUS *volaticus*, WILDFIRE RASH.

Syn. Erythema volaticum (*Sauv.*): Feu volage (*F.*): Collie Carpang (*Tamool*).

This species (Plate III. fig. 2. of BATEMAN; Pl. 1. of THE ATLAS,) is not a frequent complaint. It is characterized by small circular patches, or clusters of papulæ, grouped together, arising and exfoliating successively on different parts of the body, of a high red colour, and sometimes attended with slight feverishness. Each patch turns brown in about four days, and begins to exfoliate; and the whole series terminates in three or four weeks.

---

* Dr. Bisset, a physician of the old school, but a man of observation, notices a circumstance respecting children affected with these eruptions, which I think I have seen confirmed in a few cases. After stating that " some children are more or less affected with it till they have got all their first teeth, in spite of every endeavour to repress it, and after that period it recedes spontaneously;" he adds, " but in that case they are apt to have *carious teeth* after the eruption disappears." See his Med. Essays and Obs. § xix. p. 274.

This eruption is usually connected with a disordered state of the stomach and bowels, and is
alleviated by gentle laxatives; after which the decoction of Cinchona, " or infusion of Calumba with
Subcarbonate of Soda," or a slight chalybeate*, is
serviceable. No external application is necessary,
" unless the itching is distressing to the infant; in
which case, the patches may be sponged with vinegar
diluted with two parts of water; or they may be
touched with saliva."

SPECIES 5. STROPHULUS *candidus*, PALLID GUM
RASH.

This species (Plate III. fig. 3. of BATEMAN; Pl. 1.
of THE ATLAS,) is distinguished by papulæ of a
larger size than those of the foregoing species, having no inflammation round their base, and a smooth
and shining surface; whence they appear to be of a
lighter colour than the adjoining cuticle. They are
most frequently seen on the loins, shoulders, and
upper part of the arms; but I have observed them
also on the face and neck, when the S. confertus occupied the fore-arms: after continuing hard and elevated for about a week, they gradually disappear.
This variety of Strophulus commonly succeeds some
of the acute diseases, to which infants about a year

---

* I shall take this opportunity of recommending to the attention of
practitioners a chalybeate medicine, particularly adapted, from its taste-
less quality, to the palates of children, and possessed of more efficacy
than the vinum ferri; I mean a watery solution of the tartrite of iron,
lately introduced by an able and intelligent chemist, Mr. R. Phillips. See
his Experimental Examination of the Pharm. Londinensis, 1811. Its
qualities have been well stated by Dr. Birkbeck, in the London Medical
Review, No. xix. July, 1812.

old are liable. It has occurred also on the arms, when the face was occupied with Porrigo larvalis; and, in one case, it appeared on the arms, thighs, and neck, at the age of three years and a half, during the cutting of the double teeth. It requires no particular treatment, except to regulate the bowels with some mild aperient.

Works which may be consulted on this genus of Papulæ :—

BISSET's Medical Essays and Observations, 8vo. 1766.

PLUMBE On Diseases of the Skin, 8vo. 2d. edit. 1827.

Rayer, Traité des Maladies de la Peau, 8vo. 1826.

WILLAN On Cutaneous Diseases, 4to. 1808.

UNDERWOOD On the Diseases of Children, edited by Dr. *Merriman,* 8vo. 1827.

GENUS II. LICHEN.

Syn. Λειχην (*G.*): Exormia *lichen* (Good): Lichen, Dartre farineuse, poussée, Dartre pustuleuse miliaire, Papules (*F.*): der Zitterich, Flechte (*German*): *Lichenous Rash.*

Def. A DIFFUSE ERUPTION OF RED PAPULÆ, SOMETIMES DISTINCT, SOMETIMES IN CLUSTERS; ACCOMPANIED. WITH A TROUBLESOME SENSATION OF TINGLING OR PRICKING, AND USUALLY TERMINATING IN SCURF; RECURRENT, NOT CONTAGIOUS.*

The original acceptation of the term LICHEN is not distinctly ascertained from the writings of

---

* I have ventured to alter the definition of Dr. Willan, for the same reason which induced Dr. Good to take a similar step. In Willan's definition, which was adopted by Dr. Bateman, in the former editions of this work, the expressions " affecting adults," and " connected with internal disorder," are at variance with some of the species of the genus. T.

Hippocrates, and therefore it has been variously interpreted by succeeding writers.*   The majority have deemed it synonymous with the Impetigo of the Latins : but, as Foës, De Gorter, and other able commentators have remarked, the Impetigo described by the highest Roman authority, Celsus, is a very different disease ; while the Papula of the same author seems to accord more accurately with the Lichen of Hippocrates.†   Whence Dr. Willan decided on affixing the appellation to a papular affection.

There are seven species of this eruption :

1. L. *simplex.*	5. L. *lividus.*
2. L. *pilaris.*	6. L. *tropicus.*
3. L. *circumscriptus.*	7. L. *urticatus.*
4. L. *agrius.*	

* Hippocrates classes the Λειχηνες with Prurigo, Psora, Lepra, and Alphos, without particularizing their characteristic forms.   See his Προῤῥητικον, lib. ii. and his book Περι Παθων, where he considers them as blemishes rather than diseases.   It would seem, indeed, that the Greek writers after him looked upon the Prurigo, Lichen, Psora, and Lepra, as progressive degrees of the same affection ; the first being a simple itching, — the second, itching combined with roughness of the skin — the third, itching with branny exfoliations, — and the last, itching with actual scales.

† See Foës. Œconom. Hippocr. — De Gorter, Medicina Hippocrat. aph. xx. lib. iii.   The latter observes, respecting this aphorism, " In hoc loco, Hippocr. per Leichenas intelligit talem cutis fædationem, in qua summa cutis pustulis siccis admodum prurientibus exasperatur — sed quia humor totus fere volatilis est, non relinquit squamas ut Lepra, neque furfures ut Psora, sed siccam et asperam pustulosam cutim."   It is to be recollected that *pustula,* among the ancients, signified any elevation of the cuticle ; and therefore pustulæ siccæ are papulæ.   If the Lichen, then, be viewed in its concluding stage, when it exhibits a slight furfuraceous roughness, it may be said to have some affinity with the scaly diseases mentioned above ; and, in fact, it sometimes terminates in Psoriasis.   See Aëtius, tetrab. ii. serm. iv. cap. 16. — Actuar. lib. ii. cap. 11. — Celsus de Medicina, lib. v. cap. 28.

SPECIES 1. LICHEN *simplex*, SIMPLE LICHEN.

This species (Plate IV. fig. 1. of BATEMAN; Pl. 2. of THE ATLAS,) is an eruption of red inflamed papulæ, first appearing on the face or on the arms, and extending, in the course of three or four days, to the trunk and lower limbs. It is sometimes preceded for a few days by slight febrile irritation, which commonly ceases when the eruption appears: " but this does not always happen, and the disease occasionally occurs after great exercise in the best state of health." The eruption is accompanied with an unpleasant sensation of tingling, especially in the night : it continues nearly stationary about a week, when its colour begins to fade, and the skin soon exhibits numerous scurfy exfoliations, which remain longest about the flexures of the joints. The duration of the complaint varies considerably, however, from ten days to three weeks.

The disorder is subject to variety also in other respects. The papulæ on the face, for instance, are large and rounded, and some of them form into small tubercles, resembling those of Acne : on the breast and extremities they are more acuminated ; and on the hands they are sometimes obscurely vesicular. In some cases, the eruption is partial, affecting the face, neck, or arms only ; in some, it appears and disappears repeatedly, without leaving any scurf: in others, it is general ; and successive eruptions and exfoliations prolong the complaint for two or three months, and even longer.

The L. simplex is liable to return every spring

or summer in some individuals of irritable constitution. It appears occasionally in those who are subject to severe head-ach, and pains in the stomach, as a sort of crisis to these complaints, which are immediately relieved. It is also, sometimes, a sequela of acute fevers.[*]

This species of Lichen is often mistaken for measles, Scarlatina, and other exanthemata. But a strict attention to the Definitions, and to the course of the symptoms, will enable the observer to avoid such errors. It is sometimes also mistaken for Scabies (itch), and Prurigo, from which it is not always so easily distinguished.[†]

Species 2. Lichen *pilaris*, Hair Lichen.

This form of Lichen (Plate V. fig. 1. of Bateman; Pl. 2. of The Atlas,) is rather a modification of the preceding than a distinct species, the papulæ appearing only at the roots of the hairs of the skin. Like the former, it often alternates with complaints of the head or stomach, in irritable habits. It is not unfrequently connected with that derangement of these organs, which is induced by intemperance in the use of spirits. The great irritability of the

---

[*] See Lorry de Morbis Cutaneis, cap. iii. p. 215.

[†] See Scabies.— Prof. Lorry has stated the principal points of diagnosis with accuracy. Speaking of Lichen, under the appellation of " Papulæ," he says, " Primo a Scabie differunt, quod papulæ illæ vulgo magis confertæ sint et elatiores; 2do, quod rubicundæ magis et minus aridæ sint; 3tio, quod sæpe sanatis febribus superveniant; 4to, quod latiores sint, et sæpius recidivam patiantur quam vera et legitima Scabies; 5to, quod in furfur abeant notabile; 6to, demum quod remediis sanentur a Scabiei curatione alienis." — Loc. cit.

skin is manifest, from the facility with which the papulæ are enlarged into temporary wheals by strong friction, which the itching and tingling compel the patient to resort to. It often assumes a chronic character, and continues for years.

" The treatment of the foregoing species and this variety consists in keeping the bowels lax; in confining the diet to the lightest kinds of fresh animal food, vegetables, and ripe ascescent fruits; to the taking moderate exercise in the open air; and to an occasional use of the tepid bath. Infusion of Cinchona Bark, acidulated with any of the mineral acids; or the solution of Sulphate of Quinia in the infusion of Conserve of Roses, acidulated with diluted Sulphuric Acid, prove useful when the habit is languid."

SPECIES 3. LICHEN *circumscriptus*, CLUSTERED LICHEN.

This species (Plate V. fig. 8. of BATEMAN; Pl. 2. of THE ATLAS,) is characterized by clusters or patches of papulæ which have a well defined margin, and are of an irregularly circular form. * Some of them are stationary for a week or two, and disappear; but others extend gradually, by new papulated borders, into large figured forms,

* This variety of Lichen was not noticed in the first edition of the Order of Papulæ, published by Dr. Willan. It is the first of the two species of Papulæ described by Celsus:—" medium habet pauxillum levius: tarde serpit; idque vitium maxime rotundum incipit, eaque ratione in orbem procedit." De Medicina, lib. v. cap. 28. See also Ingrassias de Tumor. præt. Naturam, tract. 1. cap. 1.

which coalesce.   As the borders extend, the central areæ become even, but continue slightly red and scurfy.   Sometimes, before the scurf is removed, a new crop of papulæ arises, terminating like the former in exfoliations; and by these new eruptions the complaint is prolonged for several weeks.   It may be excited either by internal or external causes of irritation. *   In adults it is occasionally produced by vaccination, and may be deemed a proof of the full affection of the constitution by the virus.

Little medicinal treatment is necessary for these species of Lichen.   It is sufficient that patients avoid heating themselves by much exercise or by stimulants, and take a light diet, " avoiding all spices, wine, and alcoholic liquors;" and adhering to diluent drinks, regulating the bowels with gentle laxatives.   " Reasoning from a knowledge of the great irritability of the skin which attends this disease, we would be led to conclude, what experience has proved to be true, that all diaphoretics and medicines determining the blood to the surface are injurious in Lichen."   The diluted Sulphuric acid is a grateful tonic to the stomach during the period of exfoliation; or a light chalybeate may be

---

* Dr. Good in his " Study of Medicine," under Pratica Spasmodica, remarks, " Opium could not be had recourse to; for in every proportion, whether large or small, it threw out a lichenous rash over the surface of the body, but more especially over the extremities, possessing a heat, itching, and pricking, more intolerable than the prickly heat of the West Indies, and which was almost sufficient to produce madness. Vol. i. p. 335. — Was this Lichen or Eczema? T.

taken with advantage at the same period. All
strong external applications are improper, especially
preparations of Mercury and of Sulphur, which
produce severe irritation. The ancients recommended that the parts should be besmeared every
morning with saliva: as a substitute for this uncleanly expedient, a lotion prepared with the white
of egg, or the emulsion of Bitter almonds, will relieve the painful sensations of the patient. Lotions
of lime water, or of liquor Ammoniæ Acetatis, much
diluted, occasionally also afford relief. "The sudden repulsion of Lichen from the surface, by
imprudent exposure to cold, even in the milder
forms of the disease, is productive of febrile excitement, head-ach, and other symptoms of constitutional disorder. In this case, the use of the
warm bath is useful: but, occasionally, the fever subsides without the re-appearance of the
eruption."

SPÉCIES 4. LICHEN *agrius*, WILD LICHEN.

Syn. ἄγριος (*G.*): Papula *agria* (*Celsus*): Lichen
ferus (Good).

This severe form of Lichen (Plate IV. fig. 2.
of BATEMAN; Pl. 2. of THE ATLAS,) is ushered in
by febrile symptoms, which are commonly relieved on the appearance of the papulous eruption.
The papulæ occur in large patches, are of a high
red colour, and have a degree of inflammation
diffused around them to a considerable extent.
They are accompanied by itching, heat, and a pain-

ful tingling, which are augmented to a sensation of smarting and scalding by the heat of the bed, washing with soap, drinking wine, or using violent exercise. The symptoms undergo a daily increase and remission; for they are all greatly diminished in the morning, and recur after dinner. Some small vesicles, filled with a straw-coloured fluid, are occasionally intermixed with the papulæ; but they are not permanent.

The duration of the L. agrius is various: sometimes it continues for several weeks; and in most instances, the eruption appears and disappears repeatedly before the disease is removed. In both these cases, the cuticle of the parts affected becomes harsh, thickened, chappy, and exquisitely painful on being rubbed or handled. After repeated attacks, indeed, it is liable to terminate in a chronic pustular disease, the Impetigo.* This tendency, and the diffuse redness connecting the papulæ, distinguish the L. agrius from the preceding species, which occasionally pass into Psoriasis, as observed by the ancients.

The L. agrius is sometimes repelled by exposure to cold, upon which an acute febrile disorder en-

---

* Celsus describes his second species of Papula under the appellation of αγρια or *fera;* and has also pointed out its tendency to pass into Impetigo: — " Difficilius sanescit; nisi sublata est, in Impetiginem vertitur." (loc. cit.) His successors, the Greek writers, have also applied the same epithet to the severe form of Lichen. Galen speaks of Lichen simplex et ferus, απλες και αγριος : (Isagoge, cap. 13. See also Paul. Ægin. de Re Med. lib. iv. cap. 3.; and Oribas. ad Eunap. lib. iii. cap. 57.) and Aëtius of rough and of inflamed Lichens, τρηχεις και φλεγμαινοντες, (tetrab. iv. serm. i. cap. 134.) which appear to express the same varieties.

sues, with vomiting, head-ach, and pains in the bowels, and continues for several days. Women are more liable to this species of Lichen than men, particularly after suffering long-continued fatigue, with watching and anxiety: it sometimes occurs in spirit-drinkers.

The treatment of this form of Lichen consists in administering, at first, moderate laxatives, mercurial or saline, and afterwards, for some time, the diluted Sulphuric acid, three times a day, in the infusion of Roses, " containing in solution a few grains of sulphate of Quinia," or combined with decoction of Cinchona, " which seems to exert a specific influence in this disease ; allaying the tingling and itching, and diminishing the tendency to vesication. In obstinately-protracted cases I have seen much benefit result from the solution of Arsenic." A simple cooling unguent, as the rose pomatum, or litharge plaster softened with oil of almonds *, allays the troublesome heat or itching. All stimulating applications are, still more than in the preceding species, both painful and injurious : " and sulphureous baths, which are undoubtedly useful in several cutaneous affections, invariably increase this form of Lichen ; unless the disease have become chronic, and is disposed to pass into Impetigo. I am aware that this is contrary to the opinion of Mr. Plumbe, who remarks, that after ' the bowels have been some time kept open,' and

* Mr. Pearson recommended the following mild ointment in these cases. ℞. Emplast. Plumbi ʒij, Cera flavæ ℥ss, Olei Amygdal. dulc. ℥iss. Emplastro cum cera liquefacto adde oleum, dein agita misturam donec penitus refrixerit.

the habit reduced, 'the itching and tingling during the operation of the sulphur bath is rather severe, but it is followed by a much more tranquil state of the circulation in the cutaneous vessels, and the cure is altogether expedited by it.' " *

SPECIES 5. LICHEN *lividus,* LIVID LICHEN.

This species, (Plate V. fig. 2. of BATEMAN; Pl. 2. of THE ATLAS,) is distinguished by the dark red or livid hue of its papulæ, which appear chiefly on the extremities, and without any accompanying symptoms of fever. The papulæ are more permanent, however, than in the foregoing species: and, after their desiccation, the disorder is liable to be prolonged for many weeks, by a fresh eruption.

The affinity of this species with Purpura is evinced by the intermixture of petechiæ with the papulæ; and by the similarity of the origin and requisite treatment of the two diseases. † The nature of this species points out, that the treatment must necessarily be tonic and cordial.

SPECIES 6. LICHEN *tropicus;* " PRICKLY HEAT."

Syn. Eczesma (*Auct. Græc.*): Sudamina (*Auct. Lat.*): Essera (*Plouquet*): Chaleur piquante (*F.*): Root vout (*Belg.*): Flacherothe flecke (*Ger.*): Eshera (*Arab.*): *Prickly Heat, — Summer Rash.*

This is a hot and painful form of Lichen peculiar to tropical climates, and has been described at

---

* Practical Treatise on Diseases of the Skin, p. 196.
† See below, Order iii. Gen. 5.

great length by most of the writers on the diseases of those regions; to whose publications I shall therefore refer the reader.* " Dr. James Johnson, who suffered from this eruption in India, says, ' prickly heat, being merely a symptom, not a cause of good health, its disappearance has been erroneously accused of producing much mischief.' He ridicules the idea of its repulsion proving injurious, and remarks, ' It certainly disappears suddenly sometimes on the accession of other diseases, but I never had any reason to suppose that its disappearance occasioned them.' No external applications are useful; but some alleviation is afforded by light clothing, temperance, open bowels, and avoiding exercise in the heat of the day until the habit become assimilated to the climate."

SPECIES 7. LICHEN *urticatus;* NETTLE LICHEN. *Syn.* Lichen urticosus (*Good.*)

The first appearance of this species is in irregular, inflamed wheals, so closely resembling the spots excited by the bites of bugs or gnats, as almost to deceive the observer. The inflammation, however, subsides in a day or two, leaving small, elevated, itching papulæ, " which are spread over the upper part of the trunk of the body, and the extremities." While the first wheals are thus terminating, new

* See Hillary on the Climate and Diseases of Barbadoes, p. 5., Introd.; Moseley on the Diseases of Tropical Climates, p. 20.; Cleghorn on the Diseases of Minorca, chap. 4.; Clark on the Diseases of Seamen in Long Voyages, vol. i. p. 34.; Bontius de Medicina Indorum, cap. 18.

ones continue to appear in succession, until the whole body and limbs are spotted with papulæ, which become here and there confluent, in small patches ; " and increase both in elevation and in irritation the moment any stimulant food or exercise is taken.   It often subsides for a few days, and then re-appears more violent than ever."   This eruption is peculiar to children : it commences, in some cases, soon after birth, and sometimes later, and continues with great obstinacy for many months.   It occurs during dentition also, " recurring," says Underwood, " uniformly a little before a tooth has been cut."* Both the wheals and the papulæ are accompanied with intense itching, pricking, and tingling, which are exceedingly severe in the night, occasioning an almost total interruption of sleep, and considerable loss of flesh.

Frequent tepid bathing, particularly sea-bathing, light covering, especially in bed, with the use of small doses of sulphur, or the hydrargyrus sulphuratus niger, internally, appear to relieve the symptoms.   " Dr. Good says, that opium increases the irritability, and no other narcotic is of avail. † No benefit results from the use of sarsaparilla, nor of elm bark ; nor from any of the mercurial preparations."   The skin will not bear stimulation, and is irritated even by a bath of too high temperature. When it has occurred in feeble and emaciated children, I have seen it effectually relieved by chaly-

* Diseases of Children, 8th edit. p. 175.
† Study of Med. vol. iv. p. 559.

beate medicines, as the vinum ferri, or the solution of the tartrite before mentioned. This combination of inflamed papulæ with intense itching, unites the characters of the Lichen and Prurigo; an union, which, it must be allowed, is likewise not unfrequent in young adult persons.*

————

Genus III. PRURIGO.

Syn. κνησμός (*G.*) Pruritu (*Mercurialis*): Scabies papuliformis (*Auct. Vet.*): Intertrigo (*Lorry*): Exormia prurigo (*Good*): Prurit (*F.*): Das juckten (*Ger.*): Kejik (*Turc.*): *Pruriginous rash.*

Def. SEVERE ITCHING, INCREASED BY SUDDEN EXPOSURE TO HEAT, AFFECTING EITHER THE WHOLE SURFACE OF THE SKIN, OR A PART ONLY: IN SOME INSTANCES WITHOUT ANY APPARENT ERUPTION; IN OTHERS ACCOMPANIED WITH AN ERUPTION OF PAPULÆ NEARLY OF THE SAME COLOUR WITH THE ADJOINING CUTICLE.

* *Works which may be consulted on Lichen.*
BONTIUS de Medicina Indorum, 8vo. cap. 18.
CLARK on the Diseases of Seamen, vol. 1. p. 34.
GOOD, Study of Medicine, vol. iv. p. 530. 8vo. 1822.
CLEGHORN on the Diseases of Minorca, chap. 4. 8vo.
HILLARY on the Climate and Diseases of Barbadoes, 8vo.
JOHNSON on the Influence of Tropical Climates, 2d edit. 8vo. 1818.
LORRY, Tractatus de Morbis Cutaneis, 4to. 1777.
PLUMBE on Diseases of the Skin, 8vo. 2d edit. 1827.
RAYER, Traité Théorique et Pratique des Maladies de la Peau, 8vo. 1826.
WILLAN on Cutaneous Diseases, 4to. 1808. T.

There are four species of Prurigo : — ·

    1. P. *mitis.*   3. P. *senilis.*
    2. P. *formicans.*   4. P. *sine papulis.**

SPECIES 1. PRURIGO *mitis.* MILD PRURIGO.

This form of Prurigo (Plate VI. fig. 1. of BATEMAN ; Pl. 3. of THE ATLAS,) is accompanied by soft and smooth papulæ, somewhat larger and less acuminated than those of Lichen, and seldom appearing red or inflamed, except from violent friction. Hence an inattentive observer may overlook the papulæ altogether † : more especially as a number of small, thin, black scabs are here and there conspicuous, and arrest his attention. These originate from the concretion of a little watery humour, mixed with blood, which oozes out when the tops of the papulæ are removed, by the violent rubbing or scratching which the severe itching demands. This constant friction sometimes also produces inflamed pustules, which are merely incidental, however, when they occur at an early period of the complaint. " They appear chiefly

---

* In the former editions of this work, three species only of Prurigo are enumerated, and those which I have thrown together to form the fourth species, are described by Dr. Bateman under the term " local pruriginous affections." If we were to regard the eruption of papulæ as the chief symptom of Prurigo, these local pruriginous affections should be separated from the genus ; but as the chief characteristic is evidently the *itching*, these, in truth, may be regarded as constituting the only real species of Prurigo, whilst the three former species might, with much propriety, be transferred to Lichen. T.

† Pruritus enormes non semper densæ confertæque papulæ afferunt ; paucæ vix aspectu notandæ occurrunt, quæ hominem convellant. — Lorry de Morb. Cutan. cap. iii. art. i. par. 2.

upon the shoulders, the breast, the loins, and the thighs." The itching is much aggravated both by sudden exposure to the air, by violent exercise, and by heat; whence it is particularly distressing when the patient undresses himself, and often prevents sleep for several hours after he gets into bed.

This eruption mostly affects young persons, " usually in a good state of general health;" and it commonly occurs in the spring or the beginning of summer. It is relieved after a little time by a steady perseverance in the use of the tepid bath, or of regular ablution with warm water and mild soap, although at first this stimulus slightly aggravates the eruption. * The internal use of Sulphur, alone, or combined with Soda or a little Nitre, continued for a short time, " after bleeding and active purgation," contributes to lessen the cutaneous irritation, and may be followed by the exhibition of the mineral acids : " fully more benefit, however, is derived from a course of cooling purgatives, particularly in young and otherwise healthy people. Our own experience has taught us to place much confidence in the following formula : —

R. Magnesiæ Sulphatis ℨiij,
    Infusi Confectionis Rosæ f℥xij,
    Acidi Sulphurici diluti ♏ix ;
Misce ut fiat haustus bis die sumendus."

---

* After recommending a bath of moderate temperature, Lorry observes, " Nec mirandum, si inter balneorum usum plures papulæ prodeant. Etenim laxatis vasis, ad cutem omnia deferri æquum est. Sed nulla inde ratio est, cur minus balneis fidamus." — Loc. cit.

c 4

Under these remedies, the disorder gradually disappears; but if the washing be neglected, and a system of uncleanliness in the apparel be pursued, it will continue during several months, and may ultimately terminate in the contagious Scabies.*

Species 2. Prurigo *formicans:* Formicative Prurigo.

This affection (Plate VI. fig. 2. of Bateman, Pl. 3. of The Atlas,) differs materially from the preceding, in the obstinacy and severity of its symptoms, although its appearances are not very dissimilar. The itching accompanying it is incessant, and is combined with various other painful sensations; as of ants or other insects creeping over and stinging the skin, or of hot needles piercing it. On undressing, or standing before a fire, but, above all, on becoming warm in bed, these sensations are greatly aggravated: and friction not only produces redness, but raises large wheals, which, however, presently subside. The little black scabs which form upon the abraded papulæ are seen spotting the whole surface, while the colourless papulæ are often so minute as nearly to escape observation.

This Prurigo occurs in adults, and is not peculiar to any season. It affects the whole of the trunk and limbs, except the feet and palms of the hands;

* It is probable that the cases which have thus terminated were not genuine Prurigo. *T.*

but is most copious in those parts over which the dress is tightest. Its duration is generally considerable, sometimes extending, with short intermissions, to two years or more. It is never, however, converted, like the preceding species, into the itch, for which, however, it may be readily mistaken, nor does it become contagious; but it occasionally ends in Impetigo.

The causes of the P. formicans are not always obvious. In some instances the disease is distinctly connected with disorder in the stomach, being preceded by sickness, gastrodynia, and headach; "and these are again produced, in an augmented degree, by the sudden suppression of the eruption." In other instances, P. formicans appears to be the result of particular modes of diet, especially of the use of shell-fish and much stimulant animal food, in hot weather, with a free potation of wine, spirits, and fermented liquors, and excess in the use of condiments, pickles, and vinegar. * On the other hand, it is often observed in persons of lean habit, and sallow complexion, and in those who are affected with visceral obstructions, or reduced in strength by fatigue, watching, and low diet.

* I have known several instances of the immediate influence of the acetous acid upon the skin, especially in summer, exciting heat and tingling very soon after it was swallowed; and, in persons of peculiar cutaneous irritability, leaving more permanent effects. Dr. Withering asks, " Who has not observed the full scarlet flush upon the face after eating herrings or vinegar, after drinking acetous beer or cider?" — Treatise on Scarlet Fever, p. 62. The universal recommendation of vegetable acids and crude herbs, indeed, in these states of cutaneous irritation, in consequence of a misapplication of the term scorbutic, is in opposition to the dictates of sound observation.

The treatment of P. formicans must necessarily be varied according to the circumstances just stated; but it is not readily alleviated either by internal or external medicines. Where it appears to be connected with a state of general debility, or with some disorder of the abdominal viscera, the first object will be to remove these conditions by proper diet and exercise, together with medicines adapted to the nature of the case. Where the stomach is obviously disordered, the regulation of the diet is of material importance, especially as to the omission of those prejudicial articles above mentioned, and the substitution of a light digestible food, and of whey, milk, ass's milk, butter-milk, &c., as beverage. This regulation of the diet, indeed, is in all cases of the disease to be recommended, though there may be no apparent internal complaint from which it originates. For, in these cases, medicine alone is often extremely inert.

Combined with proper diet, the use of washed Sulphur with the Carbonate of Soda, internally, has much alleviated the painful state of sensation, and shortened the duration of the disorder: and where the habit was enfeebled, the decoctions of Sarsaparilla, Cinchona, Serpentaria, and other tonic vegetables, have proved essentially serviceable. I have seen considerable benefit derived from the internal use of the Oxygenated Muriatic acid, in this and the former species of Prurigo, both the eruption and the itching yielding during its exhibition. It may be taken in doses of a fluid drachm, and increased gradually to three times this quantity, in water or any agreeable vehicle. Strong purgatives, or a course of purgation, appear to be injurious; antimonials and mercurials are useless; and active sudorifics aggravate the complaint.

In respect to external remedies, frequent ablution with warm water, by removing the irritation of sordes, and softening the skin, contributes most materially to the patient's relief. A partial bath of the native or artificial sulphureous waters * is still more efficacious in relieving the itching : and sea-bathing has also occasionally removed the disorder. In general, the application of ointments, or of lotions, containing Sulphur, Hellebore, Mercury, Zinc, Lime-water, &c. is productive of little benefit: I have sometimes, however, found a speedy alleviation produced by a diluted wash of the Liquor ammoniæ acetatis, or of spirit, or by a combination of these, varied in strength according to the irritability of the skin. " Lotions of Calomel and Lime-water, are also frequently beneficial; and I have seen much relief obtained from the use of the following lotion : —

℞. Hydrargyri Oxymuriatis gr. iij,
    Acidi Hydrocyanici f℥j,
    Misturæ Amygdalæ amaræ f℥viij. M.

---

* This may be prepared in the following manner: Dissolve two drachms of Sulphate of Magnesia, ten grains of Supertartrate of Potass, and half a drachm of Sulphuret of Potass in twenty-four fluid ounces of warm water. It should be used at 95° of Fahrenheit. *T.*

Comfort is sometimes procured from lotions of cold spring water. Much benefit is, also, said to result from touching the prominent papulæ, previously rubbed till they bleed, with undiluted Aromatic Vinegar; and afterwards applying the following ointment liberally to the whole eruption, giving, at the same time, four or five grains of Plummer's pill every night, and five drops of the Arsenical Solution three times a day : —

> R. Sulph. Sublimati,
>   Picis Liquidi,
>   Adipis, ā. ā. lbss.
>   Cretæ ʒiv,
>   Hydrosulph. Ammoniæ ʒij. M.
> ut fiat unguentum."

SPECIES 3. PRURIGO *senilis :* INVETERATE PRURIGO.

The frequent occurrence of this species of Prurigo (Plate VI. fig. 3. of BATEMAN; Pl. 3. of THE ATLAS,) in old age, and the difficulty of curing it, have been the subject of universal observation. * The sensation of itching, in the Prurigo of that period of life, is as intolerable and more permanent than in the P. formicans; and the appearances which it exhibits are very similar, except that the

---

* See Hippoc. Aph. lib. iii. § lii. 31. where, among other diseases of old age, he mentions ξυσμοι του σωματος ὁλου. — Its obstinacy has been particularly noticed by the later Greeks. " Pruritum in senectute contingentem perfecte sanare non datur, verum subscriptis mitigare potes." Paul. Ægin. de Re Med. lib. iv. cap. 4. Actuar. Meth. Med. lib. ii. cap. 11. — See also Sennert. Pract. lib. v. p. iii. § i. cap. 8. — Mercurialis de Morb. curand. cap. 3. Heberden, Comment. cap. 76.

papulæ are for the most part larger. The comfort of the remainder of life is sometimes entirely destroyed by the occurrence of this disease.

A warm bath affords the most effectual alleviation of the patient's distress, but its influence is temporary. "The itching is said to be relieved by the sulphureous fumigating bath, when used at a temperature so low as will merely disengage the sulphurous gas." The disorder seems to be connected with a languid state of the constitution in general, and of the cutaneous circulation in particular: hence the sulphureous waters of Harrowgate, employed both internally and externally at the same time, afford on the whole the most decided benefit. A warm sea-water bath has also been found serviceable. Sometimes stimulant lotions, containing the oxymuriate of mercury, or the liquor ammoniæ acetatis, or alcohol, are productive of great relief, and occasionally render the condition of the patient comparatively comfortable, or even remove the disease. * When the surface is not much abraded, the oxymuriate will be borne to the extent of two grains to the ounce of an

---

* Dr. Heberden lays it down as an axiom, that stimulants are commonly beneficial in diseases of the skin, accompanied by itching.—
" Quod attinet ad remedia extrinsecus admovenda, illud sedulo tenendum est, acriora plerumque convenire, ubi pruritus est; sin dolor fuerit, lenia esse adhibenda," &c. (Comment. cap. 23.) This is true, perhaps, as far as it regards the unbroken or papulated skin: but itching often accompanies chops and rhagades, vesicular and even pustular diseases in a state of excoriation, and the irritable state of the surface left by the exfoliations of some of the scaly eruptions; under all which circumstances, this is an erroneous rule of practice, as I have had many opportunities of witnessing.

aqueous or weak spirituous vehicle; but it is generally necessary to begin with a much smaller proportion.

This mineral salt is likewise useful in destroying the pediculi, which are not unfrequently generated, when the Prurigo senilis runs into a state of ulceration. * Where the skin is not abraded by scratching, the oil of turpentine, much diluted with oil of almonds, may be applied with more decided effect, for the destruction of these insects.†

* The same languid state of skin which is a predisposing cause of this species of Prurigo, is also favourable to the generation of pediculi; for, as Alibert justly remarks, " la génération de ces dégoûtans animalcules tient à une foiblesse radicale et constitutionnelle de la peau, comme le développement des vers, dans le conduit intestinal, tient également à un défaut d'énergie dans les propriétés vitales de cet organe." *Descript. des Mal. de la Peau, Discours préliminaire*, p. xi. T.

† The pertinacity with which these loathsome insects often continue to infest the skin, in spite of every application that is resorted to, is surprising: but, as Dr. Willan has justly observed, the marvellous histories of fatality occasioned by lice, in the persons of Pherecydes, Antiochus, Herod, &c., are probably ascribable to mistake; the writers having confounded other insects, or their larvæ, with pediculi. Numerous instances are recorded of the generation of maggots, *i. e.* the larvæ of different species of fly (Musca), and even of other winged insects, not only in the internal cavities of the human body, but in external sores and excoriations. (For several examples of this kind I beg leave to refer to a paper of my own in the Edin. Med. and Surg. Journal for Jan. 1811, p. 41., and in the new Cyclopædia of Dr. Rees, Art. INSECTS.) In warm climates, indeed, these insects are so abundant about the persons of the sick, that the utmost care is requisite to prevent the generation of larvæ from the ova, which they deposit, not only in superficial wounds, but in the nostrils, mouth, gums, &c. Dr. Lempriere has recorded the case of an officer's lady, who had gone through an acute fever, but in whom these maggots were produced, which burrowed and found their way by the nose through the *os cribriforme*, into the cavity of the cranium, and afterwards into the brain itself, to which she owed her death. (Obs. on the Diseases of the Army in Jamaica, vol. ii. p. 182.) The worms which were generated in the patches of

SPECIES 4. PRURIGO *sine Papulis:* LOCAL PRU-
RIGO.

The local pruriginous affections are accurately
described in the first part of the general definition :
they have scarcely any affinity with the species of
Prurigo already described, except in the itching
which accompanies them, not being in general papular diseases ; a character in which all the varieties
agree.

Var. a. P. *præputii* is occasioned by an altered
or augmented secretion about the corona glandis,
and is cured by frequent simple ablution of the parts
with hot water, or with a weak saturnine lotion.

Var. b. P. *pubis* arises solely from the presence
of morpiones, or pediculi pubis, which are readily
destroyed by the white precipitated Mercury in
powder, or by mercurial ointment rubbed into the
parts affected.*

Var. c. P. *urethralis* is commonly sympathetic
of some disease about the neck of the bladder, or
of calculi in that organ : in women, however, it

Lepra, observed by Prof. Murray, proved to be larvæ of the common
house-fly. " Incredibile fere est," he says, " quanta muscarum domes-
ticarum copia continuo ad lectum advolarent, ægrumque suctu suo
torquerent, ut in clamorem usque nonnunquam erumperet." (De
Vermibus in Lepra obviis Obs. Auct. J. A. Murray, Gött. 1769. p. 25.)
In all such cases, the disease appears to have afforded only a nidus for
the ova of these domestic insects, and to have been in no other way
connected with their existence, either as cause or effect. See Scabies.

* Mr. Plumbe recommends the following ointment for this purpose:

℞. Unguenti Hydrargyri,
———— Sulphuris, ā ā, partes æquales. M.

sometimes occurs without any manifest cause, and is removable by the use of bougies, as recommended by Dr. Hunter.

Two of the next three forms of local Prurigo, namely, P. *podicis*, and *pudendi muliebris*, are more frequently the objects of medical treatment.

Var. e. P. podicis. Independently of ascarides, or hæmorrhoids, which sometimes occasion a troublesome itching about the sphincter ani, the P. *podicis* occurs in sedentary persons, and those of advanced age, in connection with an altered, highly irritating secretion from the part, and sometimes with constitutional debility. This complaint, especially in old men, is apt to extend to the scrotum, which becomes of a brown colour, and sometimes thick and scaly. The itching, in these cases, is extremely severe, especially at night, and often deprives the patient of a considerable portion of his sleep.

Var. d. P. scroti. This variety of local Prurigo is occasionally produced by friction, from violent exercise in hot weather; and sometimes it originates from the irritation of ascarides in the rectum.

Lotions, whether warm or cold, with preparations of Lead, Zinc, Lime-water, &c., have little efficacy in these affections. Those made with Vinegar, or the Acetate of Ammonia, are productive of a temporary relief; but the most useful are those made with a scruple of Calomel, or twelve grains of Oxymuriate of Mercury, and six fluid ounces of Lime-water, and used without being filtered. The mercurial ointments, especially the Unguentum Hydrargyri Nitratis, diluted are often successful applications. — Internally small doses of Calomel, with an antimonial, such as the Pilula Hydrargyri Submuriatis of the London Pharmacopœia, seem to be advantageous in correcting the morbid secretion: and the vegetable or mineral tonics should be administered in enfeebled habits. In P. podicis, much benefit is derived from the application of leeches to the verge of the anus; and in this variety, even more than in the others, great temperance should be inculcated, since stimulant diet invariably aggravates the complaint.

Var. f. P. *pudendi muliebris* is somewhat analogous to the preceding, but is occasionally a much more severe complaint. It is sometimes connected with ascarides in the rectum, and sometimes with leucorrhœa; but is most violent when it occurs soon after the cessation of the catamenia. The itching about the labia and os vaginæ is constant and almost intolerable, demanding incessantly the relief of friction and of cooling applications, so as to compel the patients to shun society, and even sometimes to excite at the same time a degree of nymphomania. This condition is generally accompanied by some fulness and redness of the parts.

" While inflammation is present, nothing is so serviceable as the application of leeches to the affected parts. The itching is moderated by the abstraction of the blood, and the other remedies act more efficaciously after the bleeding." Saturnine and saline

D

lotions, Lime-water, Lime-water with Calomel, Vinegar and oily liniments prepared with Soda or Potass, are beneficial, especially in the milder cases: but the most active remedy is a solution of the Oxymuriate of Mercury in Lime-water, in the proportion of two grains, or a little more, to the ounce. " I have seen much relief procured by a lotion composed of equal parts of the Chloro-sodaic Solution of Labaraque and water. As in the cases before mentioned, however, the presence of rhagades or excoriations will require palliation before it can be employed. M. Rayer * details a severe case of a disease of this description, which was cured by Gelatino-sulphureous Douches, recommended by M. Dupuytren. It is of importance to avoid wine, spirits, tea, coffee, pepper, and all aromatics, when the disease is severe."

Books which may be consulted on Prurigo.

DE CHAMBERET, Dissert. sur le Prurigo, 4to. 1808.
Dictionnaire des Sciences Médicales, *Art.* Prurigo.
HAFFENREFFER, Nosodoch. 12mo. 1660.
LOESCHER, De Pruritu Senilis, 8vo. 1726.
LORY, De Morbis Cutaneis, 4to. 1777.
MOURONVAL, Recherches et Obs. sur le Prurigo, 4to. 1823.
PLUMBE, on Diseases of the Skin, 2d edit. 1827.
RAYER, Traité des Maladies de la Peau, 8vo. 1820.
REIL, De Pruritu Senili, 8vo. 1803.
SOMMER, De Affectibus Pruriginosis Senum, 8vo. 1727.
WILLAN, On Cutaneous Diseases, 4to. 1798.
WILKINSON, Remarks on Cutaneous Diseases, 8vo. 1822.

* Traité des Maladies de la Peau, tome i. p. 620.

Order II.

SQUAMÆ.

SCALY DISEASES.

SYN. λεπος *(G.)*: Lepidosis (*Young. Good*): Inflammations Squameuses (*Rayer*): Kuba *or* Kouba (*Arab.*): Perjun (*Persic*): *Scaly eruptions.*

Def. AN ERUPTION OF SCALES, CONSISTING OF LAMINÆ OF MORBID CUTICLE, HARD, THICKENED, WHITISH, AND OPAQUE, DETACHING ITSELF FROM THE SKIN. SCALES, WHEN THEY INCREASE INTO IRREGULAR LAYERS, ARE DENOMINATED CRUSTS.

Those opaque and thickened laminæ of the cuticle, which are called Scales, commonly "proceed from an altered action of the vessels that secrete the cuticle, approaching to subacute inflammation;" but the degree of inflammation may be such as to affect the true skin, over which they are formed, and prove destructive to it: in the slighter forms, as for example Pityriasis, the cuticle alone, or with the rete mucosum, appears to be in a morbid condition. "When the scales fall off, they leave either a healthy surface, or a red, smooth, and glistening state of the skin, which does not soon regain its natural appearance." If the definition be carefully attended to, scales will not be confounded with the scabs succeeding confluent pustules and vesicles, and superficial ulcerations.

" A peculiar predisposition of habit is necessary for the appearance of scaly eruptions, and 'this in many instances appears to be hereditary. Women in general are more liable to them than men. The scales appear in patches, are accompanied by itching or tingling ; and owing to the diminished perspiration which they induce, the pulmonary exhalation and the secretion of urine are augmented. Scaly diseases are not contagious."

The four genera of scaly diseases are,

1. LEPRA.   3. PITYRIASIS.
2. PSORIASIS.   4. ICHTHYOSIS.

GENUS I. LEPRA. *

Syn. λεπρα (*G.*): Vitiligo (*Celsus*): Lepra Græcorum (*Auct. var.*): Leprosis, Lepriasis (*Good*): Lèpre, Léproisie (*F.*): der Aussatz (*Ger.*): Berat (*Hebrew*): Beresa (*Arab.*): Kush'tu (*Hindos.*): Vullay Koostum (*Tam.*): Tella Koostum (*Tel.*): Sweta Koostum (*Sans.*): Suffaid khere (*Duk.*): Velussu (*Malayalie*): *Lepra.*

Def. CIRCULAR PATCHES OF SMOOTH, LAMINATED SCALES, SURROUNDED BY A REDDISH AND PROMINENT CIRCLE. THE PATCHES ARE OF DIFFERENT SIZES, AND DEPRESSED IN THE CENTRE.

---

* Græce λεπρα dicitur, cujus formatio ἀπω των λεπιδων (a squamis) unde τὸ λεπρυνεσθαι, quod significat scabrum fieri et simul albescere, originem trahit. *I. Gorræus*, Schol. in Nicand. Theriac. p. 77—82.

The term LEPRA is here appropriated solely to the *Leprosy of the Greeks,* as described by the more accurate of those writers. It is characterized, as stated in the definition, by " scaly patches, of different sizes, but having always nearly a circular form."* " The parts which it chiefly attacks are below the patella, over the tibia, the elbows, the fore arms, and the surface in particular of the ulna."

There are three species of Lepra :

    1. L. *vulgaris.*
    2. L. *alphoides.*
    3. L. *nigricans.*

---

* The confusion which has every where prevailed in the use of the terms *Lepra* and *Leprosy,* seems to have originated principally with the translators of the Arabian writers after the revival of learning. The Greeks agreed in appropriating the appellation of λεπρα to a *scaly* eruption (as its etymology dictated); most of them deemed it the highest degree of *scaliness,* exceeding in this respect the Lichenes, Psora, and Alphos; and those, who were most minute in their description, stated that " it affects the skin deeply, in *circular* patches, at the same time throwing off scales like those of large fishes." (See Paul. Ægin. de Re Med. lib. iv. cap. 2.; — and Actuarius de Meth. Med. lib. ii. cap. 11.; — also Aëtius, tetrab. iv. serm. i. cap. 134.; and Galen Isagoge.) This was sufficiently clear; but those who translated the works of the Arabians into Latin, fell into the extraordinary mistake of applying the Greek term to a *tubercular* disease, which had been actually described by the Greeks under the appellation of Elephantiasis; and they applied the barbarous term *Morphæa,* together with Scabies and Impetigo, to the scaly diseases of the Greeks above enumerated. Whence their followers, who detected the error, spoke of the Lepra Arabum as well as the Lepra Græcorum; while the less accurate confounded every foul cutaneous disease under the term Leprosy. The Arabians themselves do not employ the word Lepra; but have described these different diseases under appropriate appellations. See Elephantiasis below.

SPECIES 1. LEPRA *vulgaris*, COMMON LEPRA.

Syn. Herpes furfuraceus circinatus (*Alibert*): Dartre furfuracée arrondie — Lèpre (*F.*): Weisse aussatz (*G.*): Berat lebena (*Hebrew*): Beras bejas (*Arab.*)

This species of the disease, (Plate VII. of BATE-MAN; Pl. 4. of the ATLAS,) the most ordinary in this country, commences with small, round, reddish, and shining elevations of the skin, at first smooth, but within a day or two exhibiting thin white scales on their tops. These scales gradually, sometimes rapidly, dilate to the size of half-a-crown, " are depressed in the centre," but still retain their oval or circular form, and are covered with shining scales, " not unlike mica or asbestos, but more opaque," and encircled by a dry, red, and slightly elevated border. " The scales at first are thin, somewhat resembling those of a carp, but by degrees they become laminated and denser," and in some cases accumulate, so as to form thick prominent crusts. " In mild cases of the disease, it is probable that the morbid action is confined to the scarf skin ; but when the disease is severe, the cutis vera is involved." If the scales or crusts are removed, the skin appears red and shining, being very smooth, and free from the cuticular lines in the beginning, but marked, in the advanced stages, with long deep lines and reticulations, not always coinciding with those of the adjoining surface, " but with the under surface of the desquamated layers. If the first scale which forms be forcibly detached, a small speck of blood is found in the little hollow of the scale and of the slight elevation on the skin which occupied it."

" Lepra is distinguished from Psoriasis by the regular circular form of the patches, which, in the latter disease, are always irregular; and in which, also, the borders are neither elevated nor inflamed. With one species, however, of Psoriasis, the *guttata*, Lepra may be readily confounded: but the patches are generally smaller and less regular in their figure than those of Lepra."

The Lepra most commonly commences on the extremities, where the bones lie nearest to the surface; especially below the elbow and the knee, and usually on both arms, or both legs, at the same time. From these points it gradually extends, by the formation of new and distinct patches, along the arms or thighs, to the breast and shoulders, and to the loins and sides of the abdomen. In several cases, I have observed the eruption most copious and most permanent round the whole lower belly. The hands also become affected, and in many cases the hairy scalp; but the face is seldom the seat of large patches, although some scaliness occasionally appears about the outer angles of the eyes, and on the forehead and temples, extending from the roots of the hair. In the more severe cases, the nails of the fingers and toes are often much thickened, and become opaque and of

D 4

a dirty yellowish hue, and are incurvated at the extremities; their surface is also irregular, from deep longitudinal furrows, or elevated ridges.

When the eruption of Lepra is moderate in degree and extent, it is not attended with any uneasy sensations, except a slight degree of itching after a full or an indigestible meal, or when the patient is heated by exercise, or becomes warm in bed; and a little occasional tingling in certain states of the atmosphere.* " Mr. Plumbe has remarked that a sensation of pricking always accompanies the separation of the first scales, before they have attained the size of spangles. This he attributes ' to the raising up of the edge of the scale, produced by the tumefaction and elevation of the inflamed margin, and fresh growth of the scale detaching the centre forcibly from the cutis.' "† When the patches are generally diffused, however, and there is a considerable degree of inflammation in the skin, the disease is accompanied with extreme soreness, pain, and stiffness; which I have sometimes seen so great as to render the motions of the joints impracticable, and to confine the patient to bed. Yet even under these circumstances, there is no constitutional disturbance; and if no medicine be employed, the disease of the skin may continue for months, or even years, without any material derangement of the system.

* Hippocrates remarks that some *Lepræ* itch before rain : lib. Περι Χυμων.

† Plumbe on Diseases of the Skin, 2d edit. 1827.

It is not easy to point out the causes of this disease, which appear, indeed, to be very various; for it is one of the most common affections of the skin, at least in this metropolis, and occurs at all periods, and under every circumstance of life.* It is certainly not communicable by contagion; nor does it appear to originate from confinement to certain kinds of diet, such as fish, dried or salted meats, &c. since it is not endemic in districts where these are habitually used, and occurs frequently where they are almost unknown. But, like some other cutaneous affections of a more transient character, it is certainly produced occasionally by the influence of particular articles of food and drink, which operate through the idiosyncrasy of individuals. † I have met with one gentleman, in whom spices or alcohol speedily produce it. The original attack in him occurred after eating some hot soup, containing spice, the first spoonful of which excited a violent tingling over the whole head, followed by the leprous eruption, which soon extended to the

* It is difficult, therefore, to account for the opinion expressed by the late Dr. Heberden, respecting the extreme rarity of Lepra in this country. " De vero scorbuto et lepra, nihil habeo quod dicam, cum alter rarissimus est in urbibus, altera in Anglia pene ignota; unde factum est ut hos morbos nunquam curaverim." (Comment. cap. 23.) And still more difficult to explain the statement of Dr. Cullen, whose definition of Lepra will include both the dry and humid tetters (Psoriasis and Impetigo) with the proper scaly Lepra; but who nevertheless affirms that he had never seen the disease. Nosol. Meth. class iii. gen. 88. *note.*

† Larrey ascribes the attacks of Lepra, which the French suffered in Egypt, to the unwholesome character of the pork in that country; for all those who lived upon pork for some time were attacked by a leprous eruption. *Relation Chirurgicale de l' Armée d' Orient*, 8vo. Paris, 1804. T.

limbs. In another case, in a young gentleman of nineteen, the disease commenced after taking copious draughts of cream. Vinegar, oatmeal, and other species of food, to which it has been ascribed, have probably given rise to it occasionally: but these are all anomalies, and are only referable to peculiar idiosyncrasy. * In some cases it has commenced after violent and continued exercise, by which the body had been much heated and fatigued.

Dr. Willan has imputed the origin of Lepra to cold and moisture †, and to certain dry sordes on the skin. It has seldom occurred to me, however, to witness the disease in bakers, laboratory-men, and others who work among dry powdery substances; while I have observed a considerable number of cases in young ladies, and in persons of both sexes in respectable ranks of life, by whom every attention to cleanliness was scrupulously paid. Where cold and moisture have excited the eruption of Lepra, the predisposition to it must have been peculiarly great. " Dr. Duffin has remarked, that the greater number of persons afflicted with Lepra are of a ruddy, fair complexion. The following is ⸱

* Some poisonous substances taken into the stomach have produced an eruption of Lepra. The poison of copper is stated to have speedily excited it in several persons at the same time, in one of whom it continued for a month, but disappeared in the others in about ten days. See Med. Facts and Obs. vol. iii. p. 61.

† The effects of cold and moisture on some quadrupeds tend, in some degree, to confirm this opinion. Thus Dr. Baron, having kept rabbits in a cold damp place, and fed them on green food, perceived that they became low in flesh; the abdomen became tumid, and the whole skin scaly and unhealthy. Vide Delineations of the Origin and Progress of the Changes of Structure in Man, 8vo. 1828.

his opinion of the proximate cause of the disease: ' I imagine that the primary evil lies in the secretions of the true skin, which, becoming vitiated by their local irritation, induce chronic or subacute inflammation of the vessels, that either nourish or produce the cuticle; and that they produce a superabundant supply of morbid cuticle.' * This theory is ingenious, but not altogether free from objection;" and, on the whole, it must still be admitted, that the causes of this disease are involved in much obscurity. There is obviously an hereditary predisposition to it in some individuals.

SPECIES 2. LEPRA *alphoides*, † WHITE LEPRA.

Syn. 'Αλφὸς, (*Auc. Gr.*): Alphos (*Celsus*): Lepriasis albida (*Good*): Lèpre Alphoide (*F.*): der Weisgeflecke aussatz (*German*): Boak (*Heb.*): Albohak (*Arab.*)

---

* Edin. Med. and Surg. Journ. Jan. 1826.

† The Greeks have described the *Alphos* as a milder disease, being more superficial, and less rough, than the Lepra (see Galen, de Sympt. Caus. lib. iii. — Aët. tetrab. iv. serm. i. cap. 134.) : and the description of it given by Celsus accords with the appearances of the L. alphoides above stated. " Αλφος vocatur, ubi color albus est, fere subasper, et non continuus, ut quædam quasi guttæ dispersæ videantur. Interdum etiam latius, et cum quibusdam intermissionibus, serpit." (De Medicinæ lib. v. cap. 18.) Celsus nowhere employs the term Lepra.

This scaly *Alphos*, which was deemed by Hippocrates a blemish, rather than a disease (Περι Παθων, sect. 15.), was distinguished from another *white* affection of the skin, the *Leuce*, which was not scaly, but consisted of smooth, shining patches, on which the hairs turned white and silky, and the skin itself, and even the muscular flesh underneath, lost its sensibility. The *Leuce* was a disease of an incurable nature. (Hipp. Προῤῥητικ. lib. ii.) Celsus, although pointing out this distinction, includes the Leuce and the Alphos under the same generic title, Vitiligo. (loc. cit.)

It may be remarked, that the Arabians distinguished these two affections by different generic appellations; calling the Alphos, *Albohak*, and

This is a less severe form of the disease (Plate VIII. fig. 1. of BATEMAN; Pl. 4. of THE ATLAS,) than the preceding, for it is merely a variety of it. It differs chiefly in the small size of the patches, which seldom extend beyond the diameter of a few lines, or become confluent, — in the minuteness and greater whiteness of the scales, — and in its limitation to the extremities. " It gives the parts affected a speckled appearance, formed of red patches and silvery scales irregularly dispersed." This variety of Lepra is most common in children, " and girls. under the age of fourteen. When it affects adults, the site of the scaly patches is considerably redder than the surrounding parts; and the exfoliating scales leave a smooth, red, glistening surface; which, in old cases, is intersected with fissures." It is tedious and difficult of cure, like the former, and requires similar treatment.

SPECIES 3. LEPRA *nigricans*, BLACK LEPRA.

Syn. μελας (*G.*): Melas (*Cels.*): Swarze Aussatz (*Ger.*): Berat cecha (*Heb.*): Beras asved (*Arab.*): *Black Lepra.*

---

the Leuce, *Albaras*, with the epithet *white*. Their translators have called the former *Morphæa*, and included the Leuce and Elephantiasis under the appellation of *Lepra*. By retaining these distinctions in recollection, the accounts of the older writers may be read, while the confusion arising from their misapplication of names may be avoided.

It appears probable that the *Leuce* was the Leprosy of the Jews, described in Leviticus, chap. xiii. See Greg. Horssii Obs. Med. lib. vii. p. 330. — Leon. Fuchsii Paradox, lib. ii. cap. 16. — Th. Campanellæ Ord. Medic. lib. vi. cap. 23. — Hensler, Von Abendländischen Aussatz, p. 341.

This species (Plate VIII. fig. 2. of BATEMAN; Pl. 4. of THE ATLAS,) is a more rare form of the disease, differing externally from the L. vulgaris chiefly in the dark and livid hue of its patches, which is most obvious in the margin, but even appears through the thin scales in the area of each patch. * The scales are thinner and more easily detached in this form of Lepra, and the surface remains longer tender, and is often excoriated, discharging bloody serum, till a new, hard, and irregular incrustation is formed. There is much probability in Dr. Duffin's opinion, that this form of the disease is merely the *vulgaris* in a cachectic habit.

It occurs chiefly in persons whose occupations expose them to the vicissitudes of the weather, and to a precarious diet, with fatigue and watching. It is cured by nutritive food, with moderate exercise, followed by the use of the Cinchona bark, mineral acids, and sea-bathing; and, as a local application, the Unguentum Hydrargyri Nitratis, diluted with two parts of lard.

It would be superfluous to enumerate the catalogue of useless medicines, which have been recom-

* The *Melas* of the ancients was deemed a superficial affection, resembling the Alphos, except in its colour. " Μελας colore ab hoc differt, quia niger est, et umbræ similis: cætera eadum sunt." (Celsus loc. cit.) Possibly it included the Pityriasis versicolor. See below, Genus iii. of this Order, Spec. iii.

" I cannot understand the reference to Pityriasis in this note; for, if Celsus is to be followed, it is evident, from the expression ' cætera eadem sunt,' that he intends to describe the *Melas* as a species of the same genus as the *Alphos*, that is, as a Lepra." T.

mended from ancient times for the cure of Lepra:
I shall, therefore, confine my attention to those, of
the beneficial agency of which I can speak from
experience. It is necessary to premise, however,
that there is no one remedy, nor any invariable
plan of treatment, which will succeed in Lepra,
under all the circumstances of its appearance in
different instances; and that great errors are committed by prescribing for the name of the disease.
The circumstances to which I allude more particularly, are the different degrees of cutaneous excitement, or inflammatory action, which accompany
the disease in different habits; and which, if carefully attended to, afford an important guide to the
most successful application of remedies.

In the less irritable conditions of the leprous
eruption, in which no inflammatory tendency appears, such as the L. alphoides frequently, and the
L. vulgaris occasionally, exhibits, a gently stimulant mode of treatment, at least externally, is
requisite; though in all cases of Lepra, the diet
should be light and moderate, and heating liquors
should be avoided, especially malt liquors and
spirits: for every indulgence in these points will
be felt in the aggravation of the symptoms. " When
the eruption is limited in extent, has existed for
some time, and is unattended with much itching,
pain, or irritation, little more than local remedies
are required." A frequent use of the warm bath,
at 89° to 95° Faht., with which a moderate degree
of friction may be combined, contributes to remove

the scales, and to soften the skin. " If the scales be forcibly removed before the exfoliating process is complete, the skin will bleed, which is not the case when the exfoliation is complete." If the eruption be confined to the extremities, local ablution may be sufficient, " and this is best performed by immersing the part in warm artificial Harrowgate water, as recommended by Dr. Duffin.* The following is the method of preparing this water: Dissolve ʒij of Sulphate of Magnesia, gr. x of Supertartrate of Potass, and ʒss of Sal Polychrest in fℨxxiv of hot water. The temperature of the solution when used should be 95° Fahrenheit: it should be used daily for 10 or 15 minutes each time." These cases are benefited by the use, both internally and externally, of the sulphur waters of Harrowgate, Leamington, Crofton, Moffat, and other well-known springs " in this country; and those of Barèges, de Cauterets, de Bagnères, de Bagnoles, and d'Enghien on the Continent," and by the warm sea-water bath. In fact, these gently-stimulant ablutions are often sufficient, if persevered in during several weeks, to remove the modifications of Lepra of which I am now speaking. "The sulphureous vapour baths are still more useful, particularly when combined with moderate friction."

But if the scales adhere tenaciously, or are accumulated into thick crusts, then some more active lotion must be conjoined with the warm ablution, or with the application of steam, in order to clear

* Edin. Med. and Surg. Journ. Jan. 1826. p. 23.

the surface. Lotions of diluted Alcohol, of sulphu-
rated Potass, or the decoction of Dulcamara, will
aid the exfoliation; and the thick crusts may be
softened and loosened by lotions containing a portion of the liquor Potassæ, or of the Muriatic acid.
" Blisters have been advantageously employed for
this purpose." When these are removed, the cuticle may be restored gradually to its healthy condition, by the Unguentum Picis, or the Unguentum
Hydrargyri Nitratis diluted with Saturnine Cerate,
or simple ointment; " or, which is better than any
other, an ointment composed of equal parts of
Unguentum Hydrargyri Nitratis and Unguentum
Picis :" or lotions containing a small proportion of
Oxymuriate of Mercury may be substituted. The
ointments should be applied at night, and washed
off in the morning with warm water, or a slight
saponaceous lotion, " composed of fʒiij of Liquor
Potassæ in fʒvj of water; after which the parts are
to be brushed over with a solution of Oxymurias
Hydrargyri gr. ij: Spiritus Vini fʒj. Dr. Duffin *
ascribes much of the benefit derived from the
alkaline solution to its being a perfect ablution
to the part, and requiring the aid of considerable
friction, two circumstances of great importance in
Lepra." In a few cases, the continued application
of the tar ointment has effectually cleared the skin
of the patches, and restored its texture, even when
internal remedies had little influence; but this advantage has not been permanent.

* Loco citato.

The same inert cases will be accelerated in their progress towards a cure, by the use of those internal remedies which tend to support the strength and to stimulate the cutaneous vessels. Purging is injurious, but the bowels should be kept easy by a mild pill. The Arsenical Solution*, recommended by Dr. Fowler, is the best tonic, and proves often extremely beneficial, in doses of four or five drops, which may be slowly increased to eight, and persevered in for a month or more.† "It may be given in the Decoction of Dulcamara, or of Sarsaparilla: and its efficacy is much augmented by employing for common beverage, water moderately acidulated with Nitric Acid, and sweetened. The sensible effects of the Arsenical Solution are quickening of the pulse, and an uneasy sense of stiffness in the eyelids: but when these are accompanied with griping pains, a white tongue, with its tip and edges of a florid red, anxiety in the præcordia, and frequent sighing, the remedy should be discontinued; and when it causes pains of the chest from the first, it should not be given at all." Pitch, " in doses of from six to twelve grains, and Turpentine, in doses

---

* Preparations of this mineral have a direct tendency to stimulate the cutaneous circulation, and to inflame the skin; and are, therefore, altogether inadmissible in the irritative forms of Lepra.

† This active medicine being now not only sanctioned by the profession in general, but by the Pharmacopœia of the College, it will be enough to state, that in these smaller doses, which experience has proved to be sufficient, it may be taken without any inconvenience. Another preparation, introduced by the late Dr. De Valangin, is kept at Apothecaries' Hall, under the name of Solutio Solventis Mineralis, and is equally efficacious.

of from ten to thirty grains," administered in the
form of pills, are productive of a similar good effect,
where the cutaneous circulation is very inert ; but
these medicines are liable to aggravate the eruption,
where it is connected with much irritability of the
skin. The solution of Oxymuriate of Mercury in
Alcohol, or in doses of one-fourth of a grain in a
fluid drachm of the Tincture of Cinchona, has appeared to have some efficacy in these inert states ;
and thin and delicate girls, of relaxed habit, affected
with the Lepra alphoides, have taken the Vinum
Ferri, or the tartrite before mentioned with much
advantage.*

One of the most effectual remedies for Lepra,
however, under all its varieties, is the decoction of
the twigs of the Solanum *Dulcamara*, Bitter-sweet,
which was introduced to the notice of British practitioners by Doctor, now Sir Alexander, Crichton.†
This medicine is at first administered in doses of
two or three ounces thrice every day, which are
gradually augmented, until a pint is at length con-
sumed daily. When there is a degree of torpor in
the superficial vessels, the same decoction, made
with a larger proportion of the shrub, is advantageously employed as a lotion; but if there is

* If in any case the Tinct. Lyttæ prove useful in Lepra, it would probably be in these more inert instances. But it is to be observed, that
Dr. Mead, who originally recommended this medicine, was probably
speaking, not of the scaly Lepra, but of the Leuce, or of the Elephantiasis. See his Medicina Sacra, cap. ii.

† See his communication to Dr. Willan. (Treatise on Cutaneous
Diseases, p. 145.) His formula has been adopted by the London College, and inserted into its Pharmacopœia.

any inflammatory disposition, this and every other external stimulus must be prohibited. " In a case described by Turner, after the patient, a maiden, had been salivated without effect, a cure was effected by a gentle alterative containing Ethiops Mineral, washed down with a decoction of Rumex Acutus, Sarsaparilla, and some inert roots ; with an ointment of the Hydrargyri Præcipitatus Albus, the bowels having been occasionally well purged. In all the cases I have seen, the mild alterative plan has proved the most effectual. The decoction of Dulcamara, with minute doses, *i. e.* $\frac{1}{12}$ of a grain of Oxymuriate of Mercury, or from gr. v to gr. x of Hydrargyrum c. Creta night and morning, have seldom disappointed me : but it is difficult to say what share the Dulcamara has in the cure. Among other vegetable infusions, that of the Ledum *Palustre*, Marsh Rosemary, in the proportion of ʒiv to Oij of boiling water, has a high popular reputation in the north of Europe. It is taken to the extent of a pint daily.[*] Dr. Duffin is of opinion, that both the Arsenical Solution and the Alcoholic Solution of Corrosive Sublimate produce some specific alteration on the secretions of the skin, which does not result from the employment of other stimulants; and thence their superiority in Lepra."

Where an irritable state of the disease exists, indeed, (and it is the most frequent) nothing more stimulating than tepid water, or thin gruel, or an infusion of Digitalis, made with ʒj of the leaves to

[*] Linnæus, Dissert. de Ledo Palustre. Upsal. 1775.

a quart of boiling water, can be used for the purposes of ablution; and the Arseniates, Pitch, &c.
above mentioned, must be excluded. The disease,
under this condition, will be certainly aggravated
by sea-bathing, by friction, by the external use of
the strong sulphureous waters, or of any irritant,
as I have frequently observed; but it will be alleviated by blood-letting, either general or local, followed by the use of the simple vapour bath; and by
the internal employment of Sulphur, with Soda or
Nitre, or the Hydrargyri Sulphuratus Niger with an
antimonial, especially when conjoined with the Decoction of Dulcamara or of the Ledum *Palustre*.
The Caustic Potass, or Liquor Potassæ of the
London Pharmacopœia, in the dose of twenty or
thirty drops, alone, or in combination with the Precipitated Sulphur, is likewise beneficial: and the
Tinctura Veratri, given in such doses as not to disorder the bowels, has occasionally removed this
state of the disease.

When the skin is highly inflamed, thickened, and
stiff, of a vivid red colour, intermixed with a yellowish hue, (where the cuticle is separating in large
flakes) the heat, pain, and itching, are often extremely troublesome, and the motion of the limbs
is almost impracticable. " In this state of the
habit, the irritability of the skin must be diminished
by antimonial emetics, and mercurial purgatives;
and if the excitement be considerable, general
bleeding should be resorted to before either Arsenic
or any of the remedies already mentioned can be

employed. If the local irritability be great, nau-
seating doses of Antimonials should be persisted in
for a few days, with the use of the tepid bath."
The most effectual relief is obtained, in these cases,
by gently besmearing the parts with cream, or a
little fresh and well-washed lard or butter, or cold
drawn castor oil, while the itching is relieved by a
lotion of Prussic Acid in Rose-water. " The progress of the cure, in all the species, is marked by
the scales detaching themselves in the centre of the
patches, and their edges becoming dry; and the
skin gradually ceasing to be scaly; but, in every
instance, this occurs first in the centre of the patch,
and extends to the circumference."

Books which may be consulted on Lepra.

Amœn. Acad. vol. viii. p. 285.

BONORDEN, Diss. de Lepra Squamosa, 8vo. Halæ. 1795.

Dictionnaire de Médecine, *art.* Lèpre. Paris.

DUFFIN, on Squamous Disorders. Edinburgh Med. and Surg. Journ.
No. 86.

GOOD's Study of Medicine, vol. iv. p. 574.

MECKEL, Diss. de Lepra Squamosa, 8vo. Halæ. 1795.

LORY, de Morbis Cutaneis, p. 365. 4to. Paris. 1777.

PLUMBE, on Diseases of the Skin, 8vo. 2d edit. 1827.

RAYER, Traité des Maladies de la Peau, tome i. p. 1. 8vo. Paris, 1827.

WILLAN, on Cutaneous Diseases, 4to. London, 1811.

Genus II. PSORIASIS.

Syn. Impetigo (*Sennert, Plenck, et alia*): Scabies sicca (*Etmull. Hoffm. Plater*), Hasef (*Avicenna*), Lepidosis Psoriasis (*Good, Young*): Kleinaussatz (*G.*): Dartre squammeuse sèche (*F.*): Saphat (*Hebrew*): Sahafati (*Arabic*): *Dry Scall.*

Def. Patches of dry, amorphous scales; continuous, or of intermediate outline; skin often chappy.

The Psoriasis, or *scaly tetter* *, occurs under a considerable variety of forms, exhibiting, in common with Lepra, more or less roughness and scaliness of the cuticle, with a redness underneath. It differs, however, from Lepra in several respects. Sometimes the eruption is diffuse and continuous, and sometimes in separate patches, of various sizes; but these are of an irregular figure, † without the elevated border, the inflamed margin, and the oval or circular outline of the

---

* The scaly tetter was denominated *Psora* by the Greeks, or sometimes rough and leprous Psora. (See Aetius, tetr. iv. 1. cap. 130, &c.) But the same generic term, with the epithet *ulcerating*, or *pustular*, Ψωρα ἑλκωδης, was applied to the humid tetter (Impetigo), and perhaps also to Scabies. As the appellation *Psora* has been appropriated to Scabies by many of the modern writers, Dr. Willan adopted the term *Psoriasis* (which was chiefly used to denote a scaly affection of the eyelids and of the scrotum by the ancients) for the name of the genus.

† Paul of Ægina, who treats of Lepra and Psoriasis together, points out the irregular figure of the latter as a principal distinction, that of the former being orbicular. " Λεπρα per profunditatem corporem cutem depascitur *orbiculatiore modo*, et squamus piscium squamis similes dimittit: Ψωρα autem magis in superficie hæret, et *varie figurata est*," &c. lib. iv. cap. 2. " De Lepra et Psora."

leprous patches: the surface under the scales is likewise much more tender and irritable in general than in Lepra; and the skin is often divided by rhagades or deep fissures. It is commonly accompanied by some constitutional disorder, and is liable to cease and return at certain seasons. * In Psoriasis the scales are less firmly attached than in Lepra, and do not accumulate over one another as in that disease: on the contrary, they separate with facility, leaving, as has been already mentioned, a more tender surface than in Lepra.

The causes of Psoriasis are nearly as obscure as those of Lepra. " In almost all the cases which I have seen, except those of a purely local nature, the digestive organs have been in fault; and great acidity of stomach has prevailed. It is not improbable that the arthritic diathesis, mental anxiety, and the other exciting causes mentioned in the latter part of this paragraph, always produce this state of stomach previous to the appearance of Psoriasis: and it is probable that the irritable state of the stomach, which gives rise to the imperfectly-formed gastric juice in these cases, is accompanied by a corresponding irritable condition of the skin, which, inducing sub-acute inflammation of the superficial capillaries, causes the cuticle to be secreted

---

* Celsus seems to have had this tetter in view, when describing his second species of Impetigo, and comparing it with Lichen. " Alterum genus est pejus, et simile Papulæ fere, sed asperius rubicundiusque, figuras varias habens: squamulæ ex cute decidunt: rosio major est; celerius ac latius procedit, certioribusque, quam prior, temporibus, et fit, et desinit: Rubra cognominatur." (lib. v. cap. 28.)

in the diseased state, which characterises this eruption." The disease is not contagious; with the
exception, perhaps, of the first species, which Dr.
Willan had observed to occur among children in
the same school or family, at the same time; a
circumstance, however, which I never witnessed.
An hereditary predisposition to it is manifest in
some individuals. Dr. Falconer has frequently
traced it to sudden chills, from drinking cold water
after being violently heated by exercise, — a cause
to which Lepra and other eruptive diseases are
occasionally to be imputed.* Women, and especially
those of a sanguineo-melancholic temperament,
with a dry skin and languid circulation, are most
liable to it: it affects them more particularly after
lying-in, or during a state of chlorosis. And in
children, it is not unfrequently produced by the
many sources of irritation to which they are exposed. It is also sometimes observed, in both
sexes, connected with arthritic complaints; and we
have seen it occur under states of great mental
anxiety, grief, or apprehension. In those who are
predisposed to this eruption, slight occasional
causes appear to excite it: such as, being over-
heated by exercise; the unseasonable employment
of the cold bath; a copious use of acid fruits,

* See Memoirs of the Med. Society of London, vol. iii. — In fact,
Dr. Falconer, and even the nosologists down to our own time, include
the Lepra, Scaly Tetter, and Pustular Impetigo, in their description of
Lepra. See Vogel, de Cogn. et Curand. Homin. Affect. class viii. § 699.
— Sauvages, Nosol. Meth. class. x. ord. 5. — Linn. Gen. Morbor.
class. x. ord 4 — Cullen, Nosol. class. iii. ord. 3. gen. 88.

vinegar, or crude vegetables; and some peculiar mixtures of food. The first two species of the eruption are sometimes the sequel of Lichen.

Dr. Willan has given names to eleven kinds of Psoriasis; but as several of them are local, and may be regarded as varieties of one species, affecting different parts of the body*, it is more correct to regard the genus as comprehending five species only: viz. —

1. P. *guttata.*　　　4. P. *inveterata.*
2. P. *diffusa.*　　　5. P. *localis.*
3. P. *gyrata.*

SPECIES 1. The PSORIASIS *guttata :* MINUTE DRY SCALL.

Syn. Dartre squammeuse humide et orbiculaire : Herpes squammosus madidans et orbicularis (*Alibert*).

This species (Plate IX. fig. 1. of BATEMAN, Pl. 5. of THE ATLAS,) is a sort of connecting link between the genus of Psoriasis and Lepra, the little patches being distinct, and small (seldom exceeding two or three lines in diameter), but with an irregular circumference, and the other peculiar characters just described. They "first appear in the form of small, solid, red elevations, resembling flat pimples, which are soon covered with small dry scales :" this occurs on almost every part of the body, and even on the face: but in the latter situation they exhibit only

---

* In this arrangement we have followed Dr. Good : see *Study of Medicine,* vol. iv. p. 593.

a redness and roughness, without scales. "The patches increase in size, but seldom exceed half an inch in diameter; and these, in the decline of the disease, first become healthy in the centre, and on this account often assume the appearance of circles, or segments of circles." The patches frequently coalesce. This eruption is most common in the spring, at which season it is liable to recur for several years. It is preceded by general pains, and slight feverishness. In children it often spreads rapidly over the body in two or three days; but in adults its progress is gradual and slow.

SPECIES 2. The PSORIASIS *diffusa:* SPREADING DRY SCALL. *

Syn. Dartre squammeuse humide, — Dartre squammeuse orbiculaire (*Alibert*).

This species (Plate IX. fig. 2.; X. 1. and 2.; XI. XIII. 1. of BATEMAN; Pl. 6. of THE ATLAS,) presents a considerable variety of appearances. In most cases it " commences like Psoriasis *guttata*, but soon coalesces" into large patches, which are irregularly circumscribed, and exhibit a rough, red, and chappy superficies, with very slight scaliness interspersed. This surface is exceedingly tender and irritable, and is affected with a sensation of burning and intense itching, both of which are

* Correct representations of this affection are given in Alibert's 13th and 14th plates; the former exhibiting it on the neck and ear (" Dartre squammeuse humide"), — the latter in a patch on the cheek (" Dartre squammeuse orbiculaire.") Liv. iii.

much augmented on approaching a fire, on becoming warm in bed, or even on exposure to the direct rays of the sun; "and in some cases which have come under my care, a humid state of the atmosphere has always augmented the irritation and itching;" but they are relieved by the impression of cool air. Sometimes these extensive eruptions appear at once; but, in other instances, they are the result of numerous minute elevations of the cuticle, upon which small distinct scales, adhering by a central point, are soon formed, and which become gradually united by the inflammation of the intervening cuticle. As the disorder proceeds, the redness increases, and the skin appears thickened and elevated, with deep intersecting lines or furrows, which contain a powdery substance, or very minute scurf. The heat and painful sensations are much aggravated by the least friction, which also produces excoriation, and multiplies the sore and painful rhagades. — This form of the disease is most frequent about the face and ears, and the back of the hands; the fingers are sometimes nearly surrounded with a loose scaly incrustation, and the nails crack and exfoliate: but it occasionally occurs on other parts of the body, either at the same time, or in succession. "Rayer remarks, that it is not uncommon to see P. *guttata* in the trunk of the body, whilst the limbs are affected with the species under consideration." *
It commonly begins with some general indisposi-

* Traité Théorique et Pratique des Mal. de la Peau, tome ii. p. 51.

tion; and a degree of erethism, with occasional
sharp pains in the stomach, is sometimes kept up,
during several weeks, by the constant irritation
which it excites. Its duration is from one to four
months, and sometimes much longer; and it is
liable to return, in successive years, in the spring
or autumn, and sometimes in both seasons.

" This species of Psoriasis occasionally occurs in
a severe degree in children from two months to
two years of age. It commences like the P. *guttata*; but the inflammation gradually extends
around the patches, and these rapidly coalesce,
resembling in some degree the Impetiginous Eczema, which is, however, a vesicular disease. The
scales are rather whiter, and approach nearer to
the character of Lepra than those of the common
form of P. *diffusa*, (see ATLAS, Plate 6.) I cannot agree with Willan in regarding it as a distinct
species. Dr. Underwood remarks, that he had
' seen it chiefly during a cold season.' It is certainly connected with dentition, often subsiding as
this is perfected, or after the gums are lanced. It
is described in the following manner by Dr. Underwood: ' It appears in some parts in very
small eruptions, like the points of pins, with watery
heads; and in other parts as large as peas, and
sometimes in foul blotches, which, after breaking,
form sores, and broad ugly scabs. These die away,
and the like appear successively, in other parts,
sometimes for two or three months, leaving the
skin of a dirty adust hue.' He considers that it

is contagious. The practice he recommends is to wash the parts with a lotion composed of f℥ij of Liquor Potassæ in a pint of water; giving, at the same time, Hydrargyrum cum Creta, or Hydrargyrum c. Sulphure and the juice of Sium *nodiflorum.* He says, 'an ointment consisting of the Unguentum Sulphuris and Unguentum Hydrargyrari Nitratis with a greater or less proportion of the latter, has hitherto never failed.' "*

In other cases, the P. diffusa commences in separate patches, of an uncertain size and form, which become confluent until they nearly cover the whole limb. Local instances apparently of this species also occur; but as they arise from local irritations, they will be described under P. *localis.*

SPECIES 3. The Psoriasis *gyrata,* GYRATED DRY SCALL. ·

In this species (Plate XII. of BATEMAN; Pl. 5. of THE ATLAS,) the patches are in stripes of a tortuous or serpentine form, resembling worms or leeches, or sometimes bending into rings. It is apt to be confounded with the vesicular and pustular ring-worm (Herpes and Impetigo).

SPECIES 4. PSORIASIS *inveterata,* INVETERATE DRY SCALL.

Syn. Psoriasis agria (*Auct. Vet.*): Dartre squammeuse lichenoide: Herpes squammosus lichenoides (*Alibert*).

---

* Treatise on Diseases of Children, 8th edit. p. 184.

This species (Plate XIII. fig. 2. of BATEMAN; Pl. 5. of THE ATLAS,) is the most severe modification of the complaint, beginning in separate irregular patches, which extend and become confluent until at length they cover the whole surface of the body, except a part of the face, or sometimes the palms of the hands and soles of the feet, with an universal scaliness, interspersed with deep furrows, and a harsh, stiff, and thickened state of the skin. The production of scales is so rapid, that large quantities are found every morning in the patient's bed.* The nails become convex, thickened, and opaque, and are frequently renewed; and, at an advanced period, especially in old people, extensive excoriations sometimes occur, frequently caused by the attrition of the clothes, chiefly on the thighs, nates, and scrotum; and these are followed by a discharge of lymph, followed by a hard dry cuticle, which separates in large pieces. Sometimes small suppurating patches are interspersed, which occasionally are crowded in patches, intersected with deep fissures and excoriations. In this extreme degree, it approaches very closely to the inveterate degree of Lepra vulgaris in all respects; the only difference being in the form of the patches before they coalesce. It is sometimes the ultimate state of the Psoriasis diffusa; and occasionally a sequel of the Prurigo senilis.

* In a case detailed by Turner (Treatise on Diseases of the Skin), this was one of the symptoms; yet many of the other symptoms of that case leads to the supposition that the disease was Ichthyosis simplex. T.

As the disease declines, the new cuticle is at first red, harsh, and sometimes shriveled, and does not acquire its natural texture for several weeks.

SPECIES 5. PSORIASIS *localis :* LOCAL DRY SCALL.

This species comprehends several varieties, which exhibit appearances closely resembling some of the foregoing species, but which are seldom accompanied with constitutional affections.

Var. a. P. *labialis.* SCALL OF THE LIPS. This affects the prolabium, especially of the under lip, the tender cuticle of which is thickened, cracks, and exfoliates, sometimes for a long period of time : the scales usually adhere more firmly than on other parts, and are only detached when the new cuticle under them is completed, which in its turn cracks and is thrown off in the same manner; and this occurs successively whilst the disease remains.

Var. b. P. *lotorum.* WASHERWOMEN'S SCALL. This variety (Plate X. fig. 2. of BATEMAN ; Pl. 6. of THE ATLAS,) appears on the wrists and forearms of washerwomen, from the irritation of soap. The inflammation is considerable, and the cuticle, which becomes brittle, separates in large irregular plates in rapid succession.

Var. c. P. *palmaria,** SCALL OF THE PALM.

Syn. Dartre squammeuse centrifuge : Herpes squammosus centrifugus (*Alibert*).

---

* Well represented in M. Alibert's 15th plate, under the title of " Dartre squammeuse centrifuge."

This variety (Plate XIV. of BATEMAN; Pl. 6. of THE ATLAS,) is an obstinate tetter, confined to the palm of the hand and wrist, which are rough, hot, and itchy, of a dirty hue, and cleft by deep furrows, that bleed when the fingers are stretched. A variety of P. *diffusa* closely resembles P. *palmaria*; but it is not a local affection, and the disease in the commencement is accompanied with pustules or favi; and may be readily mistaken for Eczema. The itching is intolerable whenever the hands are exposed to heat; the palm is harsh and dry, and rhagades rapidly form. The soles of the feet are often the seat of this local Psoriasis.

Var. d. P. *ophthalmica,* OPTHALMIC SCALL. In this the scaliness occurs chiefly about the angles of the eyes, producing an itching, inflammation, and thickening of the eyelids, with a watery discharge.* In children this variety is often productive of the loss of the eyelids.

Var. e. P. *pistoria,* BAKER'S SCALL OR ITCH. This variety (Plate XI. of BATEMAN; Pl. 6. of THE ATLAS,) chiefly attacks the back of the hands of bakers, and those who work with dry powder. The hands tumefy, and are covered with rough, scaly patches, interspersed with rhagades. The nails sometimes thicken, become curved, and are cast off; but those which replace them are generally attacked by the disease, and run the same course.

* Galen distinguished the Psoriasis from the Psorophthalmia. " Psoriasis autem exterius est; Psorophthalmia internam palpebram, superiorem præcique afficit." Galen de Oculo, cap. 7.

Var. f. P. *præputii,* SCALL OF THE PREPUCE.

This variety often accompanies the P. palmaria, is characterised by painful fissures and thickening of the part, and is usually attended with phymosis.

Var. g. P. *scrotalis,* SCALL OF THE SCROTUM. In this variety the scaliness, heat, itching, and redness, are followed by a hard, brittle texture of the skin, and by painful chaps and excoriations.

The same general plan of treatment is applicable to the different modifications of Psoriasis; the period of its duration, and the degree of irritability, being carefully attended to. The popular practice, which hinges upon the old humoral hypothesis, consists chiefly in attempts to expel imaginary humours by evacuations, or to correct them by what are called antiscorbutics. But bleeding and repeated purging are injurious; and the vegetable juices, which an absurd notion of the *scorbutic* nature of Psoriasis suggested, appear to be totally inefficacious. A more recent empiricism, which resorts to mercury in all affections of a chronic nature and of some obscurity, is not more successful: in fact, all these varieties of scaly tetter are ultimately aggravated by perseverance in a course of mercurials. " In Psoriasis *diffusa,* however, benefit is derived from Plummer's pill, in doses of five grains every night; whilst Cinchona and Soda, as we shall have to notice afterwards, are given during the day. We have, also, seen considerable benefit derived from

F

Hydrargyrum cum Creta in Psoriasis *guttata*, carried to the point of slightly touching the gums."

In the commencement of the eruption, when it appears suddenly, and the constitution is obviously disordered, a moderate antiphlogistic treatment must be pursued. A gentle purgative should be administered, and the diet made light, by abstracting every thing stimulant. This regimen, indeed, is requisite throughout the course of the disease, which is immediately aggravated in sympathy with irritation of the stomach, whether by spices, fermented liquors, pickles, or vegetable acids; whence the disuse of these articles contributes materially to its cure.

But if the constitutional disturbance has subsided, the use of the fixed alkali, combined with Sulphur Lotum, " or the Sulphuret of Potass, is useful: the Sulphuret, however, is apt to nauseate; and therefore is seldom continued long by the patients of private practitioners. The waters of Harrowgate, Barèges, &c. are beneficial when the skin is inert, but hurtful in irritable states of the nervous system." These, in conjunction with an infusion of Cinchona, together with tepid washing with simple water, or milk and water, will gradually remove the complaint. If the scaly patches have extended over a considerable part of the body, and have assumed a more inert and chronic character, it must be viewed in a similar light with the Lepra, and the remedies recommended for the first and second species of that disease must be resorted to. " Alibert mentions that an inveterate case of Psoriasis diffusa, chiefly affecting the thighs, was much benefited by the use of a strong infusion of Saponaria *officinalis*, during the use of which he says, ' que les symptômes diminuoient d'intensité, que le prurit sur-tout s'éteignoit entièrement.' " *

" In Psoriasis *inveterata*, the use of the Arsenical Solution has, in many instances, been found highly beneficial when the dose has been gradually carried to an extent, which would be dangerous in other states of the habit. Thus in a case successfully treated by Mr. Gaskoyne †, the dose was gradually increased to thirty-eight drops twice a day ; and it was not until the desired change occurred in the eruption, that the colicky pains and other symptoms of an overdose of Arsenic presented themselves. Candour obliges me to acknowledge that, notwithstanding the powerful influence of Arsenic in Psoriasis *inveterata*, I have met with cases which resisted it, even when administered in the largest doses. In some instances Erysipelas has accompanied the use of the Arsenical Solution ; in which case the administration of the remedy should be suspended until the Erysipelas be removed, and afterwards renewed in smaller doses."

" From my own experience, I can confidently assert, that the medicine on which the greatest confidence may be placed, in Psoriasis *diffusa* and

* Mal. de la Peau, p. 95.
† Plumbe's Practical Treatise, 2d edit. p. 170.

in the milder cases of P. *inveterata*, is the Liquor Potassæ. I usually commence with thirty drops of the solution in two fluid ounces of the Bitter Almond Emulsion, twice a day; and gradually increase the dose of the solution to eighty or even one hundred drops. If the patient be delicate, the infusion of Yellow Cinchona Bark or of Cascarilla is substituted for the Almond Emulsion. I have frequently found the Hydrargyrum cum Creta, in doses of six or eight grains, given at bed-time, an useful adjunct to the Solution of Potash."

The shooting and burning pain and itching, in the early and more inflammatory stages of Psoriasis, induce the patient to seek anxiously for relief from local external applications; but he is mortified to find that even the mildest substances prove irritants, and aggravate his distress. A decoction of bran, a little cream, or oil of almonds, sometimes produce ease; but any admixture, even of the Oxide of Zinc, or preparations of Lead, with these liniments, is commonly detrimental. " Dr. Morrison treated several cases of Psoriasis successfully by friction, at the same time excluding the atmospheric air. His plan is to dip a sponge in tepid water, and after squeezing it hard, to cover it with oatmeal. With this the affected parts are briskly rubbed for a considerable time, renewing the oatmeal on the sponge; and after this operation, when the parts have been well washed and dried, applying neatsfoot oil over them with a varnishing brush. This operation is to be repeated twice or thrice a day, according to the urgency of the case."* "Caution, however, is requisite in the use of external remedies. Alibert mentions the case of a lady affected with Psoriasis *inveterata* all over the abdomen; and who, to absorb the discharge, covered the eruption with hot flour. The eruption disappeared after eight days; but left behind it great irritability of stomach, an unquenchable thirst; ' sa salive est devenue épaisse, fétide, et comme platreuse. Pour comble d'infortune, ses yeux sont totalement perdus.' "†

" Much benefit often results from the use of the tepid bath; but in general it is not used long enough each time of employing it. Alibert mentions a case of Psoriasis *diffusa* cured by tepid baths alone, "pris tous les jours, et pendant l'espace de deux heures."‡

But the more local, and less inflammatory, eruptions of Psoriasis are considerably alleviated by local expedients. " A bath, with the Sulphuret of Potass, twice a week, has been found useful. In chronic cases the sulphureous fumigating baths are extremely beneficial." The P. *palmaria* is deprived of its dryness and itching by exposure to the vapour of hot water, and by the application of the Unguentum Hydrargyri Nitratis, diluted with the Unguentum Cetacei or Ceræ, according to the degree of irritation in the skin. " It has yielded to blisters

---

* Edinburgh Med. and Surg. Journ. vol. xvi. p. 525.
† Mal. de la Peau, p. 84.
‡ Ibid. p. 97.

after resisting both internal and external remedies for upwards of a year.* The following ointment, recommended by M. Chevalier, has been found useful:

Chlorure of Lime, 3 gros
Turbith Mineral, 2 gros
Oil of Almonds, 6 gros
Lard, 2 onces. Mix.†

Sea-bathing, continued for many weeks, has been found an effectual remedy. The P. *scrotalis* and P. *ophthalmica* are also relieved by the same application, or the Unguentum Hydrargyri Præcipitati albi: but great care is requisite, in the former case, to keep the parts clean by frequent ablution, and to prevent attrition. In the Psoriasis of the lips, nothing acrid can be borne; and much of the cure depends upon securing the parts from irritation, even from heat and cold, by a constant covering of some mild ointment or plaster. In all these cases some of the internal remedies above mentioned must be at the same time employed, according to the period and other circumstances of the disease.

Books which may be consulted on Psoriasis.

ALIBERT, Maladies de la Peau, fol.
DUFFIN, on Squamous Disorders, Edin. Med. & Surg. Journ. No. 86.
Edinburgh Med. and Surg. Journ. vol. xvi. p. 526.
GOOD's Study of Medicine, vol. iv. 2d edit. 1822.
PLUMBE's Practical Treatise on Diseases of the Skin, 2d edit. 1827.
RAYER, Traité Théorique et Pratique des Mal. de la Peau, t. 2. p. 51.
WILLAN on Cutaneous Diseases, 4to. 1808.

* Med. Repos. vol. iii. *New Series*, p. 58.
† Journ. de Chimie Méd. Mars, 1826.

Genus III. PITYRIASIS.

Syn. πιτυρίασις (*G. et Auct. Vet.*): Lepidosis Pityriasis (*Young, Good*): Schuppen (*Ger.*): *Dandriff.*

Def. IRREGULAR PATCHES OF THIN BRAN-LIKE SCALES, WHICH REPEATEDLY EXFOLIATE AND RECUR, BUT WHICH NEVER FORM CRUSTS, NOR ARE ACCOMPANIED WITH EXCORIATIONS. IT IS NOT CONTAGIOUS.*

There are four species of Pityriasis : —

1. P. *capitis.*   3. P. *versicolor.*
2. P. *rubra.*   4. P. *nigra.*

SPECIES 1. PITYRIASIS *capitis,* DANDRIFF OF THE HEAD.

Syn. Dartre furfuracée volante. — Herpes furfuraceus volitans (*Alibert*): Shoondoo (*Tam.*): Buffa (*Duk.*): Tsoondoo (*Tel.*): Crusta capitis numatorum (*Plenck*): der Kneis, Haufstschappen (*Ger.*)

---

* These negative characters distinguish this eruption, especially when it affects the scalp, from the furfuraceous Porrigo; a distinction which the last-mentioned circumstance rendered important and necessary. The ablest of the later Greek writers, Alexander and Paul, have described the disorder, as consisting of " slight scaly and branny exfoliations, without ulceration." (See Alex. Trall. lib. i. cap. 4. — Paul. Ægin. lib. iii. cap. 3.) Yet all the translators have rendered Πιτυριασις by the word *Porrigo;* which, according to Celsus, comprehended the ulcerating pustules, or achores, of the Greeks (de Med. lib. vi. cap. 2.). The use of the term Pityriasis, therefore, to designate a dry and furfuraceous eruption, as distinct from the ulcerating Porrigo, is sanctioned by authority, as well as by etymology, and pathological observation.

This affection (Plate XV. fig. 1. of BATEMAN), which in infants is called simply *dandriff*, appears in a slight whitish scurf along the top of the fore- head and temples, but in larger, flat, separate semi- transparent scales on the occiput.   A similar affec- tion occurs on the scalp of aged persons.*

It is only necessary to enforce a regular ablution of the scalp with tepid soap and water, or with an alkaline or weak spirituous lotion; for which pur- pose the hair must be removed, if it be not thin. If this be neglected, the affection may ultimately degenerate into Porrigo.

SPECIES 2.   The PITYRIASIS *rubra*, RED DAN- DRIFF.

This species occurs most frequently in advanced life, and is the result of a slight inflammation of the portions of the skin affected, somewhat resem- bling in this respect the Psoriasis *diffusa*.   The cuticle is at first only red and rough, but soon be- comes mealy or scurfy, and exfoliates, leaving a similar red cuticle underneath, which undergoes the like process; the scaliness becoming greater, as the exfoliation is repeated.   This complaint is attended with a dry and unperspiring surface, a troublesome itching †, and a feeling of stiffness.

* A good representation of Pityriasis on the occiput of an adult is given by Alibert, pl. 11., which he calls " Dartre furfuracée volante."

† Alibert, nevertheless, remarks, " dans les Dartres furfuracées, le prurit est presque nul, parceque les papilles de la peau y sont très-peu intéressées."   Vide Mal. de la Peau, p. 81.   T.

There is also a general languor and restlessness. When the redness and scales disappear, the patches are left of a yellowish or sallow hue. But the whole process is liable to be repeated at short intervals, and the disease to be thus greatly prolonged.

The P. *rubra* is removed by a combination of antimonials with the decoction of woods, and the warm sea-water bath. I have also seen it materially relieved by small doses of the Tinctura Veratri. Where the irritability of the skin is not very great, a gentle restringent lotion or ointment, containing a portion of Borax or Alum, and Superacetate of Lead, may be applied to the parts affected with advantage.

SPECIES 3. The PITYRIASIS *versicolor*, VARIEGATED DANDRIFF.

This species (Plate XV. fig. 2. of BATEMAN) is most remarkable for the chequered and variegated discoloration of the cuticle which it exhibits. It appears mostly about the breast and epigastrium, and sometimes on the arms and shoulders, in brown patches of different shades, variously branching and coalescing, and interspersed with portions of the natural hue.* In a few instances, it has extended

* These patches scarcely ever appear, like Ephelides and freckles, on the face and hands, but chiefly on covered parts, as is remarked by Sennertus, who has given an accurate description of this eruption, under the appellation of " Maculæ hepaticæ," latinizing the popular German term, *Leberflechte.* He considers it as the *Melas,* or dark variety of Vitiligo. See his Pract. Med. lib. v. part iii. § 1. cap. 7.

over the whole back and abdomen, even to the thighs, and slightly affected the face. There is generally a slight scurfy roughness on the discoloured parts; but this is in some cases scarcely perceptible, and there is no elevation or distinct border to the patches. Dr. Willan states, that the P. versicolor "is not merely a cuticular disease; for, when the cuticle is abraded from any of the patches, the sallow colour remains, as before, in the skin, or rete mucosum." This, however, is not universal: for I have seen several instances of the eruption, in which the discoloured cuticle peeled off at intervals, in a thickened state, and a new cuticle was found underneath, of a red hue, as is usual under large exfoliations. "Mr. Plumbe mentions a variety of this species in which no sensible elevation is perceptible to the finger when it is rubbed over the discoloration; but when the part is forcibly rubbed with a dry cloth, large films of thin delicate cuticle are detached, and the cutis which is bared remains tender, and becomes more inflamed."*

The P. versicolor is usually of little moment; for it is rarely accompanied by internal disorder, or by any troublesome sensations, if we except a slight itching on growing warm in bed, after strong exercise, or drinking warm or strong liquors. In those instances, however, where the eruption is very extensive, the itching and irritation connected

---

* Plumbe's Practical Treatise, 3d. edit, p. 202.

with it are sometimes extremely distressing, depriving the patients of their natural rest. In these cases the digestive organs are also commonly disordered. But even when the eruption is not troublesome, great uneasiness is often occasioned by its appearance; since its brown and almost coppery hue frequently suggests, even to medical practitioners, the idea of a syphilitic origin. But a little experience will soon enable the observer to recognise the eruption, independently of the total absence of any tendency to ulceration, however long its duration may be, and of every other concomitant symptom of syphilis.

The causes of this Pityriasis are not well ascertained. It occurs most frequently in those who have resided in hot climates, especially in its troublesome form. In one young gentleman it began after a year's residence in the Greek islands: it is also not uncommon in military and seafaring people. The most extensive eruption that I have seen, occurred in a custom-house officer, after drinking spirits freely during a day of fasting in a boat on the Thames. Fruit, mushrooms, sudden alternations of heat and cold, violent exercise with flannel next to the skin, have been mentioned as probable causes of this eruption.

Internal medicines have not appeared to have much influence on this eruption, as Dr. Willan has stated. The Oxygenated Muriatic Acid, however, I think, is possessed of some efficacy; and if the affection were of sufficient importance to induce the

patient to persevere in swallowing medicine, the
Pitch pills * would probably be serviceable.   By
active external stimulants the disorder is often removed ; as by lotions of strong spirit, containing
the Muriatic Acid, or the Caustic Potass : one
drachm of the former, or two or three of the
Liquor Potassæ, may be added to half a pint of distilled water.   Sea-bathing is likewise beneficial,
both as a remedy and as a preventive of its recurrence.   The more extensive and irritable eruptions
of Pityriasis approximate somewhat in their character to the Psoriasis, and are alleviated by the
same treatment.

SPECIES 4.   PITYRIASIS *nigra*. BLACK DANDRIFF.
Subsequent to the period of his publication,
Dr. Willan had observed a variety of Pityriasis in
children born in India, and brought to this country,
which commenced in a partially papulated state of
the skin, and terminated in a black discoloration,
with slight furfuraceous exfoliations.   It sometimes
affected half a limb, as the arm or leg ; sometimes
the fingers and toes. †

" The disease termed PINTA, or *Blue stain*,
which prevails in Mexico, appears to be a variety of Pityriasis *nigra*.   It commences with
slight febrile symptoms, which last a few days

---

* See below, page 82.

† M. Alibert has figured an eruption on the hand, which seems referable to this species, and which he denominates a " scorbutic Ephelis."
(See his plate 27, *bis*.)   It appears to be the result of a degree of misery
and filth, as little known in this country as the disease.

only; and, on subsiding, leave the face, breast, and limbs covered with yellowish maculæ, which change to a blue, and, in advanced stages, to a black colour. The skin assumes a rough and scaly appearance, and exhales a very offensive perspiration: but the general health is not affected. It is said to be infectious. It is relieved by light cathartics and active diaphoretics."*

Books which may be consulted on Pityriasis.

ALIBERT, Précis Théorique et Pratique sur les Mal. de la Peau, 2 tomes 8vo. 1822.
BIDOUX, Reflex. Pratiques sur les Mal. de la Peau, 8vo. 1826.
GOOD, Study of Medicine, vol. iv.
PLUMBE, On Diseases of the Skin, 2d edit. 1827.
RAYER, Traité des Maladies de la Peau.
SENNERTUS, Pract. Med. lib. v. part. iii. 8vo.
WILLAN on Cutaneous Diseases, 4to. 1805.

GENUS IV. ICHTHYOSIS.

Syn. Lepra Ichthyosis (*Sauv.*): Lepidosis Ichthyosis (*Young*): Lepidosis Ichthyasis (*Good*): Ichthyose(*F.*): der Fischsckuppen-penansatz (*G.*): *Fish Skin.*

Def. A PAPILLARY, INDURATED, HORNY CONDITION OF THE SKIN TO A GREATER OR LESS EXTENT.

The ICHTHYOSIS, or *fish-skin disease,* is characterized by a thickened, hard, rough, and in some

---

* American Med. Review, vol. ii.

cases almost horny texture of the integuments of
the body, with some tendency to scaliness, but
without the deciduous exfoliations, the distinct and
partial patches, or the constitutional disorder, which
belong to Lepra and Psoriasis.

"The disease appears to be seated in the papillæ
of the skin, which elongate into horny cones, and
sometimes spread so as to acquire broad irregular
tops. Dr Good supposes that the incrustation, as
he terms it, is formed by the cutaneous excretories
throwing out an excess of calcareous matter, which
is deposited in the cutis, rete mucosum, and cuticle *; but in our opinion, the disease is in the
papillæ, which assume a state nearly resembling
that which constitutes the common wart."

There are two species of Ichthyosis :

    1. I. *simplex.*   2. I. *cornea.* †

SPECIES 1. ICHTHYOSIS *simplex :* SIMPLE FISH-
SKIN.

Syn. Ichthyosis simplex (*Good*) : Ichthyose
nacrée (*F.*).

In its commencement this disease (Plates XVI.
and XVII. of BATEMAN ; Pl. 7. of THE ATLAS,)
exhibits merely a thickened, harsh, and discoloured
state of the cuticle, which appears, at a little distance, as if it were soiled with mud. When fur-

---

* Study of Medicine, vol. iv. p. 598.

  † Both Willan and Bateman have erred in placing Ichthyosis in the
order *squamæ :* notwithstanding the minuteness of the morbid papillæ, it
certainly is more allied to the Tubercula. T.

ther advanced, the thickness, hardness, and roughness become much greater, and of a minute warty
character, and the colour is nearly black. The
roughness, which is so great as to give a sensation
to the finger passing over it, like the surface of a
file, or the roughest shagreen, is occasioned by
innumerable rugged lines and points, into which
the surface is divided. These hard prominences,
being apparently elevations of the common lozenges
of the cuticle, necessarily differ in their form and
arrangement in different parts of the body, according to the variations of the cuticular lines, as well
as in different stages and cases of the complaint.
Some of them appear to be of uniform thickness
from their roots upwards; while others have
a short narrow neck, and broad irregular tops.
The former occur where the skin, when healthy, is
soft and thin; the latter where it is coarser, as
about the olecranon and patella, and thence along
the outside of the arms and thighs. On some parts
of the extremities, however, especially about the
ankles, and sometimes on the trunk of the body,
these excrescences are scaly, flat, and large, and
occasionally imbricated, like the scales of carp:
" but it is probable that this imbricated state may
depend on the pressure of the clothes." In other
cases, they have appeared separate, being intersected by whitish furrows.

This unsightly disease appears in large continuous patches, which sometimes cover the greater
part of the body, except the flexures of the joints,

the inner and upper part of the thighs, and the
furrow along the spine. " These patches are
sometimes gradually lost in the healthy skin; at
other times, they terminate abruptly." The face is
seldom severely affected; but in one case, in a
young lady, the face was the exclusive seat of the
disorder, a large patch covering each cheek, and
communicating across the nose. (Plate XVIII. of
BATEMAN.)* The mammæ, in females, are some-

* The Editor consulted Dr. Bateman respecting the case of a young
lady so exactly similar to that which is represented in the 18th Plate of
Bateman's Delineations, that, were he not certain of the contrary, he
would imagine that plate to be a representation of the same case. The
following are the particulars of the case : —

The patient was about fifteen years of age in the spring of the year
1810, when the disease was first observed. She had previously been
subject to headaches, flatulence, disordered bowels, cold feet, and flushing of the cheeks. The first symptom was little more, to use her own
words, than a soiled appearance of the cheeks, which was easily washed
off with warm water and soap; and it was not until the autumn of
1812, that this soiling began to increase and adhere more firmly; and
in the course of a few months it became so considerable, that the parents of the patient consulted the late Dr. James Gregory of Edinburgh.
After the use of some acrid applications, which produced inflammation
and ulceration, Dr. Gregory succeeded in clearing the skin in ten days.
This improvement, however, was of short duration: the disease returned; when Steel and Aloetics, Mercury carried to salivation, warm
sea-water baths, shaving off the incrustation, an ointment composed of
Carbonate of Soda, Spirit of Turpentine, Sugar, and Resin Ointment; a
strong lotion with Oxymuriate of Mercury, and various other means
were successively employed to clear the skin, for three years, but without success; when she came to London for further advice.

The eruption at this period extended over both cheeks, and across
the bridge of the nose: it was of a dirty olive-brown hue, and greatly
disfigured a face which was naturally very beautiful. It had much the
appearance and the harshness of shagreen. Under Dr. Bateman's care,
the patient took Pitch pills, and employed various internal and external
remedies, but without any permanent benefit, for six months; when,
becoming tired of medicine, she resolved to return to Scotland uncured,

times encased in this rugged cuticle. The whole
skin, indeed, is in an extremely dry and unperspir-
able condition, and on the palms of the hands, and
the soles of the feet, it is much thickened and
brittle. The disease often commences in childhood,
and even in early infancy. " In some instances it
is hereditary* : but even when this is the case, the
disease does not show itself in all the children of
the same family."

This affection has been found to be very little
under the control of medicine † : stimulating ointments and plasters have been industriously employed, with no material effect; and the disorder

---

The Editor, however, having persuaded her to remain in the metropolis,
after the empirical trial of many remedies, succeeded in completely
removing the eruption, by means of a decoction of the root of the sharp-
pointed Dock, Rumex *acutus*, taken internally. In eight days the skin
acquired its natural texture and appearance; but, the use of the decoction having been discontinued, at the end of ten days more the eruption
re-appeared; it was again removed by the decoction; and in this manner it was combated at successive intervals for several months, always
returning a short time after the decoction was discontinued. Conceiv-
ing that the return of the eruption depended on a habit acquired by
the skin from the long continuance of the disease, the face was blistered
with the Cantharides plaster immediately after the eruption was again
cleared off, and the cure became permanent. T.

* Rayer regards Ichthyosis as a congenital disease; and cases con-
firming this opinion have been published by Dr. Girdlestone (Med. and
Phys. Journ. vol. viii.), and Mr. Martin (Med. Chirurg. Trans. vol. ix.
p. 52.) T.

† For examples of Ichthyosis the reader may refer to Panarolus (Pen-
tecoste v. obs. 9.); Van der Wiel (obs. xxxv. cent. 2.); Marcel. Do-
natus (Mirabil. lib. i. 3.; or Schenck, Obs. Medic. Rarior. p. 699., where
the same case is related); and Philos. Transact. vol. xiv. no. 160. —
and vol. xliv. for 1755. See also the 37th plate of Alibert, in which
the I. *simplex* is well represented. His appellation is " Ichthyose
nacrée."

has been known to continue for several years, with
occasional variations. — Dr. Willan trusted to the
following palliation by external management:
" When a portion of the hard scaly coating is removed," he says, " it is not soon produced again.
The easiest mode of removing the scales," says Dr.
Willan, " is to pick them off carefully with the
nails from any part of the body, while it is im-
mersed in hot water. — The layer of cuticle, which
remains after this operation, is harsh and dry; and
the skin did not, in the cases I have noted, recover
its usual texture and softness: but the formation
of the scales was prevented by a frequent use of
the warm-bath, with moderate friction."—" In the
limited practice of the Editor, this method of proceeding has never proved beneficial; indeed, it is
not likely that the removal of the corneous cuticle
would be of any use whilst the disease which first
produced it remains unsubdued. Blistering has
been found serviceable, particularly when the
disease is of long standing. Mr. Plumbe relates
two cases in which the incrustation, which was
confined to the leg, was removed by the application
of pressure by means of adhesive straps and bandages, and keeping the part constantly cool with
a lotion applied over these. At the end of four
or five days the straps were removed, when ' the
eruption was found liberated from its attachment
to the cutis, and came off in large flakes nearly
through its whole extent, exposing a white and
ill-formed cuticle, which might be scraped off

without pain.' By persevering in this plan the skin gradually acquired a healthy texture." *

I have known the skin cleared of this harsh eruption by bathing in the sulphureous waters, and rubbing it with a flannel or rough cloth, after it had been softened by the bath; but the cuticle underneath did not recover its usual condition; it remained bright and shining: and the eruption recurred. " The sulphurous fumigating baths are more certain in clearing the skin, and more permanent in their effects." Internally the use of pitch has in some instances been beneficial, having occasioned the rough cuticle to crack, and fall off, and left a sound soft skin underneath. This medicine, made into pills with flour, or any farinaceous powder, may be taken to a great extent, not only without injury, but with advantage to the general health; and affords one of the most effectual means of controlling the languid circulation, and the inert and arid condition of the skin. † Upon the same principle, the Arsenical Solution has been employed in Ichthyosis: in one case, in a little girl affected with a moderate degree of the disease on the scalp, shoulders, and arms, this medicine produced a complete change of

* Practical Treatise on Diseases of the Skin, 1st edit. p. 334.

† A lady took for a considerable time from three drachms to half an ounce of pitch daily, with the most salutary effect both on her skin and general health. She had commenced with four pills, of five grains each, three times a day, and gradually augmented the dose. — It may be remarked, that the unpleasant pitchy flavour of the pills is materially diminished, if they are kept for some time after being made up.

the condition of the cuticle, which acquired its natural texture; but in two others no benefit was derived from it. The decoction of the inner bark of the elm has been said to be a specific for Ichthyosis, by Plenck; but this originated in a misconception as to the use of the term.* " The most beneficial internal remedy certainly is the decoction of the root of the sharp-pointed Dock, Rumex *acutus*, either alone or conjoined with Arsenic. It is prepared by slicing one ounce of the recent root, and boiling it in two pints of water down to one pint, and then straining. The dose is a wine-glass full three times a day. Sometimes it purges rather too briskly, which should be checked by the addition of a few drops of tincture of Opium to each dose of the decoction."†

Species 2. Ichthyosis *cornea*. Horny Fish Skin.

Syn. Ichthyiasis cornigera (*Good*): Cornua cutanea (*Plenck*): Appendices cornés (*Rayer*): Corne, Ichthyose cornée (*F.*)

Several cases of a rigid and horny state of the

---

* The definition of Ichthyosis given by Plenck, as well as the description of " Lepra ichthyosis," by Dr. Lettsom, on whose authority Plenck has mentioned this remedy, obviously refers to the Lepra vulgaris. See Plenck, Doctrina de Morb. Cutan. p. 89.—Lettsom, Med. Memoirs of the Gen. Dispensary, sect. iii. p. 152.

† A case of Ichthyosis, detailed by Turner under the idea that it was Lepra Græcorum, was cured by Mercury, Antimony, and a diet drink, in which this Rumex acutus was a principal ingredient.—Treatise on the Diseases of the Skin, 4th edit. p. 30. T.

integuments, sometimes partial, but sometimes extending nearly over the whole body, have been recorded by authors *; and occasionally such a condition of the cuticle has been accompanied with the actual production of excrescences of a horny texture. These, however, are rare occurrences; and all the cases on record have been congenital.

The ordinary formation of horny excrescences in the human body, of which many examples have been described from the time of the Arabians downwards, is, however, unconnected with any general rigidity of the cuticle. These excrescences have been improperly called horns; for they are purely of cuticular growth, having no connexion with the bones or other parts beneath, and consisting of a laminated callous substance, contorted and irregular in form, and not unlike isinglass in appearance and texture. † They originate from two or three different diseased conditions of the cuticle; as from warts, encysted tumours, steatomata, &c. Morgagni has mentioned

---

* See Philos. Trans. no. 176. no. 297. and vol. xlviii. pt. ii. p. 580. — Also Zacut. Lusitan. Prax. Hist. obs. 188. — Ephem. Acad. Nat. Cur. dec. i. p. 89. — Alibert has figured a singular case of " Ichthyose cornée," (plate 38.) which resembles the case of the " porcupine man," described by Mr. Baker, Philos. Trans. vol. xlix. p. 1.

† " Cornua certe, quæ hoc mererentur nomen, nunquam vidi;" says M. Lorry, " sed varias excrescentias in corpore et cute humana innascentes, et extra cutem forma singulari succrescentes, quis non vidit?" De Morbis Cutan. p. 520. Yet our credulous countryman, Turner, declines treating of horns, because, he affirms, " they are generally much deeper rooted than in the skin, arising from the cartilages or ligaments, or the bones themselves." On Diseases of the Skin, p. 1. ch. xii. at the end.

the growth of a horn on the sinciput of an old
man, the basis of which was a wart; and other
authors have noticed the same fact. *   In the most
numerous instances, however, they have arisen
from the cavity of encysted tumours, of very slow
growth, which were lodged under the cuticle of
the scalp, or over the spine, after the discharge
of their contained fluid. †   In one case, a horn of
this sort was the result of inflammation and discharge from a small steatomatous tumour of many
years' continuance. ‡   Nearly the whole of these
examples have occurred in women of advanced
age.

If these excrescences are sawed or broken off,
they invariably sprout again.   Excision, with the
complete destruction of the cyst, or morbid se-

---

* Morgagni de Sedib. et Caus. Morbor. epist. lxv. art. 2.—Avicenna,
who noticed the growth of horns on the joints, considered them as
verrucous. Canon iv. fen. 7. tract. iii. cap. 14. See also Lorry, p. 519.
—† Plenck de Morb. Cut. p. 98.

† See two cases of this sort described by Mr. (now Sir Everard)
Home in the Philosophical Transactions, vol. lxxxi. p. 1.; and references to nine other cases of similar origin, in which the horny excrescences were from four or five to twelve inches long: one of them eleven
inches in length, and two inches and a half in circumference, is preserved in the British Museum. See also Medical Facts and Observations, vol. iii. — Eph. Acad. Nat. Curios. dec. i. an. i. obs. 30.; and
dec. iii. an. v. app. — Hist. de la Soc. Roy. de Méd. de Paris, for 1776,
p. 516.— Bartholin. Hist. Anat. Rar. cent. i. 78.

‡ See Memoirs of the Medical Society of London, vol. iv. app.
p. 591.   The reader will find other examples of horny excrescences in the works of Ingrassias, de Tumor. præt. Naturam, tom. i.
p. 336.: Fabric. Hildan. cent. ii. obs. 25, 26., and many more referred
to by Haller, Elem. Physiol. tom. v. p. 30. note. Malpighi has figured
similar excrescences, originating from a morbid growth of the nails.
Opera Posthuma, p. 99. and tab. xix. fig. 3 — 6.

creting surface, is the only effectual remedy, when they have appeared, and a preventive during the growth of the primary tumour.

Works which may be consulted on Ichthyosis.

ALIBERT, Dis. des Maladies de la Peau, fol. 1806.
ARCHIVES GENERALES de Médecine, tom. v.
FOLLET, Rech. sur l'Ichthyose cornée, 4to. 1815.
GOOD's Study of Medicine, vol. iv.
JOULHIA (P. G.) Diss. sur l'Ichthyose nacrée, 4to. 1819.
HIST. de la Soc. Roy. de Paris, for 1776.
LORRY, de Morbis Cutaneis, 4to.
MEDICO-CHIRURGICAL Trans. of London, vol. ix.
MEM. della Societa Italiana, tom. xvi.
MEDICAL FACTS and Observations, vol. iii.
PHILOSOPHICAL TRANSACTIONS, vol. xiv. xlviii, xlix. and lxxxi.
RAYER, Traité des Maladies de la Peau, tom. 2.
SCHENCK, Obs. Med. Rarior, p. 699.
WILLAN on Cutaneous Diseases, 4to. 1805.

Order III.

EXANTHEMATA.

SYN. εξανθηματα (*G.*): Exanthematica (*Good*): Exanthème, Exanthémateux (*F.*): Inflammations exanthémateuses (*Rayer*): Rashes.

Def. SUPERFICIAL RED PATCHES, VARIOUSLY FI-
GURED, AND DIFFUSED IRREGULARLY OVER THE
BODY, LEAVING INTERSTICES OF A NATURAL COLOUR,
AND TERMINATING IN CUTICULAR EXFOLIATIONS.

The term EXANTHEMATA, *efflorescence,* appears
to have been used by the Greek writers in a very
general sense, equivalent to that of our word *eruption* * ; and it has been employed, in this acceptation, by many modern authors. The nosologists,
however, have limited it to those eruptions which
are accompanied with fever †, and which have their
regular periods of efflorescence and decline. In

---

* Hippocrates applies the term to numerous eruptions, which he
often classes together, as to Lichen, Lepra, Leuce (Prædict. lib. ii. ad
finem); to miliary vesicles, and wheals (Epid. i. in the case of Silenus,
some of which were prominent, like vari); and to eruptions resembling
burns, flea-bites, bug-bites, &c. (Coac. Prænot. 441. 39. ed. Foës.—
Epidem. lib. 7. p. 359. 28. &c.): he speaks also of τα αμυχωδεα εξανθισμαῖα,
or excoriations (Coac. Prænot. 444.); and applies the verb even to
ulcers; — εξανθεει ἑλκεα ες την κεφαλην (de Morbo Sacro, § iii. p. 88.)
He has likewise εξανθησεις ἑλκωδεες, (aph. 20. lib. iii.)

† Cullen confines the term to comprehend those eruptions only
which arise from the application of a specific contagion, " which first
produces fever, and afterwards an eruption upon the surface of the
body." First Lines, § DLXXXV. T.

this arrangement, it is appropriated solely to those appearances which are usually called RASHES; namely, to patches of superficial redness of the skin, of various extent and intensity, occasioned by an unusual determination of blood into the cutaneous vessels, sometimes with partial extravasation. It has no reference, therefore, to the existence of fever or contagion, or to the duration and progress of the complaint. The heat and tumefaction of the affected parts vary; and pain is not always present. The genera are acute diseases, which run their course within a certain space of time; and sometimes the accompanying fever assumes the intermittent character; at other times the typhoid. The first and second and the last genus only of this order are contagious.

The order comprehends seven genera:

1. RUBEOLA,	5. PURPURA,*
2. SCARLATINA,	6. ERYTHEMA,
3. URTICARIA,	7. ERYSIPELAS.†
4. ROSEOLA,	

GENUS I. RUBEOLA.‡

Syn. Morbilli; Blactiæ (*Auct. variæ*): Febris morbillosa (*Hoffman*): Phœnicismus (*Plouquet*):

---

* Purpura is here misplaced by Bateman.

† I have ventured to remove Erysipelas from the Bullæ, and to place it here, for reasons which shall be afterwards stated.

‡ The continental writers in general have designated this disease by the term *Morbilli,* the *minor plague;* an appellation borrowed from the

Typhus morbillosus (*Crichton*): Enanthesis rubeola (*Good*): Fièvre morbilleuse, Rougeole, Roseole (*F.*): die Kindsfecken (*German*): Hasbet (*Arab.*): Kyzamak (*Turkish*): Serukje (*Persian*): Chin ummay (*Tam.*): Chin umma (*Tel.*): Gobrie (*Duk.*): Khrusvāmasoorikāle (*Sans.*): Chumpak (*Malay*): *Measles.*

Def. AN ERUPTION OF CRIMSON STIGMATA, OR DOTS, GROUPED IN IRREGULAR CIRCLES OR CRESCENTS, CONTINUING FOR FOUR DAYS, AND TERMINATING IN MINUTE FURFURACEOUS SCALES; PRECEDED BY FEVER, SNEEZING, HOARSENESS, AND A SEROUS DISCHARGE FROM THE EYES AND NOSTRILS.

" Measles is a contagious disease, rarely appearing more than once during life. It is preceded by catarrhal fever," during which a rash appears usually on the fourth, but sometimes on the third, fifth, or sixth day, and, after a continuance of four days, gradually declines with the fever. The disease commences from ten to fourteen days after the contagion has been received. " It attacks chiefly children ; but no period of life is exempt* ; and it appears in all climates." This genus comprehends three species :

Italians, among whom *il Morbo* (the disease) signified *the Plague* (see Sennert. Med. Pract. lib. iv. cap. 12.) The terms Rubeola, Rubeoli, Roseola, Rossalia, Rossania, &c. had been applied, with little discrimination, to measles, scarlet fever, Eczema, &c. until Sauvages fixed the acceptation of the first of them.

* Instances have occurred of children having the disease before birth, in conjunction with the mothers. T.

1. R. *vulgaris*.
2. R. *sine catarrho, seu spuria*.
3. R. *nigra*.

SPECIES 1. RUBEOLA *vulgaris*. COMMON MEASLES.
Syn. Morbilli regulares (*Syden.*): Rougeole vulgaire (*F.*): *Measles*.

The precursory fever of the measles is accompanied, especially on the third and fourth days, with a tenderness and some inflammation of the eyes, and a slight turgescence of the eyelids, together with a serous discharge both from the eyes and nostrils, which excites frequent sneezing. There is likewise a teasing dry cough, with some degree of hoarseness and difficulty of breathing, " for some days before the eruption appears, sometimes seven or even fourteen," and often accompanied with sighing and a roughness or slight soreness of the throat. " There is occasionally great pain of the back, and sometimes of the epigastrium." These symptoms are generally more severe in children than in adults, and are sometimes accompanied with drowsiness and slight delirium in the night : " and the more severe the preceding symptoms are, the worse is the disease. The surface of the tongue at this time is generally white, with the edges of a vivid red."

The rash (Plate XIX. of BATEMAN; Pl. 8. of THE ATLAS,) on the fourth day, begins to appear like the bites of fleas, gradually clustering into irregular crescent-shaped patches about the forehead and below the chin, then on the nose and over the rest of the face; and on the following morning it is visible on the neck and breast, spreading towards evening over the trunk of the body, and lastly over the extremities. During this day the fever is generally increased, as is also the restlessness; but the eyes are less impatient of light: the efflorescence in the face is most vivid: " on the following day (the fifth), the eruption is fading on the face, but increasing on the neck and chest:" on the sixth day it begins to fade and subside on the neck, while the patches on the body are highly red. " At this period, also, if the fauces be examined, some patches of obscure redness, resembling the eruption on the skin, are observed upon them." The eruption is accompanied with itching and heat of the skin. The patches on the body and the extremities begin to fade on the seventh day; and the patches on the back of the hand, which usually appear last (sometimes on the sixth or even the seventh day of the fever), do not always decline till the eighth. On the ninth day slight discolorations only remain, which vanish before the end of the tenth, leaving a slight pulverulent or brown desquamation.

It is important, with a view to diagnosis, to attend accurately to the form of the rash, that it may not be confounded with Scarlatina and Roseola. It first shows itself in distinct, red, and nearly circular spots, somewhat less than the ordinary areolæ of flea-bites.* As these increase in number, they coalesce, forming small patches, of an irregular figure, but approaching nearest to that of semicircles or crescents.† These patches, which give no sensation of roughness to the finger, are intermixed with the single circular dots, and with interstices of the natural colour of the skin: on the face, they are slightly raised, so as to give the sensation of inequality of surface to the finger passed over the cuticle: but no suppuration occurs. The whole face, indeed, is often sensibly swelled, at the height of the eruption; and occasionally the tumefaction of the eyelids is so great as to close the eyes for a day or two, as in the small-pox ‡: but on the other parts of the body the patches are not sensibly elevated. In many persons, however, as Dr. Willan has remarked, miliary vesicles appear (see ATLAS, Pl. 8.) during the height of the efflorescence, on the neck, breast, and arms; and papulæ often occur on the wrists, hands, and fingers. The decline of the eruption is accompanied with more troublesome itching than is experienced during its rise.

Measles, before the eruption appears, may be mistaken for severe catarrh; but it is of little mo-

* See the excellent history of measles detailed by Sydenham, Obs. Med. sect. iv. cap. 5.

† This observation, which is peculiar to Dr. Willan, is important; for, though entirely overlooked by ordinary observers, it is commonly very manifest, and therefore a valuable diagnostic guide.

‡ See Macbride, Introd. to Med. part ii. chap. 14. — Heberden, Med. Trans. of the Coll. of Phys. vol. iii. art. xxvi., and Comment. de Morb. cap. 63.

ment, as the treatment is the same. The catarrhal
symptoms, and even the fever, are somewhat augmented on the appearance of the eruption; but the
latter usually ceases when the eruption declines,
which is generally on the fourth or fifth day; but,
a day or two days before, the vivid redness changes
to a brownish red. At this period a diarrhœa commonly supervenes, if it have not occurred earlier,
and affords relief to the other symptoms. This,
however, is the period when the danger, which is a
consequence rather than a concomitant of measles,
commences: for now the catarrh is occasionally
aggravated to acute inflammation of the lungs, of
more obstinacy than ordinary pneumonia, on which
hectic sometimes supervenes, and ultimately hy-
drothorax, spitting of blood, or, in scrophulous
habits, confirmed consumption.

Other inflammatory affections, indicative of a cachectic condition of the system, are liable to occur
at the close of the disease, and prove tedious and
troublesome. In some, severe attacks of ear-ache,
with deafness; in others, inflammation of the eyes
and eyelids of a more unmanageable character than
the common ophthalmia; and in others, swellings
of the lymphatic glands take place. Sometimes
the mesenteric glands become diseased, and marasmus ensues: and sometimes chronic eruptions on
the skin, especially Ecthymata, Rupia, Herpes, and
porriginous pustules, with tumid lip, discharges
behind the ears, and tedious suppurations, are the
sequelæ of the disease. " Measles frequently occurs

as an epidemic, sometimes benign, at other times
proving very fatal. The disease, however, is seldom severe, unless in children at a very early age;
or during dentition. In adults predisposed to pulmonary affections, it is to be dreaded; and it is
also frequently severe in pregnant women. The
intensity of the pulmonary inflammation, and
symptoms of meningitis accompanying the eruption,
always authorize a doubtful prognosis. The season of the year when measles is most commonly
epidemic is early in spring." The eruptive stage of
measles in general is seldom attended with danger,
and, therefore, requires little medicinal treatment.
It is chiefly necessary to open the bowels, to confine
the patient to a light vegetable diet, with cold,
sub-acid, aqueous drinks, and to maintain a cool
regular temperature of the room, which should be
moderately obscured. I have seen fatal effects
result from the exposure of the patient to cold air
during the eruption. An emetic is sometimes useful at the commencement of the disease. The
usual diaphoretics and emulsions have little influence over the fever or catarrh; and the inhal-
ation of steam, or the use of the pediluvium, is not
more efficient * : but a steady refrigerant regimen,
while it is grateful to the feelings of the patient,
contributes to repress present fever, restlessness,
and delirium, and to diminish the inflammatory
tendency of the disease in the cerebral membranes,

* Dr. Macbride (loc. cit.) and Dr. Willan have recommended the two
last as palliatives.

the lungs, eyes, &c. on the decline of the eruption. *

Almost all practitioners have concurred in the
recommendation of blood-letting in measles ; some
employing it at the height of the eruption, which
they deem the most inflammatory period, and some
at the close of it, when pneumonic inflammation
more commonly supervenes; while others consider it as safe and beneficial at any period in or
after the disease, where the symptoms are very distressing.† Dr. Heberden, indeed, contends that
" bleeding, together with such medicines as the
occasional symptoms would require in any other

---

* I am indebted to Mr. Magrath of Plymouth, through the medium
of my friend Dr. Lockyer, of the same place, for some important in-
struction, respecting the safety and efficacy of the *cold effusion* during
the fever and eruption of measles. Mr. Magrath favoured me with a
perusal of the official reports of the treatment of a great number of
patients in the hospital of the Mill prison, in which the practice was
highly successful. He affirms that he has never witnessed any of the
untoward circumstances which are usually apprehended from cold, such
as the retrocession of the eruption, increase of the catarrhal symptoms,
&c.; but, on the contrary, he is persuaded that the inflammatory affections of the chest, which are apt to supervene, on the decline of the
rash, are prevented by the suppression of the early excitement, to the
violence of which they are chiefly to be attributed. This accords
strictly with well-established experience of the operation of cold in
scarlet fever and small-pox. See an interesting case in illustration of
the safety and advantages of this practice in measles, communicated to
me by Mr. Magrath, in the Edin. Med. and Surg. Journal, for April
1814, p. 258.

" I have seen the most marked benefit result from the cold effusion in
Scarlatina; but I should be extremely cautious of ordering it in measles,
on account of the pneumonic symptoms. I have had occasion to witness a fatal result from the imprudent exposure of the body, in a case
of measles, to cold air. T.

† See Morton de Morbillis. — Sydenham, loc. cit. — Heberden, loc.
cit.

fever, is the whole of the medical care requisite in the measles :" and he considers that this cannot be dispensed with even during the flow of the menses ; he should have added, provided the cough is hard, and the breathing much oppressed. Dr. Willan has placed this matter in the most judicious point of view. The mere oppression of the respiration, with a labouring pulse, on the first or second day of the eruption, is common to other eruptive fevers, and usually disappears in the course of twenty-four hours. When, therefore, it is not accompanied by a hard cough, and pains in the chest, it may, even in adults, be safely left to the natural termination. On the other hand, when the eruption has disappeared, and these symptoms, together with difficulty of breathing, have become severe, bleeding, either from the arm or by leeches, and cupping, may be repeatedly necessary, aided by blisters, and demulcents, with anodynes. " In applying leeches on very young and on delicate children, they should be placed on parts only which will admit of the application of pressure should the bleeding not readily stop ; for much danger has often resulted from placing them on soft parts. When the eruption retrocedes suddenly, and the pneumonic symptoms increase, the tepid bath must be employed ; with sinapisms to the chest after bleeding. Opiates, although recommended by several authors *, do not allay the violence of the cough during the

* Riverius, Obs. Cent. 11. n. 45. — Sydenham Opusc. p. 247. Young on Opium, sect. 36.

H

eruptive fever ; and tend to augment the heat and restlessness."

A diarrhœa frequently occurs at the close of the measles, which appears to alleviate the pneumonic symptoms, and to prevent some of the troublesome sequelæ of the disease before noticed. Hence this evacuation should not be interrupted, at least for a few days ; and laxatives should be administered, where it does not take place, as the most advantageous mode of allaying and preventing inflammatory symptoms. If the usual diarrhœa should be protracted, however, the patient will require the support of light but nutritious diet, and cordials. *
" When the severity of the symptoms has required that the depleting plan be carried to a great extent, the patient is often left in such a state of debility as to require bark with a nourishing diet, and even the use of wine, provided there be no reason to dread a return of the inflammatory symptoms."

Species 2. Rubeola *sine catarrho, seu spuria vel Incocta.* Imperfect Measles.

This is a peculiarity, scarcely amounting to a species, observed by Dr. Willan, in a few rare instances, during an epidemic Rubeola, which is only important as it leaves the susceptibility of receiving the febrile measles after its occurrence.

Dr. F. Home attempted to communicate measles by inoculating with the blood of the parts on which the eruption appeared; but the results of his experiments were unsatisfactory. Vide Med. Facts and Experiments. Lond. 1758.

The course and appearance of the eruption (Plate XX. of BATEMAN; Pl. 8. of THE ATLAS,) are nearly the same as in the R. *vulgaris;* but no catarrh, ophthalmia, or fever accompanies it. An interval of many months, even two years, has been observed between this variety and the subse-quent febrile Rubeola: but the latter more fre-quently takes place about three or four days after the non-febrile eruption.*

SPECIES 3. RUBEOLA *nigra.* BLACK MEASLES.

Dr. Willan applied this epithet to an unusual ap-pearance of the measles about the seventh or eighth day, when the rash becomes suddenly livid, with a mixture of yellow (Plate XXI. of BATEMAN;

---

* The correctness of all the statements of writers before the close of the last century, in regard to the recurrence of febrile measles, is very questionable; since the eruption had been confounded with that of Scarlatina down to this period. — Tozzetti, a physician of Florence; — Schacht, (Inst. Med. lib. i. cap. 12.);—Meza, (Compend. Med. fascic. i. cap. 20.),— and de Haen (de Divis. Febrium, cap. vi. § vi. p. 106.) affirm that they have seen the measles more than once in the same individual; while Rosenstein (on the Dis. of Children, chap. xiv.) affirms, that during forty years he had never seen such a recurrence, and Morton, that, in the same period of practice, he had witnessed it but once. But Morton himself deemed Scarlatina and Measles only varieties of the same disease! (De Morbillis et Scarlatina, cap. 4.)

It cannot now be doubted, however, that exceptions occasionally occur in respect to measles, as well as to small-pox and other contagious diseases which in general affect individuals but once during life. Since my first edition was printed, I have met with two papers by Dr. Baillie, in the 3d vol. of the Trans. of a Society for the Improv. of Med. and Chir. Knowledge (p. 258), which prove decisively that measles may occur a second time in the same individual, accompanied by their pe-culiar febrile and catarrhal symptoms. His authority will not be ques-tioned.

Pl. 8. of The Atlas,) "accompanied with languor and quickness of pulse. It occurs chiefly in persons of debilitated habits." It is generally devoid of inconvenience or danger, and is removed in a week or ten days by a light infusion of Cinchona bark with the mineral acids. " The symptoms, nevertheless, sometimes present the most alarming aspect: for example, in a case which came under the care of the Editor in 1804, the relaxation was so great, that the cuticle rubbed off, like a moist cobweb, when the wrist was compressed in feeling the pulse. The Cinchona, with the diluted Sulphuric Acid, wine and cordials, were freely administered; and the patient, a child eight years of age, recovered, has since enjoyed good health, and is now (1828) alive."

Works which may be consulted on Measles.

De Bacher, de Morbillis. 1790.
Fabricius, Diss. de Variolis et Morbillis. 1628.
Frank, Historia de Cur. Hom. Morb. l. iii. p. 245.
Good's Study of Medicine, vol. ii.
Heberden, Com. in Morb. Hist. et Cur.
Home's Facts and Experiments.
Lee, de Rubeola, 1779.
Lorry, in Mém. de la Société de Médecine, 1776.
Morton de Morbillis et Scarlatina.
Med. Trans. of the Coll. of Physicians, vol. iii.
Percival's Essays.
Rayer, Traité des Maladies de la Peau, vol. i.
Roberdiere, Recherches sur la Rougeole. 1776.
Roux, Traité sur la Rougeole. 1807.
Rush, Medical Inquiries, vol. ii. N. S.
Sims's Observations.
Sennertus, Diss. xiii. de Variolis, Morbillis, &c. 1628.
Sydenham, Opera Univ. 3d Edit.

Trans. of a Society for the Improv. of Med. and Chirurg. Knowledge, vol. iii.

WATSON, Med. Obs. and Inquiries, vol. iv. n. 22.

WILSON on Febrile Diseases, vol. ii.

WILLAN on Cutaneous Diseases.

YOUNG on Opium, sect. 36.

UNDERWOOD, on the Diseases of Children.

The limits of this Synopsis will not allow me to enter fully into the interesting inquiry, respecting the existence of the contagious eruptive fevers in the time of the Greek and Roman physicians. The general inference in favour of the negative has arisen from the defect of such unequivocal descriptions of these formidable maladies, as might have been expected in the writings of those, who have accurately delineated many other diseases of less moment, with which we are now familiar. But it appears to me, on the one hand, that this defect is perfectly explicable upon the ground of their absolute devotion to the humoral pathology, and of their systematic adoption of the dogmata of their predecessors; and, on the other, that there is a sufficient, though scattered, evidence in their works, to sanction the opposite conclusion. I shall here therefore briefly state the reasons of my belief in the affirmative of this question.

It is almost superfluous to remark, that, from Galen, who adopted and extended the doctrine of the four humours mentioned by Hippocrates, through the whole series of Greek writers, down to

Actuarias, the same opinions were received with the utmost servility. They supposed that they had reached the perfection of medical observation, when they had named the hypothetical humours which were believed to be in fault. They contented themselves, therefore, with classing together all the eruptive fevers as pestilential, and with referring the various eruptions, that accompanied them, to different combinations of the humours. Such eruptions were frequently mentioned by Hippocrates and Galen, under the appellation of erysipelata, herpetes, phlyctænæ, phlyzacia, ecthymata, erythemata, exanthemata, &c. as the concomitants of malignant and epidemic fevers. Hippocrates has generalized some of these observations, and has deduced especially the following prognostic, respecting the eruptions of inflamed pustules (phlyzacia), which seems referable only to the small-pox. " Quibus per *febres continuas* φλυζακια *toto corpore nascuntur*, lethale est, nisi superveniat apostema, quod fiat præcipue circa aures." [*]

But omitting, for the sake of brevity, the detached passages relating to this subject, it will be sufficient, I think, to refer to a remarkable chapter of Herodotus, " On the treatment of eruptions (εξανθηματα) occurring in fevers," which has been preserved by Aëtius. [†] This Herodotus was an eminent physician of the pneumatic sect at Rome, in the reign of Trajan, more than half a century

---

[*] See his Coac. Prænot. n. 114. ed. Foës. See also Epidem. lib. iii.
[†] See his Tetrabib. ii. serm. i. cap. 129.

before Galen settled in that city. He describes
first the herpetic eruptions "which appear about
the mouth at the crisis of simple fevers," and subsequently the wheals of the febrile Urticaria, the
miliary vesicles, and, I conceive, with considerable
precision, the rashes of measles and scarlatina, and
the pustules of smallpox. After mentioning the
labial Herpes, which occurs at the termination of
catarrhal and other slight fevers, he says, "But in
the early stages of fevers, which are *not simple,* but
the result of vicious humours, there arise *over the*
whole body patches like flea-bites; and, in the
malignant and *pestilential* fevers, these *ulcerate,* and
some of them have an affinity with carbuncles : all
these eruptions are signs of the redundancy of
corrupt and corrosive humours in the habit; but
those *which appear on the face* are the most malignant of all." He then proceeds to describe the
prognostics to be derived from the different appearances of these eruptions, almost in the same
terms which the Arabian writers on the smallpox
and measles subsequently used; and he was obviously acquainted with the danger of the highly
confluent, and red or livid forms of these eruptions.
" They are worse if numerous, than if few," &c.—
" Moreover," he remarks, " those which are extremely red are of the worst kind; but those which
are livid, black, and tumid, like flesh that has been
stained, are still more fatal; and these are copious
on the face and breast, abdomen, sides, and back."
He considers these cases as so desperate, that he

advises the practitioner not to hazard his reputation
by any active interference, lest the blame of their
fatality should be imputed to his attempts. " For
those eruptions," he asks, " which arise from
beneath, in a mortifying state of the surface, what
can they denote but that the life is passing from
within ?"

Now it seems unquestionable, that these, and
much more ample details, delivered in the language
of experience, are applicable exclusively to the
contagious eruptive fevers ; *i. e.* to smallpox, measles, and scarlatina. For we are not acquainted
with any other *continued fevers*, that are malignant
and *pestilential*, in the early stages of which *eruptions* appear *all over the body*, beginning *like flea-
bites*, and sometimes *ulcerating*, i. e. suppurating,
specially on the face, except the diseases just
mentioned.

But the difficulty and rarity of original observation, even under more favourable circumstances,
will be sufficiently manifest, if we trace the history
of medical opinions upon the subject of the same
diseases in later times.

It might be supposed that, after the existence
of these eruptive fevers had been so clearly pointed
out by the Arabians, their distinctive characters
would have been speedily ascertained, even by
ordinary observers. But the fact was directly the
reverse. Almost a thousand years elapsed, during
which the smallpox, measles, and scarlet fever
continued to commit their ravages, and physicians

continued to record them; while the individuals, who were spared by one of these maladies, were seen to suffer successively from attacks of the others: nevertheless, they were still viewed through the eyes of the Arabians, and were universally deemed varieties of one and the same disease, until near the beginning of the eighteenth century: and it was not till towards the close of that age of enlightened observation, that the distinct character and independent origin of these three contagious disorders were universally perceived and acknowledged.

We not only find the able and learned Sennertus, in the middle of the seventeenth century, discussing the question, "Why the disease in some constitutions assumes the form of smallpox, and in others that of measles?"* but in the posthumous work of Diemerbroeck, an intelligent Dutch professor, published in 1687, it is affirmed that smallpox and measles differ only in degree. " Differunt (scil. morbilli) a variolis accidentaliter, vel quoad magis et minus."† And still later, the same assertion was made by J. Christ. Lange, a learned professor at Leipsic. " Præterea tam morbilli quam variolæ sunt eruptiones in eo duntaxat discrepantes, quod vel minus vel magis appareant," &c.‡ But we must descend still nearer our own times, before we discover the complete unravelling of the subject,

* Medicin. Pract. lib. iv. cap. 12.
† Tractat. de Variolis et Morbilis, cap. 14.
‡ Miscell. Med. Curios. § xxxiv.

in the separation of scarlatina and measles, as distinct genera; although, as varieties, they had been pointed out even by Haly Abbas. *   Our countryman Morton maintained the identity of these two exanthemata, and considered their relative connexion the same as that of the distinct and confluent smallpox.† And so late as the year 1769, Sir William Watson did not distinguish the measles from the scarlet fever.‡ The publication of Dr. Withering's Essay on Scarlet Fever, in 1778, or rather of the second edition of that work in 1793, may be considered perhaps as the date of the correct diagnosis of this disease.   So difficult is the task of observation, — so tardy the development of truth. §

Surely, then, the imperfection of the knowledge of the ancients, respecting the nature of these eruptive fevers, affords no just inference against their existence: while, on the contrary, the brief but repeated notices, which they have transmitted to us, of eruptions resembling nothing that we are now acquainted with, except the contagious maladies in question, lead to the fair and legitimate conclusion, that the diseases of mankind, like their

* Theorice, lib. viii. cap. 14.

† De Morbillis et Scarlatina, exercit. iii.

‡ See his paper in the Med. Obs. and Inquiries, vol. iv. p. 152.

§ It is not the least curious circumstance in the history of medical discoveries, that the vulgar have, in many instances, led the way; and have actually given distinctive appellations to many varieties of disease, before medical philosophers had learned to distinguish them. This is strongly exemplified in the history of chicken-pox (see the 2d note on Varicella below); and also in Scabies, cow-pox, &c.

physical and moral constitution, have not undergone any great and unaccountable change; and that the eruptive fevers have prevailed from the earliest ages.

———

Genus II. SCARLATINA.*

Syn. Purpura (*Schulz, Junck*): Rossalia (*Ingrass et auct. Neap.*): Rosalia (*Auct. Hisp.*): Febris Scarlatina (*Syden. Morton, et auct. Ang.*): Mal de la Rosa (*Thiery*): Febris rubra (*Heberd.*): Typhus Scarlatinus (*Cricht.*): Enathesis Rosalia (*Good*): Fièvre rouge, scarlatine (*F.*): der Scharlachaufschlag (*Ger.*): Scarlet Fever.

Def. A CONTAGIOUS FEVER, ACCOMPANIED WITH A SCARLET RASH, APPEARING THE SECOND DAY ON THE FACE AND NECK; SPREADING PROGRESSIVELY OVER THE BODY; AND TERMINATING ABOUT THE SEVENTH DAY, AFTER WHICH THE CUTICLE EXFOLIATES.

The *scarlet fever* is characterized by a close and diffuse efflorescence, of a high scarlet colour, which appears on the surface of the body, or within the

* This barbarous term, which appears to have been of British origin, having found admission into all the systems of nosology, Dr. Willan did not deem it expedient to reject it.

With regard to the origin of the term Scarlatina, Dr. Good says that Dr. Willan is mistaken; " for the term itself is Italian, and was long in use as a vernacular name, on the shores of the Levant, before it was imported into our own country."—Study of Medicine, vol. ii. T.

mouth and fauces, usually on the second day of fever, and terminates in about five days.

Scarlatina sometimes appears as an epidemic; but, in general, it is propagated, like the smallpox, measles, and chicken-pox, by a specific contagion; and, like them, it affects individuals but once during life.* But it commences after a shorter interval from exposure to the contagion than the disorders just mentioned; namely, on the third, fourth, or fifth day.† Adults, however, are not so suscep-

* This fact is now fully ascertained. Dr. Withering, when he pub-lished the first edition of his tract, was of opinion, that the ulcerated sore-throat might occur in those who had undergone the Scarlatina anginosa: but, in the subsequent edition, he expresses his conviction that he was in error. Among two thousand cases, Dr. Willan never saw the recurrence of the disease, under any of its forms. (See also Rosenstein on the Dis. of Child. cap. xvi.) Dr. Binns, indeed, mentions two instances of such recurrence at distant periods: but, at all events, these can only be looked upon as exceptions to the general fact, such as occur both in small-pox and measles.

That such cases occur is undoubted. In the autumn of 1826, I at-tended a gentleman who was labouring under Scarlatina *anginosa*; and who informed me that this was the third time he had been attacked by the disease. Expressing some doubt regarding the correctness of his information, he gave me an accurate history of each attack, and stated that in both the prior cases he had suffered severely from the ulceration of the throat, and that in both there was extensive desquamation of the cuticle. The second attack was at the distance of three years after the first; the third five years after the second. T.

A further analogy is also observable between these diseases and Scar-latina; *viz.* the poison may operate locally, and even excite some se-condary constitutional indisposition, in persons who have previously gone through the fever. Thus such persons, if much exposed to the contagion of Scarlatina, are liable to severe affections of the throat unaccompanied by the rash on the skin.

† See Withering on the Scarlet Fever and Sore-throat, p. 61. — Heberden, Comment. de Morb. cap. 7. De Angina et Febre rubra, p. 20. — Dr. Blackburne states the interval to be " from four to six days." (On Scarlet Fever, p. 34.) In one family Dr. Maton says the intervals varied from seventeen to twenty-six days; but Dr. Good cor-rectly refers this to idiosyncrasy.

tible of the contagion as children, and, in them, the disease does not always appear so soon : women also are less susceptible than men. Many medical practitioners, who have attended great numbers of patients affected with every species of scarlatina, have never experienced any of its effects.

There are three species of Scarlatina :

   1. S. *simplex*,
   2. S. *anginosa*,
   3. S. *maligna*.*

SPECIES 1. The SCARLATINA *simplex*, SIMPLE SCARLET FEVER.

Syn. Scarlatina febris (*Sydenham*): Scarlatina maligna (*Macbr.*): Rosalia simplex (*Good*): Roseole (*F.*).

 This species (Plate XXII. of BATEMAN; Pl. 9. of THE ATLAS,) consists merely of the rash, with a moderate degree of fever. The day after the slight febrile symptoms have appeared, the efflorescence begins to show itself about the neck and face, in innumerable red points, which, within the space of twenty-four hours, are seen over the whole surface of the body. These, as they multiply, coalesce into small patches, but on the following day (the

---

* Many authors regard Cynanche *maligna* as a species of Scarlatina, although no rash appears on the skin; and with this opinion Dr. Bateman, in the former editions of this work, accords; observing that the rash, which characterizes the three species above named, appears " in the fourth only in the mouth and throat, to which, therefore, the appellation of Scarlatina has never been applied." T.

third) form a diffuse and continuous efflorescence over the limbs, especially round the fingers. On the trunk, however, the rash is seldom universal, but is distributed in diffuse irregular patches, the scarlet hue being most vivid about the flexures of the joints and the loins. On the breast and extremities, in consequence of the great determination of blood to the miliary glands and papillæ of the skin, the surface is somewhat rough, like the cutis anserina : several papulæ are scattered on these parts : " occasionally minute vesicles are visible, sometimes apparently filled with a pellucid serum, at other times empty *:" and when these desquamate, a peculiar scaly state of skin remains. On the following (the fourth) day the eruption remains at its acme ; and on the fifth it begins to decline, disappearing by interstices, and leaving the small patches as at first.† On the sixth day it is indistinct, and is wholly gone before the end of the seventh. Between the eighth and twelfth days a scurfy desquamation of the cuticle takes place.

The efflorescence spreads over the surface of the

* Sauvage considers this circumstance sufficient to constitute a distinct species, under the name Scarlatina *variolodes*. T.

† At this period, and on the evening of the second day, some attention is requisite to distinguish the scarlet rash from Rubeola : the observation of the crescent-like form of the patches of the latter, and the more diffuse and irregular shape of the former, will be a material guide. This re-appearance of the rash in patches is noticed by Sennertus. " In statu vero, universum corpus rubrum et quasi ignitum apparet, ac si universali erysipelate laboraret. In *declinatione*, rubor ille imminuit, et maculæ rubræ latæ, *ut in principio*, apparent," &c. (De Febribus, lib. iv. cap. xii.) See also Etmuller. Opera, tom. ii. p. 416. where this circumstance is accurately stated.

mouth and fauces, and even into the nostrils, and is occasionally visible over the tunica albuginea of the eye: the papillæ of the tongue too, which are considerably elongated, extend their scarlet points through the white fur which covers it. The face is often considerably swelled. There is usually great restlessness, and sometimes slight delirium, which appear to be much connected with the great heat of the surface, and continue in various degrees of severity, together with the fever, from three to seven days. A few patients escape with very little fever, almost without indisposition.

" The disease with which Scarlatina is most likely to be confounded, is the Roseola: but it is readily detected by noticing the manner in which the eruption appears. In Scarlatina it first attacks the face and then extends to the trunk of the body, passing off by the extremities, whereas in Roseola the extremities are first affected."

It is scarcely necessary to speak of the treatment of a disease, which has been pronounced, by great medical authority, fatal only " through the officiousness of the doctor." * The principal business of the practitioner, therefore, is to prevent the useless and pernicious expedients of nurses ; but, above all, to insist upon the coolness of the patient's apartment, and the lightness of his bed-clothes; and to restrict him to the use of cool drinks and

---

* " Æger non rarò nulla alia de causa, quam nimiâ medici diligentiâ ad plures migrat." (Sydenham, § vi. cap. 2.)

of light diet, without animal food.   Moderate laxatives are also to be recommended.

SPECIES 2. SCARLATINA *anginosa*, SCARLET FEVER WITH SORE THROAT.

Syn. Scarlatina cynanchica (*Cullen*): Rosalia paristhmitica (*Good.*)

In this variety of Scarlatina (Plate XXIII. fig. 2. of BATEMAN; Pl. 9. of THE ATLAS,) the precursory febrile symptoms are more violent, and an inflammation of the fauces appears, together with the cutaneous efflorescence, and goes through its progress of increase and decline with it. Occasionally, however, the affection of the throat commences with the fever, and sometimes not until the eruption is at its height.

With the first febrile symptoms, a sensation of stiffness and a dull pain on moving are felt in the muscles of the neck; and on the second day the throat is rough and straitened, the voice thick, and deglutition painful. On this and the two following days, the symptoms of fever are often severe; the breathing is oppressed; the heat of the skin is more intense than in any other fever of this climate, rising to 106°, 108°, or even 112° of Fahrenheit's thermometer *; there is sickness, with headach, great restlessness, and delirium; and the pulse is frequent, but feeble: there is also an extreme languor and faintness.   The tongue, as well as the whole

---

* See Dr. Currie's " Reports on the Effects of Water," &c. vol. ii. p. 428. Sennert observes, " Calor ferventissimus." Loc. cit.

interior of the mouth and fauces, is of a high red colour, especially at the sides and extremity, and the papillæ protrude their elongated and inflamed points over its whole surface. (Plate XXIII. fig. 1. of BATEMAN; Pl. 9. of THE ATLAS.)

The rash does not always appear on the second day, as in Scarlatina simplex, but not unfrequently on the third; nor does it so constantly extend over the whole surface, but comes out in scattered patches, which seldom fail to appear about the elbows. " On the third and fourth day, symptoms of Coryza, frequently, show themselves: but the matter is less acrid and fœtid than that discharged in Scarlatina maligna." Sometimes too it vanishes the day after its appearance, and re-appears partially at uncertain times, but without any corresponding changes in the general disorder: the whole duration of the complaint is thus lengthened, and the desquamation is less regular. When the rash is slight, indeed, or speedily disappears, no obvious desquamation often ensues; while, in other instances, exfoliations continue to separate to the end of the third week, or even later, and large pieces of the entire cuticle fall of, especially from the palms of the hands and the soles of the feet.

The tumour and inflammation of the throat often disappear, with the declining efflorescence of the skin, on the fifth and sixth day of the fever, without having exhibited any tendency to ulceration. Slight superficial ulcerations, however, not unfrequently form on the tonsils, velum pendulum, or at the back of the pharynx, sometimes early, and sometimes late. Little whitish sloughs are seen, intermixed with the mottled redness; and when they are numerous, the throat is much clogged up with a tough viscid phlegm, which is secreted among them. When these are removed, after the decline of the fever, some excoriations remain, which soon heal.

The S. anginosa is not unfrequently followed by a state of great debility, under which children are affected with various troublesome disorders, similar to those which more commonly supervene after the cessation of Rubeola. * But there is one affection peculiar to the decline of Scarlatina, which occurs especially when the eruption has been extensive; namely, anasarca of the face and extremities. This dropsical effusion is commonly confined to these parts, and therefore unattended with danger: it usually appears in the second week after the declension of the rash, and continues for a fortnight or longer. But in a small number of cases, when the anasarca had become pretty general, a sudden effusion has taken place into the cavity of the chest, or into the ventricles of the brain, and occasioned the death of the patient in a few hours, of which I have witnessed two instances. † " One sequel of

---

* See above, p. 94. — Also Heberden, Comment. cap. vii. p. 20.

† There is some difference of opinion as to the dangerous tendency of the dropsical state, which succeeds the scarlet fever. Dr. Willan never saw any considerable effusion take place into the internal cavities; and several other writers look upon this dropsy as altogether harmless. (See Cullen, First Lines, § 664. — Dr. Jas. Sims on Scarlatina

the disease is a fœtid purulent discharge from the
ears, which is scarcely ever cured, and frequently
terminates in permanent deafness. Keeping the
meatus clean, by syringing it with warm water
containing a small proportion of the Chloro-sodiac
solution of Labaraque, and dropping into it a few
drops of the following mixture, is the best mode of
correcting the fœtor and lessening the discharge :

R. Bals. Peruv. fʒii.
Fellis Bovinæ fʒi. Misce."

The principles, by which the treatment of Scarlatina anginosa should be regulated, have been
satisfactorily established within the last few years ;
especially since the influence of diminished temperature, in febrile diseases, was demonstrated by
the late Dr. Currie, of Liverpool, and the effects
of purgative medicines have been better understood.
For we have thus acquired two instruments, which
are singly of the utmost value in the management
of fever, and when combined are greatly auxiliary
to each other.

As a general rule, the Scarlatina anginosa must
be submitted, from its commencement, to a strict
antiphlogistic treatment. The extraordinary heat,
the great restlessness, anxiety, and distress, and
the other symptoms of high excitement, which ac-

---

ang. in Mem. of the Med. Soc. vol. i.) Other practitioners, however,
have mentioned the occurrence of these effusions as of dangerous tendency, and not unfrequently fatal. (See Plenciz, Tract. de Scarlatina;
Frank de curand. Hom. Morbis, p. iii. § 295.; Vogel, de cognosc. et
curand. Aff. § 154.

company the efflorescence, do not, indeed, require blood-letting, as was formerly supposed; on the contrary, that evacuation would, in most cases, occasion a hurtful waste of strength. But in respect to the moderate but free evacuation of the bowels, the use of cold drinks, and of external cold, and the interdiction of all stimulant and cordial ingesta, under this state of excitement, experience has clearly decided.

The best writers on this disease agree in recommending the exhibition of an emetic in the beginning of the fever; which some have deemed it advisable to repeat, at intervals of forty-eight, or twenty-four hours, or even at shorter periods, according to the urgency of the symptoms.* An emetic is, doubtless, a safe, and perhaps an useful medicine, at the very onset of the disease: but this active employment of emetics seems to be supported neither by experience nor by principle.† Some practitioners, indeed, combined the emetic with Calomel, and ascribed a considerable portion of the advantage to the laxative operation.‡ Dr. Hamilton more lately has affirmed, that moderate purgatives of Calomel, with Rhubarb or Jalap, are not only extremely beneficial, in the early stages

---

* See Dr. Withering's Treatise before quoted.

† There appears to be a considerable inconsistency in Dr. Withering's recommendation of " larger doses" and " powerful vomits," in order " to secure a *certain violence* of action upon the system," and in the apprehension of the danger of their acting as purgatives, which he at the same time expresses, and principally from hypothetical considerations. (Loc. cit. p. 78—81.)

‡ Dr. Rush.

of Scarlatina; but that they may supersede the use of emetics.* My own observation accords with this view of the subject. I. have never witnessed any injurious effect from trusting to moderate purging, and have frequently seen the disease proceed with uniform security, where the affection of the throat was very considerable, under the use of laxatives alone, with the cool treatment to be mentioned immediately.

The value of moderate purgation, indeed, has been admitted by several cautious physicians. Dr. Willan, although stating that "purgatives have nearly the same debilitating effects as blood-letting," observes, nevertheless, that " the occasional stimulus of a small dose, as two or three grains, of Calomel, is very useful;" and in the beginning of the disease he combined with it an equal portion of antimonial powder. The same combination, he informs us, was freely administered by a physician at Ipswich, in 1772, in larger doses; and of three hundred patients, thus treated, none died. (P. 357, note.) Dr. Binns † candidly acknowledges his obligations to a medical acquaintance, " for his removal of a prejudice against laxatives in the early stage of the disease, imbibed from various authors, and confirmed by the dreadful consequences he had seen, when a diarrhœa came on in

* See his Treatise on Purgative Med.

† See his able account of the management of Scarlatina, when it prevailed in the large school at Ackworth, in Dr. Willan's treatise, p. 357.

this fever." But so far from producing injury, he was afterwards satisfied, that the laxatives actually tended to prevent the diarrhœa which he dreaded.*
" When the stomach is very irritable, Calomel, in doses of from five to seven grains, uncombined with either antimonial or purgative, sooner allays this morbid irritability than any other medicine, whilst at the same time it stimulates the peristaltic motion of the bowels."

Many practitioners recommend the use of anti-monials, and of saline and camphorated diapho-retics, in order to excite perspiration, during the first days of this fever ; and some have advised the exhibition of opium in small doses, to alleviate the great inquietude and wakefulness that accompany it. But a little observation will prove, that such medicines fail altogether to produce either diapho-resis or rest, under the hot and scarlet condition of

---

* It can scarcely be matter of surprise, that purgatives should have been deemed highly injurious in fevers, by those practitioners who were unacquainted with the cool treatment. For the extreme degree of de-pression and exhaustion which the hot regimen occasioned, was a suf-ficient cause for a just apprehension of the ill effects of purgation. Mr. White informs us, when speaking of the miliary fevers of puerperal women (which occurred under the depressing influence of that regi-men), that " a few loose stools, in some cases spontaneous, in others produced by art, have sunk patients beyond recovery." (Treatise on the Management of Pregnant and Lying-in Women, chap. 8.)

We may remark, on the other hand, that the same artificial exhaus-tion created a necessity for the copious use of wine and other stimu-lants, in these fevers, to prevent the patients from sinking irrecoverably. And hence a great two-fold mistake, in the treatment of fevers, was propagated ; viz. the fear of purgatives, and the excessive administra-tion of stimulants. See Miliaria, infra.

the skin; and that, on the contrary, they aggravate the heat and dryness of the surface, and
increase the thirst, the restlessness, the quickness
of pulse, and every other distressing symptom.*
In truth, the temperature is considerably too high
to admit of a diaphoresis; and the only "safe" or
effectual "method" of producing it (which was a
desideratum with Dr. Withering, consists in *reducing
the heat*, by the application of external cold, upon
the principles established by Dr. Currie.

We are possessed of no physical agent, as far as
my experience has taught me, (not excepting even
the use of blood-letting in acute inflammation) by
which the functions of the animal œconomy are
controlled with so much certainty, safety, and
promptitude, as by the application of cold water
to the skin, under the augmented heat of Scarlatina, and of some other fevers. " The patient is
to be taken out of bed, stripped naked, and placed

* See Huxham on the malignant ulcerous Sore-throat; Fothergill;
Grant; Plenciz, &c. — Dr. Huxham, however, acknowledges the great
difficulty of producing sweating by any means. Dr. Withering writes
" *Sudorifics, Cordials, Alexipharmics*. The medicines generally signified
by these denominations have but little to do in the cure of Scarlatina.
The patients are not disposed to sweat, when the scarlet rash prevails
upon the skin, nor do I know of any *safe method* by which we could
attempt to excite a diaphoresis, even if we should expect it to be advantageous," p. 81. Dr. Willan (p. 359) and Dr. Blackburne (Facts
and Obs., &c. on Scarlatina, p. 27.) make the same observation in
stronger terms.

With respect to opium, Dr. Withering observes, " I never saw it
effect the purpose for which it was given; on the contrary, it visibly
increased the distress of the patient," p. 91. Dr. Cotton has a similar
remark. (See his " Obs. on a particular Kind of Scarlet Fever, that
prevailed at St. Alban's," 1749. p. 16.)

in an empty tub : a bucket or two of cold water is then to be suddenly emptied over the head ; and, the body being quickly dried, he is to be again placed in bed. If the sensation of chilliness remain, a little warm wine and water is to be administered." This expedient combines in itself all the medicinal properties which are indicated in this state of disease, and which we should scarcely *à priori* expect it to possess : for it is not only the most effectual *febrifuge* (the " febrifugum magnum," as a reverend author long ago called it *,) but it is, in fact, the only *sudorific* and *anodyne*, which will not disappoint the expectation of the practitioner under these circumstances. I have had the satisfaction, in numerous instances, of witnessing the immediate improvement of the symptoms, and the rapid change in the countenance of the patient, produced by washing the skin. Invariably, in the course of a few minutes, the pulse has been diminished in frequency, the thirst has abated, the tongue has become moist, a general free perspiration has broken forth, the skin has become soft and cool, and the eyes have brightened ; and these indications of relief have been speedily followed by a calm and refreshing sleep. In all these respects, the condition of the patient presented a complete contrast to that which preceded

---

* Dr. Hancocke, rector of St. Margaret's, Lothbury, published a pamphlet in 1722, entitled " *Febrifugum Magnum* ; or, Common Water the best Cure for all Fevers," &c. which contains many sound observations and valuable facts, detailed in the quaint language of the time.

the cold washing; and his languor was exchanged for a considerable share of vigour. The morbid heat, it is true, when thus removed, is liable to return, and with it the distressing symptoms; but a repetition of the remedy is followed by the same beneficial effects as at first. *

Partly from the difficulty of managing the cold affusion, and partly from its formidable character in the estimation of mothers and nurses, imbued with the old prejudices, I have generally contented myself with recommending the *washing* of the skin with *cold water*, or water and vinegar, more or less frequently and extensively, according to the urgency of the heat. In the beginning of the disease, the affusion of a vessel of cold water over the naked body is, doubtless, the most efficacious: but, by a little management, all the benefits of a reduction of the morbid temperature that can be expected at a subsequent period, may be obtained

---

* After the extensive evidence, which a period of more than twenty years has furnished, in proof of the uniform efficacy and security of the external use of cold water, in Scarlatina, and in other febrile diseases connected with high morbid heat of the skin, it is to be lamented that some practitioners still look upon the practice as an *experiment*, and repeat the remnants of exploded hypotheses, about repelling morbid matter, stopping pores, &c. as reasons for resisting the testimony of some of the greatest ornaments of the medical profession. For my own part, I have been in the constant habit of resorting to the practice at every opportunity in Scarlatina (and also in typhoid fevers, during my superintendence of the Fever Institution for the last ten years), attending to the simple rules laid down by Dr. Currie, and I have never witnessed any inconvenience, much less any injury from it; but an uniformity in its beneficial operation, of which no other physical expedient, with which I am acquainted, affords an example.

by the simple washing. In less violent cases, washing the hands and arms, or the face and neck, is of material advantage.*

It is, of course, necessary to enjoin the cool regimen, as directed for the Scarlatina simplex; to attend to the ventilation and moderate temperature of the apartment; and to administer the drink cold.† Acidulated drinks are grateful, and by coagulating the mucus secreted in the fauces, are beneficial to those parts. Dr. Willan and Dr. Stanger have recommended the oxygenated muriatic acid, in doses of half a drachm for adults, and ten or twelve drops for children, diluted in water, as an agreeable refrigerant.

When there is a considerable degree of inflammation and tumefaction of the tonsils, rendering the act of deglutition difficult, the application of a blister to the external fauces has proved extremely

---

* For the direction of those who may not be acquainted with the principles of this practice, if any such remain in the profession, it may be stated, in the words of Dr. Currie, that the cold washing is invariably safe and beneficial, " when the heat of the body is steadily above the natural temperature — when there is no sense of chilliness present, — and no general or profuse perspiration." But I have found the following direction to the nurses amply sufficient; viz. to apply it, ' whenever the skin is *hot* and *dry*.' Dr. Stanger, in treating Scarlatina among the children of the Foundling Hospital, found no other precaution necessary. " Its effects in cooling the skin, diminishing the frequency of the pulse, abating thirst, and disposing to sleep, were very remarkable. Finding this application so highly beneficial," he adds, " I employed it at every period of the fever, provided the skin were hot and dry." See a *note* in Dr. Willan's Treatise, p. 360.

† Cold drink is, like the washing, always salutary in the same hot and dry state of the skin, and tends, like it, to promote perspiration.

beneficial.* Acidulated gargles, " containing a
a moderate proportion of the Tincture of Capsicum," likewise afford a material relief, and probably
contribute to obviate the diarrhœa, by preventing
the acrid mucus from being swallowed.

Wine, Cinchona, and other cordials and tonics,
are not only useless, but injurious, until after the
efflorescence has declined, together with the febrile
symptoms. During the hot feverish state, the cold
washing is, in fact, the best *cordial;* for, by allaying the excessive febrile action, it removes the
cause of the extreme languor and depression, and
thus prevents the tendency to those symptoms of
malignancy and putrescency, to obviate which the
bark and wine have been supposed to be particularly required. The convalescence, likewise, is
more rapid, and the tendency to dropsical effusions is less, when the violence of the febrile symptoms has been restrained by this expedient. It is
advisable, however, with a view to accelerate the
convalescence, and to prevent anasarca, to resort
to the Cinchona, with mineral acids, and a little
wine, as soon as the fever and rash have entirely
disappeared. The same medicines, combined with
diuretics, and small purgative doses of Calomel, are
generally efficacious remedies for the dropsy, when
it supervenes.

* Drs. Willan, Heberden, Rush, Clark, and Sims have concurred in
the same observation. But Dr. Withering was of opinion that blisters
were injurious, when the brain was affected; and that they were less
advantageous when the inflammation was confined to the fauces than
in other quinsies.

SPECIES 3. SCARLATINA *maligna*, MALIGNANT
SCARLET FEVER.

Syn. Cynanche maligna (*Cullen*): Angina maligna (*Auct. var.*): Empresma paristhmitis (*Good*):
Angine maligne (*F.*)

This form of Scarlatina, (Plate XXIII. fig. 3. of
BATEMAN; Pl. 9. of THE ATLAS.) although it commences like the preceding, shows in a day or two
symptoms of its peculiar severity. The efflorescence
is usually faint, excepting in a few irregular patches,
and the whole of it soon assumes a dark or livid
red colour. It appears late, and is very uncertain
in its duration; in some instances, it suddenly disappears a few hours after it is seen, and comes out
again at the end of a week, continuing two or
three days. The skin is of a less steady and intense heat: the pulse is small, feeble, and irregular: the functions of the sensorium are much
disordered; sometimes there is early delirium, and
sometimes coma, alternating with fretfulness and
violence. The eyes are dull and suffused with
redness, the cheeks exhibit a dark red flush, the
mouth is incrusted with a blackish or brown fur,
and there is a black streak in the centre of the
tongue. The ulcers in the throat are covered with
dark sloughs, and surrounded by a livid base; and
a large quantity of viscid phlegm clogs up the
fauces, impeding the respiration, and occasioning
a rattling noise, as well as increasing the difficulty
and pain of deglutition. An acrid, often fœtid
discharge also distils from the nostrils, producing

soreness, chops, and even blisters of the upper lip. These symptoms are often accompanied by severe diarrhœa, and by petechiæ and vibices on the skin, with hæmorrhagy from the mouth, throat, bowels, or other parts, which, of course, but too often lead to a fatal termination. This generally takes place in the second or third week; but, in a few instances, the patients have suddenly sunk as early as the second, third, or fourth day, probably from the occurrence of gangrene in the fauces, œsophagus, or other portions of the alimentary canal* : and sometimes, at a later period of the disease, when the symptoms had been previously moderate, the malignant changes have suddenly commenced, and proved rapidly fatal. Even those who escape through these dangers, have often to struggle against many distressing symptoms, for a considerable length of time; such as ulcerations spreading from the throat to the contiguous parts, suppuration of the glands, tedious cough and dyspnœa, excoriations about the nates, &c. with hectic fever.

The treatment of Scarlatina maligna must necessarily be different from that prescribed for the preceding species, and is unfortunately much less efficient. The active remedies, which operate so favourably in the S. anginosa, especially the cold washing, are altogether out of place here : even the effect of a cathartic is admitted by the unpre-

---

* " Hæc gangrena œsophagum, asperamque arteriam, sæpe ante occupat, quàm illam percipere, illique mederi queamus." Navier, in Com. de Reb. p. i. vol. iv. 338.

judiced to be often deleterious, by rapidly sinking the powers of the constitution; " but, nevertheless, much advantage is obtained from Calomel, given to the extent of eight or ten grains for a dose, and permitting it to pass off without the aid of a cathartic:" blisters, also, are not always applied with impunity. On the whole, the practice of administering gentle emetics appears to be beneficial, especially at the very onset of the disease. It is of great importance to remove frequently, but in a gentle way, the viscid offensive matter that encumbers the fauces, and which, if swallowed, produces considerable irritation in the stomach and bowels. For this purpose, warm restringent gargles are useful: such as the decoction of Contrayerva, with Oxymel of Squills, or Muriatic Acid; an infusion of Capsicum, or an acidulated decoction of Cinchona. " No gargle is more useful than the following :—

> ℞. Solutionis Confect. Rosæ f℥vj,
> Tinct. Capsici fℨij,
> Acidi Muriatici diluti f℥ss,
> M. et cola ut Ft. Gargarisma sæpe utendum.

The Chloro-sodaic solution of Labarraque, in the proportion of f℥xij of the solution to f℥vss of water, and ℨiv of honey, forms, also, an excellent gargle. The same solution, in the proportion of f℥vj to f℥v of water, without the addition of honey, if frequently thrown into the nostrils by means of a gum elastic bottle mounted with a tube, soon removes the Coryza; after which the malignant character of the disease vanishes, and the case is reduced to one of Scarlatina *anginosa*." Tincture of Myrrh, camphorated spirit, and other stimulant liquids, may be likewise employed with advantage. Fumigations, by means of the vapour of Myrrh and Vinegar, but particularly by the Nitrous Acid Gas, (separated from powdered Nitre by the strong Sulphuric Acid) contribute materially to cleanse the fauces. The latter vapours, or the Nitro-muriatic Acid Gas (chlorine) (separated from a mixture of equal parts of powdered Nitre and of Sea Salt by the strong Sulphuric Acid), often supersede the necessity of gargles.

As the disease advances, and the symptoms of malignancy or extreme debility increase, it becomes necessary to support the patient by moderate cordials, Wine, Opium, and the mineral acids, with light nourishment. In this, as in other violent fevers accompanied with much sinking of the vital powers, it was formerly the custom to prescribe the Cinchona copiously. But while the tongue is loaded, the face flushed, and the skin parched, I believe this drug to be always prejudicial. Much of this malignancy, indeed, may be often counteracted by proper ventilation; and where the cutaneous heat is great, and the surface dry, gentle tepid washings, especially in the early stages of the disease, contribute much to prevent the future depression. Subsequently, where there is great languor of the circulation in the skin, warm bathing or fomenting, or even the application of the warm vinegar and spirits, has been attended with benefit.

Similar treatment, both local and general, will be required in that variety of the disease, in which the throat is ulcerated, without any efflorescence on the skin, according to the degree of its virulence.

The Scarlatina rapidly infects children, whenever it is introduced among those who have not already undergone its influence in some one of its forms; insomuch that the most rigid separation of the diseased from the healthy, in schools or large families, has not always prevented its propagation. It is not accurately ascertained, at what period a convalescent ceases to be capable of communicating the infection: in some cases, the infectious power certainly remained above a fortnight after the decline of the efflorescence; and there seems to be little doubt that, so long as the least desquamation of the cuticle continues, the contagion may be propagated.*

* Dr. Hahnemann, and several continental physicians, recommend the administration of Extract of Belladonna in minute doses, during the prevalence of Scarlatina, to prevent the infection from being received. Two grains of the Extract are dissolved in f$\mathfrak{z}$j of Cinnamon Water; and $\mathfrak{m}$ ij of this solution are given night and morning to a child under one year of age; and in larger doses, according to the age of the children! It requires more faith than we possess to credit the assertions which have been given to the public on this subject. But we have no doubt, that by carrying the dose of Belladonna so far as to produce a scarlet efflorescence on the skin, the contagion might be warded off.   T.

Works which may be consulted on Scarlatina.

ARCHIVES Générales de Méd. tom. v. 8vo. Paris.

ARMSTRONG, Practical Illustrations of Scarlet Fever, 1818.

BEDDOES, Contributions to Med. and Phys. Knowledge, 1799.

BLACKBURNE, Facts and Observations, &c. 1803.

BREMSER, Diss. de Scarlatina anginosa, 1800.

COTTON, Observ. on particular Kind of Scarlet Fever, 1749.

COVENTRY, And. De Scarlatina Cynanch. 1783.

Edinburgh Med. and Surg. Journ. vols. iii. xiv. xvi. xvii. xviii.

HAHNEMAN, (S.), Heilung und Verhütang des Scharlach Fiebers, 8vo. 1801.

HAKEN, (T.) De Febre Scarlatina, 1781.

HUFFELAND, Journ. de Pract. Hulkunde, *passim.*

MAC MICHAEL, New View of Scarlet Fever.

PLENCIZ, de Scarlatina Tractatus.

SIMS, Memoirs of the Med. Society, vol. i.

SYDENHAM, Opera Universa, § vi. cap. 2.

WILSON on Febrile Diseases.

WILLAN, A Treatise of Scarlatina, 1815.

WITHERING's Account of Scarlet Fever and Sore Throat, 1703.

VIEUSSEUX, de l'Anasarque à la Suite de la Scarlatine.

ZIMMERMAN, De Scarlatina, &c.

GENUS III. URTICARIA.

Syn. Uredo (*Lin.*): Purpura urticata (*Junck*): Scarlatina urticata (*Sauv.*): Febris urticata (*Vogel*): Essera, Aspritudo (*Auct. Var.*): Der Brennessel-ausschlag (*German*): Fièvre ortiée, Porcelaine (*F*): Benat allil (*Arab.*), *Nettle-rash.*

Def. ITCHING, NETTLE-STING WHEALS APPEARING ABOUT THE SECOND DAY AFTER A SLIGHT FEBRILE ATTACK; FADING AND REVIVING, AND WANDERING FROM PART TO PART.

The *nettle-rash* is distinguished by those elevations of the cuticle, which are usually denominated wheals. (Def. 9.) They have a white top, often surrounded by diffuse redness. The

K

complaint is not contagious. It may be confounded with Erythema nodosum; but this does
not disappear and again re-appear, nor has the
elevated part the aspect of the sting of the nettle.
It more closely resembles Roseola, but this never
rises into wheals. Dr. Willan particularly noticed
six species of Urticaria :

1. U. *febrilis.*   4. U. *conferta.*
2. U. *evanida.*   5. U. *subcutanea.*
3. U. *perstans.*   6. U. *tuberosa.*

SPECIES 1. URTICARIA *febrilis* * : FEBRILE NETTLE-
RASH.

Syn. Purpura urticata *(Juncker)*: Febris erysipelatosa *(Sydenh.)*: Exanthemata urticata *(Burserius)*: Scarlatina urticata *(Sauv.)*

The rash, in this variety of Urticaria, (Plate
XXIV. fig. 2. of BATEMAN; Pl. 10. of THE ATLAS,)
is preceded for two days or more by feverish symptoms, with cramps of the limbs, headach, pain and
sickness of the stomach, and considerable languor,
anxiety, and drowsiness, and sometimes even by
syncope. The wheals appear in the midst of irregular patches of a vivid red efflorescence, some-

---

* This form of the disorder has been accurately described by Juncker
and others under the name of " Purpura Urticata." (See his Conspect.
Med. Pract. tab. 64.; also Lochner, Eph. Nat. Cur. cent. 6. obs. 96.;
and Schacht, Inst. Med. Pract. cap. xi. § vi.) Sydenham has likewise
described it, under the title of " Febris Erysipetalosa;" (Obs. Med. § v.
cap. 6.) and Sauvages, as a variety of Scarlatina, spec. 2. S. urticata.
But Vogel pointed out its distinction from Purpura, Erysipelas, and
Scarlatina. (De cogn. et curand. Morb. § 158. " de Febre Urticata.")
See also Burserius " de Exanthemata Urticato," tom. ii. cap. 5.; and
Frank, " de Curand. Hom. Morb." lib. iii. § 306.

times nearly of a crimson colour, on different, even very distant parts of the body, and accompanied by an extreme degree of itching and tingling, especially during the night, or on exposing the parts affected by undressing. *

The eruption appears and disappears irregularly on most parts of the body, and may be excited on any part of the skin by strong friction or scratching.† The surrounding efflorescence fades during the day, and the wheals subside; but both return in the evening, with slight fever. The patches are often elevated, with a hard border; so that, when they are numerous, the face, or the limb chiefly affected, appears tense and enlarged.

The febrile nettle-rash continues about a week ‡, with considerable distress to the patient, in consequence of the heat, itching, and restlessness with which it is accompanied: the disorder of the stomach, however, is relieved by the appearance of the eruption; but it returns if the eruption disappears. A slight exfoliation of the cuticle generally succeeds.

This eruption occurs chiefly in summer; is often connected with teething or disordered bowels in children, in whom, however, it is attended with less fever than in adults, and often disappears in a few hours; and among adults, affects persons of

---

* " Illud enim singulare habent, quod in frigido magis emergant, et in calido evanescant." Vogel. See also Burserius, § 96.; and Frank, § 309.

† See Sydenham; and Frank, § 307.

‡ " Febris primo septenario inter sudores decedit." Vogel.

full habit, who indulge in the gratifications of the table, or suffer from domestic afflictions and other causes of anxiety. It sometimes occurs as a symptom of other diseases, cancer uteri for instance, as mentioned by Dr. C. M. Clarke. *

Modifications of the febrile nettle-rash, indeed, are produced by certain articles of food, which, in particular constitutions, are offensive to the stomach; especially by shell-fish, such as lobsters, crabs, and shrimps, but above all by muscles.† In a few individuals, in consequence of a peculiar idiosyncrasy, other substances, when eaten, are followed by the same immediate affection of the skin; such as white of egg, mushrooms, honey, oatmeal, almonds, and the kernels of stone-fruit, raspberries, strawberries, green cucumber with the skin upon it‡, &c. In some persons, the internal use of Valerian has produced the nettle-rash.§ The operation of these substances is sometimes almost instan-

* Observ. on Diseases of Females, which are attended with discharges. By C. M. Clarke, 8vo. London, 1814.

† On some parts of the coast of Yorkshire, where muscles are abundant, a belief is prevalent among the people, that they are poisonous, and they are consequently never eaten. This opinion is most probably the result of traditional observation, in regard to the frequent occurrence of Urticaria, after they were swallowed. A case, indeed, is mentioned by Ammans and Valentinus, in which a man died so suddenly after eating muscles, that suspicion of having administered poison fell upon his wife. (See Behrens, " Diss. de Affectionibus a comestis Mytilis.")

‡ Dr. Winterbottom, who is subject to this affection after eating sweet almonds, observes that he takes them with impunity, when they are blanched. See Med. Facts and Obs. vol. v. where the symptoms are minutely described.

§ Dr. Heberden, Med. Transact. vol. ii. p. 176.—Frank, § 310.

taneous *, and the symptoms are extremely violent for several hours; but they generally cease altogether in a day or two. Not unfrequently in delicate and irritable females febrile nettle-rash arises from overloading the stomach. The eruption, however, is not always accompanied with wheals, but sometimes is a mere efflorescence, not unlike that of Scarlatina. It is generally attended by great disorder of the stomach, with violent pains in the epigastrium, and other parts of the body, sickness, languors, fainting, with great heat, itching, stiffness, and often much swelling of the skin. In a few instances, it is said to have been fatal.†

An emetic of Ipecacuanha, if there be suspicion that the disease arises from any thing which has been taken into the stomach, but, if the offending cause be putrid fish, the Sulphate of Zinc, or that of Copper, is to be preferred as an emetic, on account of the quickness of its operation. This, followed by a brisk cathartic, or, in ordinary cases, by a gentle laxative, with light and cooling diet, (with total abstinence from fermented liquors, and from sudorific medicines,) constitute the sole treatment which appears to be requisite for the safe conduct of these disorders to their period of decline; at which

* See Moehring de Mytilorum Veneno. ægrot. iii. in Haller's Disput. tom. iii. p. 191.

† " Licet etiam ea symptomata, quamcunque gravia, intra unum alterumque diem, sine vitæ periculo deflagrare, aut extingui soleant; tamen non desunt exempla rariora, nobis quidem non visa, ubi mortem arcessiverunt." Werlhoff, Pref. to the Diss. of Dr. Behrens, subjoined to his treatise " De Variolis et Anthracibus," Hanov. 1735; also Van Swieten, Comment. ad aph. 723.

time the Cinchona, with diluted Sulphuric Acid,
is beneficial. In children, when the disease does
not soon spontaneously disappear, it is best managed
by the Compound Powder of Contrayerva, or any
other absorbent powder; at the same time keeping the bowels in a lax state. As local applications to allay the sensation of stinging and tingling,
which accompanies the wheals, a lotion consisting
of one part of Alcohol with three of water, or of
two parts of vinegar, and three of water, will be
found beneficial.

SPECIES 2. The URTICARIA *evanida*, EVANESCENT
NETTLE-RASH.

This species (Plate XXIV. fig. 1. of BATEMAN;
Pl. 10. of THE ATLAS,) is a chronic affection, in
which the wheals are not stationary, but appear
and disappear frequently, according to the temperature of the air, or the exposure of the patient,
and vary with the exercise which he uses, &c. It
is not accompanied by fever, and seldom by any
other derangement of health. The wheals are
sometimes round; and sometimes longitudinal, like
those which are produced by the stroke of a
whip; they may be excited on any part of the
body, in a few seconds, by friction or scratching;
but these presently subside again. * They are
sometimes slightly red at the base; but never

* I knew a young lady, enjoying good health, who could at any time
instantaneously excite long, white, and elevated wheals on her skin, by
drawing the nails along it with some degree of pressure: but the wheals
soon subsided, and she was not subject to them from any other cause.

surrounded by an extensive blush. A violent itching, with a sensation of tingling or stinging, accompanies the eruption; which, as in the febrile species, is most troublesome on undressing, and getting into bed.

The disorder is extremely various in its duration. The eruptions, as Dr. Heberden remarks, last only a few days in some persons; while in others they continue, with very short intervals, for many months, and even for several years. * Persons affected with it are liable to suffer headach, languor, flying pains, and disorders of the stomach. It attacks people of all ages and both sexes; but more especially those of sanguine temperament, and females more frequently than males.

As it is often obviously connected with irritability of the stomach, or some peculiar idiosyncrasy; so, when it continues long, Dr. Willan justly suggests the probability, that it originates from some article of diet, which disturbs digestion. Hence, he says, " I have desired several persons, affected with chronic Urticaria, to omit first one, and then another article of food or drink, and have thus been frequently able to trace the cause of the symptoms. This appeared to be different in different persons. In some it was malt-liquor; in others, spirit, or spirit and water; in some, white wine; in others, vinegar; in some, fruit; in others, sugar; in some,

---

The same cutaneous irritability co-exists occasionally with Impetigo, and other chronic affections of the skin, which have no relation to Urticaria.

* Med. Trans. p. 175. See also his Commentar. cap. 36. De Essera.

fish; in others, unprepared vegetables." He acknowledges, however, that in some cases, a total alteration of diet did not produce the least alleviation of the complaint. In such cases, occasional laxatives, and the mineral acids, have been found the most advantageous remedies. Sometimes, where the indigestion was considerable, I have found Soda or the Caustic Potass, combined with Aromatic bitters, such as Cascarilla, afford relief. Dr. Underwood recommends the following,

> ℞. Hydrarg. Sulph. Rubri ʒss,
> Radicis Serpentariæ, in pulvere, Ɔj,
> Syrupi q. s. ut fiat bolus,
> Bis die sumendus; superbibendo haust: Infusi florum Sambuci.

The complaint is generally too extensive to be completely alleviated by lotions of Spirit, Vinegar, or Lemon juice, &c. which afford local relief. But the warm bath is beneficial; and a persevering course of sea-bathing, for a considerable time, has generally been found an effectual remedy.

SPECIES 3. URTICARIA *perstans*, STATIONARY NETTLE-RASH.

This differs from the preceding species, principally in the stationary condition of the wheals, which remain after the redness, at first surrounding them, has disappeared. They continue hard and elevated, with occasional itching, when the patient is heated, for two or three weeks, and gradually subside, leaving a reddish spot for some days. The treatment directed for the foregoing species is here beneficial.

SPECIES 4. URTICARIA *conferta*, CONFLUENT NETTLE-RASH.

In this species the wheals are more numerous, and in many places coalesce, so as to appear of very irregular forms: they are also sometimes considerably inflamed at the base; and the itching is incessant. This variety of the complaint chiefly affects persons above forty years of age, who have a dry and swarthy skin; and seems to originate from violent exercise, or from indulgence in rich food and spirituous liquors. Hence the patients find little relief from medicine, unless they use at the same time a light cooling diet, and abstain from malt-liquor, white wines, and spirits. Alterative medicines, or tonics, are sometimes useful, if this plan of diet be conjoined with them; and warm bathing affords a temporary relief. The eruption often continues many weeks.

SPECIES 5. URTICARIA *subcutanea*, SUBCUTANEOUS NETTLE-RASH.

This is a sort of lurking nettle-rash, which is marked by a violent and almost constant tingling in the skin, and which, from sudden changes of temperature, mental emotions, &c. is often increased to severe stinging pains, as if needles or sharp instruments were penetrating the surface. These sensations are at first limited to one spot on the leg or arm; but afterwards extend to other parts. It is only at distant intervals that an actual eruption of wheals takes place, which continue two or three days, without producing any change in the other distressing symptoms. In persons so affected, the stomach is frequently attacked with pain, and the muscles of the legs are subject to cramps. It is relieved by repeated warm-bathing in sea-water, and gentle friction.

SPECIES 6. URTICARIA *tuberosa*, TUMID NETTLE-RASH.

This species, which was named by Dr. Frank, is marked by a rapid increase of some of the wheals to a large size *, forming hard tuberosities, which seem to extend deeply, and occasion inability of motion, and deep-seated pain. They appear chiefly on the limbs and loins, and are very hot and painful for some hours: they usually occur at night, and wholly subside before morning †, leaving the patient weak, languid, and sore, as if he had been bruised, or much fatigued. It seems to be excited by excesses in diet, over-heating by exercise, and the too free use of spirits, and is often tedious and obstinate. A regular light diet and a course of warm-bathing are to be recom-

---

* " Tumores vero, palmæ latitudinem habentes, et colore rubro sed obscuro instructi, cum pruritu ad animi deliquium usque intolerabili, universam corporis, sed femorum imprimis, superficiem occupare cernuntur." Frank, loc. cit. § 399. tom. iii. p. 108.

† Some writers have hence considered this eruption as the Epinyctis of the ancients: but Sennertus corrects this mistake. The epinyctides contained a bloody sanies, according to Galen, Aëtius, and Paul: and Celsus says, " reperitur inter exulceratio mucosa."

mended, with occasional gentle laxatives, where the organs of digestion appear to be deranged. *

Books which may be consulted on Urticaria.

BURROWS, London Med. Repository, vol. iii. p. 445.

CRAMER, Diss. de Purpuræ Urticatæ et Scarlat. Febris discrimine. Hal. 1759.

FRANK, de Curand. Hom. Morbis, lib. iii.

GRAUER, Progr. de Febre Urticata, &c. 1774.

HEBERDEN, Med. Trans. vol. 1.

JOURNAL de Médecine, Années 1759 et 1762.

KOCK, Progr. de Febre Urticata, Lips. 1792.

MOERING, Epist. de Mytilorum Veneno, 4to. 1747.

PLUMBE, on Diseases of the Skin, 2d edit. 1827.

RAYER, Traité des Maladies de la Peau, 1826.

WILLAN on Cutaneous Diseases, 1818.

WINTERBOTTOM, Med. Facts and Observ. vol. v. No. 6.

GENUS IV. ROSEOLA.

Syn. Rubeola (*Auct. vet.*) : Exanthesis Roseola, (*Good*): Roseole, Fausse rougeole, Eruption anomale rosace (*F.*), *Rose-rash.*

Def. A ROSE-COLOURED EFFLORESCENCE, VARIOUSLY FIGURED, MOSTLY CIRCULAR AND OVAL, WITHOUT WHEALS OR PAPULÆ, OCCASIONALLY FADING AND REVIVING : NOT CONTAGIOUS.

The efflorescence to which Dr. Willan appropriated the title of Roseola, is of little importance in a practical view † ; for it is mostly symptomatic,

---

* Frank, loc. cit. § 312.

† Fuller (in his Exanthematologia, p. 128.) speaks of this sort of rose-rash, as a flushing all over the body, like fine crimson, which is void of danger, and "rather a ludicrous spectacle, than an ill symptom." The appellation of Roseola is to be found in the works of some of the early modern writers; but it was applied somewhat indiscriminately to scarlet fever, measles, &c. (See above, p. 58. *note*.)

occurring in connection with dentition, dyspepsia, and different febrile complaints, and requiring no deviation from the treatment respectively adapted to them. It is necessary, however, that practitioners should be acquainted with its appearances, in order to avoid the error of confounding it with the idiopathic exanthemata. It has been occasionally mistaken both for measles, erythema, urticaria, and scarlet fever; and from this want of discrimination, probably, the supposition that scarlatina was not limited, like the other eruptive fevers, to one attack during life, has been maintained by many persons up to the present time. * There is no difficulty in distinguishing it from erythema and urticaria; from measles it is known by the absence of the catarrhal symptoms; and from scarlatina by the course of the rash, which, contrary to what occurs in scarlatina, begins at the extremities and terminates upon the face and trunk of the body.

There are seven species of Roseola:

1. R. *œstiva.*
2. R. *autumnalis.*
3. R. *annulata.*
4. R. *infantilis.*
5. R. *variolosa.*
6. R. *vaccina.*
7. R. *miliaris.*

* Instances have occurred in which undoubted Scarlatina has attacked the same individual more than once. I witnessed a severe instance which was the third attack of the disease in the same individual. T.

SPECIES 1. ROSEOLA *æstiva*, SUMMER ROSE-RASH.

This species (Plate XXV. fig. 1. of BATEMAN; Pl. 11. of THE ATLAS,) is sometimes preceded for a few days by slight febrile indisposition. It appears first on the arms, face, and neck, and, in the course of a day or two, is distributed over the rest of the body, producing a considerable degree of itching and tingling. The mode of distribution is into separate small patches, of various figure, not crescent-shaped, but larger and of more irregular forms, and paler than in the measles, with numerous interstices of the natural skin. It is at first red, but soon assumes the deep roseate hue peculiar to it. The fauces are tinged with the same colour, and a slight roughness of the tonsils is felt in swallowing. The rash continues vivid through the second day, after which it declines in brightness; slight specks only, of a dark red hue, remaining on the fourth day, which, together with the constitutional affection, wholly disappear on the fifth.

Not unfrequently, however, the efflorescence is partial, extending only over portions of the face, neck, and upper part of the breast and shoulders, in patches, very slightly elevated, and itching considerably, but without the tingling which accompanies nettle-rash. In this form the complaint continues a week or longer, the rash appearing and disappearing several times; sometimes without any apparent cause, and sometimes from sudden mental emotions, or from taking wine, spices, or warm liquors. The retrocession is usually accompanied with disorder of the stomach, headach, and faintness; which are immediately relieved on its appearance.

This variety of Roseola commonly occurs in summer, in females of irritable constitution; and is ascribed to sudden alternations of heat and cold, especially to drinking cold liquors after violent exercise. It is sometimes connected with the bowel-complaints of the season.

Light diet, and acidulated drinks, with occasional laxatives, alleviate the symptoms. The complaint is liable to retrocession, it is affirmed, from the influence of very chill air, or the application of cold water, which occasions considerable disorder of the head and alimentary canal; but I have not seen any instance of this kind.

SPECIES 2. ROSEOLA *autumnalis*, AUTUMNAL ROSE-RASH.

This species (Plate XXV. fig. 2. of BATEMAN; Pl. 11. of THE ATLAS,) occurs in children, in the autumn, in distinct circular or oval patches, which gradually increase to about the size of a shilling, and are of a dark damask-rose hue. They appear chiefly on the arms, and continue about a week, sometimes terminating by desquamation. There is little itching, tingling, or constitutional affection, connected with this efflorescence; and its decline seems to be expedited by the use of Sulphuric Acid internally, exhibited in the infusion of Conserve of Roses, or the infusion of Gentian, in combination with small doses of Sulphate of Magnesia. *

* The following cases are certainly severe instances of this species of Roseola, although Dr. Bateman, who details them, regarded them as different from any of the species described by Dr. Willan. I have quoted them to show the height to which the febrile symptoms may extend.

"The two cases, set down under the head of Roseola, were febrile diseases, and one of them was of considerable severity and duration. In both these instances the rash appeared on the second day of fever, and continued beyond the ninth day, the fever then declining with it. In the more severe case, the rash bore a considerable resemblance to that of rubeola, consisting of numerous small, slightly-elevated spots, of a pale red colour, not acuminated, covering the face, extremities, and trunk; but, although here and there confluent, not forming into crescents, like the measles, nor approaching to the raspberry hue. The patient complained during the whole period of great general distress; the skin was exceedingly hot, although the perspirations were considerable, and there was even a tendency to delirium. On the ninth day the eruption began to disappear, and the fever to diminish; but she was left in a state of great debility and languor, and recovered slowly. Purgatives, diaphoretics, and acids were principally employed; but it is probable that a cooler bed and apartment, than the parents of the girl chose to maintain, would have materially alleviated the complaint. The second patient, a younger girl, only eleven years of age, exhibited on the second day of a moderate fever, accompanied by sickness, a diffuse rose-red rash on the legs, of an erythematous form, slightly elevated, but of an uneven surface, the most elevated parts being reddest: on the fourth and fifth days (the fever, with slight headach continuing), a similar rash appeared on the arms; and on the sixth day, when the eruption on the legs began to fade, a large circular patch of the same bright red rash showed itself upon each cheek. These patches were extremely vivid, when the patient was first seen on the seventh day, at which time the eruption on the arms was less bright, and that on the legs was much faded, the elevated parts only remaining red, and giving a mottled appearance to the skin. Some remains of the rash continued on the face on the eleventh day, when she visited the Dispensary, free from fever; and a slight roughness, from imperfect desquamation, was found on the arms. She had taken some laxative

SPECIES 3. The ROSEOLA *annulata*, ANNULAR ROSE-RASH.

This species (Plate XXVI. fig. 1. of BATEMAN; Pl. 11. of THE ATLAS,) appears on almost every part of the body, in rose-coloured rings, with central areas of the usual colour of the skin; sometimes accompanied with feverish symptoms, in which case its duration is short; at other times, without any constitutional disorder, when it continues for a considerable and uncertain period. The rings at first are from a line to two lines in diameter; but they gradually dilate, leaving a larger·central

---

before she applied to the charity, and was treated with Infusum Rosæ and Magnesiæ Sulphas, followed by the decoction of Cinchona and Sulphuric Acid.

"These febrile rashes, of which there is a considerable variety †, are not often either dangerous or severe, and chiefly deserve to be noticed with a view to the diagnosis from the contagious eruptive fevers, scarlatina and measles. I lately attended a case, resembling the former of these in appearance, although not in the severity of the concomitant fever, which excited a great alarm in the family, from the belief that it was scarlet-fever; a supposition which was strengthened by the occurrence of a slight sore throat. But a careful attention to the form, distribution, and progress of the eruption, as well as to the concomitant circumstances, will generally enable an observer, accustomed to analyse those appearances, to decide promptly as to their difference from the contagious fevers just mentioned. The causes of them are by no means easily traced; in the latter of the two cases above described, the disorder was supposed to have been occasioned by having been excessively heated, by working at a mangle, a week before the symptoms appeared." Vide Edin. Med. and Surg. Journ. vol. viii. p. 224.

---

† Neither of these cases accorded accurately with the species of Roseola described by Dr. Willan, as having most frequently occurred to his observation. But it were not easy to follow these rashes through all their varieties. They agreed with his general definition: "a rose-coloured efflorescence, variously figured, without wheals or papulæ, and not contagious." — Ord. III. Genus VI.

space, sometimes to the diameter of half an inch. The efflorescence is less vivid (and, in the chronic form, usually fades) in the morning, but increases in the evening or night, and produces a heat and itching, or prickling, in the skin. If it disappear or becomes very faint in colour for several days, the stomach is disordered, and languor, giddiness, and pain of the limbs ensue, — symptoms which are relieved by the warm bath.

Sea-bathing and the mineral acids afford much relief in the chronic form of this rash.

SPECIES 4. The ROSEOLA *infantilis*, INFANTILE ROSE-RASH.

This form of Rose-rash (Plate XXVI. fig. 2. of BATEMAN; Pl. 11. of THE ATLAS,) is closer, leaving smaller interstices than the R. *æstiva* above described, and occurring in infants during the irritation of dentition, of disordered bowels, and in fevers. It is very irregular in its appearances, sometimes continuing only for a night; sometimes appearing and disappearing for several successive days, with violent disorder; and sometimes arising in single patches, in different parts of the body successively.

Where the rash is pretty generally diffused, it is often mistaken, as Dr. Underwood has remarked *, for measles and scarlatina. Whence it is necessary that practitioners should be acquainted with it;

---

* On the Diseases of Children, vol. i. p. 87.

although it requires no specific treatment, but is
" alleviated by testaceous powders, or the Pulvis
Contrayervæ Compositus and Nitre," and other remedies adapted to bowel-complaints, painful dentition, and various febrile affections, with which it is
connected.

SPECIES 5. ROSEOLA *variolosa*, VARIOLOUS ROSE-
RASH.

This rash (Plate XXVII. fig. 1, 2. of BATEMAN;
Pl. 11. of THE ATLAS,) occurs previous to the
eruption both of the natural and inoculated smallpox, but not often before the former. It appears
in about one case in fifteen, in the inoculated disease, on the second day of the eruptive fever, which
is generally the ninth or tenth after inoculation.
It is first seen on the arms, breast, and face;
and on the following day it extends over the trunk
of the body and the extremities. " In general, like
rash in R. æstiva and autumnalis, it appears first
on the extremities, and gradually advances to the
trunk and face, taking the opposite course of
scarlatina, which generally terminates on the extremities." * Its distribution is various : sometimes

* This course of the eruption is well exemplified in the following instance, which occurred previous to the eruption in a case of
smallpox after vaccination. 30th June 1826, I was called to see
Miss ——, who was supposed to be labouring under scarlatina. The
hands, the forearms, the feet, the legs half way up, and the mammæ
around the nipples, are covered with the rose eruption: but there
are scarcely any patches on the thorax, and none on the face nor on
the trunk of the body. The fever is moderate, the pulse soft, and the
tongue moist: there is a slight blush over the fauces, and a pustule on

in oblong irregular patches, sometimes diffused with numerous interstices (see Pl. 10. of THE ATLAS); and, in a few cases, it forms an almost continuous redness over the body, being in some parts slightly elevated. It continues about three days, on the second or last of which, the variolous pustules may be distinguished, in the general redness, by their rounded elevation, by their hardness, and by the whiteness of their tops : and as soon as these appear, the rose-rash declines.

This rash is generally deemed, by inoculators, a certain prognostic of a small and favourable eruption of the smallpox ; but such does not always follow. * It is not easily repelled by cold air or cold drinks, against which the old inoculators enforced many prohibitions and cautions.

These roseolous efflorescences, antecedent to the

---

the left tonsil. 1st July: The rash is nearly gone from the legs and arms, and beginning to appear on the face and neck and trunk; the variolous pustules which have appeared, are few and distinct; the pulse is soft; there is no feeling of sore-throat. 2d July: The rash is entirely gone, and the pustules are advancing. T.

* Dr. R. Walker, indeed, speaking of the natural smallpox, says, " In every bad kind of smallpox, the eruption is ushered in by a scarlet rash, which appears first upon the face, neck, and breast, and sometimes spreads over the whole body; it is observed some part of the second day, and within twelve hours, sooner or later, the pimples emerge from these inflamed parts of the skin." See his " Inquiry into the Smallpox, Medical and Political," chap. viii. Edin. 1790.—But Dr. Willan remarks, that it is an universal efflorescence, of a dark red colour, with violent fever, that indicates a confluent eruption and a fatal disease. See also Morton de Variol. et Morb. p. 186. — Rayer, speaking of the usual prognostic of a mild disease, when Variola is preceded by Roseola, remarks, " Mes observations, du moins, me conduisent à penser précisément le contraire." *Traité Théorique et Pratique des Maladies de la Peau*, tom. i, p. 47.

eruption of smallpox, were observed by the first writers on the disease; and both by them and subsequent authors were deemed measles, which were said to be converted into smallpox.

Species 6. Roseola *vaccina;* Vaccine Rose Rash.

An efflorescence (Plate XXVII. fig. 3. of Bateman; Pl. 10. of The Atlas,) which appears generally in a congeries of dots and small patches, but sometimes diffuse, like the variolous Roseola, takes place in some children on the ninth and tenth day of vaccination, at the place of inoculation, and at the same time with the areola that is formed round the vesicle; and thence it spreads irregularly over the whole surface of the body. But this does not occur nearly so often as after variolous inoculation. It is usually attended with a very quick pulse, white tongue, and great restlessness.

Species 7. Roseola *miliaris,* Miliary Rose Rash.

This rash often accompanies an eruption of miliary vesicles, with fever.

In simple continued fevers*, whether the bilious fever of summer, in this climate, or the typhus or contagious fever, an efflorescence resembling the Roseola *æstiva* occasionally takes place, of a hue, however, more approaching to that of measles. I

---

* These roseolous spots are also sometimes connected with intermittents. See Pechlin. Obs. Phys. Med. lib. ii. 18.

have seen this efflorescence in three cases of mild
fever, in the House of Recovery, at a late period
of its course; in two of which it was slight, and
remained from two to three days. In the third
case, it appeared on the ninth day of fever, in a
young woman, after a sound sleep and a moderate
perspiration, in patches of a bright rose-pink colour, of an irregular oval form, somewhat elevated, and smooth on the surface, affecting the
arms and breast, but most copious on the inside of
the humerus. It was unaccompanied by any itching
or other uneasy sensation. All the febrile symptoms were alleviated on that day, and she did not
keep her bed afterwards. On the following day
the efflorescence had extended, the patches having
become larger and confluent; but the colour, especially in the areas of the patches, had declined,
and acquired a purplish hue in some parts, while
the margins continued red and slightly elevated.
The whole colour on the third day had a livid
tendency; and on the fourth there were scarcely
any perceptible remains of it, or of the febrile
symptoms.

A roseolous efflorescence is sometimes connected
with attacks of gout, and of the febrile rheumatism. I lately attended a gentleman of gouty
habit, in whom a Roseola, accompanied with considerable fever, and with extreme languor and
depression of spirits, total loss of appetite, and
torpid bowels, subsisted a week upon the lower
extremities, and also upon the forehead and vertex

of the scalp. On the seventh day, the latter terminated by desquamation, and at midnight his knuckles and right foot were attacked with arthritic inflammation.

Books which may be consulted on Roseola.

BAUMANN. Diss. de Roseolis saltantibus. Altd. 1700.

EDINBURGH MED. AND SURG. JOURN. vol. viii. p. 245.

HEIM, Journ. de Méd. de Huffland, 1812.

ORLOV, Programma de Rubeolarum et Morbil. discrimine, 4to. 1783.

PLUMBE, On Diseases of the Skin, 2d edit. 1827.

SEÏLER, Diss. de Morbilles inter et Rubeolas differentia verâ, 4to. 1805.

GENUS V. PURPURA.

Syn. Πορφύρα (*G.*): Scorbutus, Petechiæ sine febre (*Auct. var.*): Purpura (*Riverius*): Hæmorrhœa petechialis (*Adair*): Porphyra (*Good*): Hæmorrhagies souscutanées (*Rayer*): *Scurvy.*

Def. AN ERUPTION OF SMALL, DISTINCT, PURPLE SPECKS AND PATCHES, ATTENDED WITH LANGUOR, GENERAL DEBILITY, AND PAINS IN THE LIMBS.

The specks and patches, mentioned in this definition, are *petechiæ* and *ecchymomata*, or *vibices*, occasioned, not, as in the preceding exanthemata, by an increased determination of blood into the cutaneous vessels, but by an extravasation, from the extremities of these vessels, under the cuticle.*

* Rayer objects, with justice, to Purpura being placed among the Exanthemata. — *Traité Théorique et Pratique des Maladies de la Peau,* Introduction, p. xii. T.

The Purpura*, in this arrangement, is therefore intended to include every variety of petechial eruption, and of spontaneous ecchymosis ; not only the chronic form of it, which is unaccompanied by fever, and which has received various denominations (such as Hæmorrhœa petechialis, Petechiæ sine febre †, land-scurvy, &c.), but also that which accompanies typhoid and other malignant fevers.

The chronic Purpura appears under three or four

---

* The term Purpura was applied to *petechial* spots only by Riverius, Diemerbroeck, Sauvages, Cusson, and some others. But it has been employed by different writers in so many other acceptations, that some ambiguity would perhaps have been avoided by discarding it altogether: for some authors have used it as an appellation for measles, others for scarlet fever, for Miliaria, Strophulus, Lichen, Nettle-rash, and the petechiæ of malignant fevers. The title of *Hæmorrhœa petechialis*, which was given to the chronic form of the eruption by Dr. Adair, in his inaugural thesis in 1789, and which I adopted in my own dissertation upon the same subject in 1801, would perhaps have been more unexceptionable. But, in deference to Dr. Willan, I retain this term.

† This appellation is generally ascribed to Dr. Graaf (see his Diss. Inaug. *De Petech. sine Febre*, Gött. 1775); but it was employed half a century before his time by Rombergius (see Ephem. Nat. Cur. decad. iii. ann. 9 & 10, obs. 108 ; and Acta Phys. Med. Acad. Nat. Curio . vol. ix. obs. 21. p. 95). The term was adopted by many writers as expressive of the most remarkable feature of the disease ; for petechiæ had been generally deemed symptomatic of fevers only. Whence also J. A. Raymann, who has given a good history of the disease, called the spots " petechiæ *mendaces*," in contradistinction from the febrile petechiæ, which he denominated " *sinceræ*." (See the Acta Phys. Med. for 1751, just quoted, p. 87. — See also Duncan's Med. Cases and Obs. p. 90 ; Med. Comment. vol. xv. and xx. and Annals of Med. vol. ii. — Dr. Ferris's case, Med. Facts and Obs. vol. ii. 1791. — Dr. Zetterstrœm's Diss. Inaug. Upsal, 1797). Amatus Lusitanus had also marked the absence of fever, about the year 1550, when he described the disease under the similar title of " Morbus pulicaris *sine febre ;*" Curat. Med. cent. iii. obs. 70) as had Cusson, who called it " Purpura *apyreta*." — Pezoldus (obs. 6) and Zwingerus (Pædoiatreia Pract. p. 622) treated of it under the appellation of " maculæ nigræ *sine febre*."

varieties of form; the first and second of which, however, seem to differ chiefly in the degree of severity of their symptoms.

There are five species of Purpura : —

1. P. *simplex.*   4. P. *senilis.*
2. P. *hæmorrhagica.*   5. P. *contagiosa.*
3. P. *urticans.*

SPECIES 1. PURPURA *simplex*, PETECHIAL SCURVY.

Syn. Petechiæ sine febre (*Auct. var.*): Phæ-nigmus petechialis (*Sauv.*): Profusio subcutanea (*Young*): Porphyra simplex, *var. pulicosa* (*Good*): Rothe punkt (*Ger.*): Pétéchies sans fièvre (*F.*): *Petechial Scurvy.*

In this species (Plate XXVIII. fig. 1. of BATE-MAN; Pl. 12. of THE ATLAS,) there is an appear-ance of petechiæ, without much disorder of the constitution, except languor, and loss of the mus-cular strength, with a pale or sallow complexion, and often with pain in the limbs. " The tongue is covered with a yellow fur, the bowels are consti-pated, the appetite is diminished, and not unfre-quently there is nausea and head-ache." The petechiæ are most numerous on the breast, and on the inside of the arms and legs, and are of various sizes, from he most minute point to that of a flea-bite, and commonly circular. They may be dis-tinguished from recent flea-bites, partly by their more livid or purple colour, and partly, because, in the latter, there is a distinct central puncture

(Pl. 12. of The Atlas,) the redness around which disappears on pressure.   There is no itching, nor other sensation attending the petechiæ.

Species 2.   Purpura *Hæmorrhagica* *, Land Scurvy.

Syn. 'Iλεoς αἱματιτης (*Hippoc.*): Hæmorrhagia universalis (*Wolf.*): Stomacace universalis (*Sauv.*): Porphyra hæmorrhagica (*Good*): Hémacelinose (*Rayer*): Pourpre, Hémorrhagie pétéchiale (*F.*): *Land Scurvy.*

This species (Plate XXVIII. fig. 2. of Bateman; Pl. 12. of The Atlas,) is considerably more severe than the former; the petechiæ are often of a larger size, and are interspersed with vibices and ecchymoses, or livid stripes and patches, resembling the marks left by the strokes of a whip, or by violent bruises.   They commonly appear first on the legs, and at uncertain periods afterwards, on the thighs, arms, and trunk of the body; the hands being more rarely spotted with them, and the face generally free.   They are usually of a bright red colour when they first appear, but soon become purple or livid; and when about to disappear, they change to a brown or yellowish hue: so that, as

---

* This term is not very correctly employed in this place; since it implies that these more extensive eruptions, or rather extravasations of Purpura are always accompanied by hæmorrhages; which is not the fact.

By a sort of solecism, Sauvages has described this form of the disease under the title of Stomacace *universalis*, class ix. gen. 3.   The Purpura simplex he terms Phœnigmus petechialis, class x. gen. 32.

new eruptions arise, and the absorption of the old ones slowly proceeds, this variety of colour is commonly seen in the different spots at the same time. The cuticle over them appears smooth and shining, but is not sensibly elevated: in a few cases, however, the cuticle has been seen raised into a sort of vesicles, containing black blood.* This more frequently happens in the spots which appear on the tongue, gums, palate, and inside of the cheeks and lips, where the cuticle is extremely thin, and breaks from the slightest force, discharging the effused blood. The gentlest pressure on the skin, even such as is applied in feeling the pulse, will often produce a purple blotch, like that which is left after a severe bruise.

The same state of the habit which gives rise to these effusions under the cuticle †, produces likewise copious discharges of blood, especially from the internal parts, which are defended by more delicate coverings. These hæmorrhages are often very profuse, and not easily restrained, and therefore sometimes prove suddenly fatal. But in other cases they are less copious; sometimes returning every day at stated periods, and sometimes less

* See Reil, Memorab. Clinic. vol. i. — Comment. in Reb. Med. &c. gestis, Leipsic. vol. vi. — Dr. Willan's Reports on the Dis. of London, p. 167.—Wolff. in Act. Nat. Cur. (before quoted) vol. vii. obs. 131. and Rogert, in Act. Reg. Soc. Med. Hauniensis, vol. i. p. 185.

† It has been a question whether the vessels are dilated or ruptured: — it is certain that in hæmorrhage from the gums, and from some internal organs, as, for instance, the bladder, the blood comes from the whole surface, not from any organic lesion in one or more points. T.

frequently and at irregular intervals; and sometimes there is a slow and almost incessant oozing
of blood. The bleeding occurs from the gums,
nostrils, throat, inside of the cheeks, tongue, and
lips, and sometimes from the lining membrane of
the eyelids, the urethra, and the external ear; and
also from the internal cavities of the lungs, stomach, bowels, uterus, kidneys, and bladder. There
is the utmost variety, however, in different instances, as to the period of the disease, in which
the hæmorrhages commence and cease, and as to
the proportion which they bear to the cutaneous
efflorescence.

This singular disease is often preceded for some
weeks by great lassitude, faintness, and pains in the
limbs, which render the patients incapable of any
exertion; but, not unfrequently, it appears suddenly,
in the midst of apparent good health.* It is always
accompanied with extreme debility and depression
of spirits: the pulse is commonly small and feeble,
and sometimes hard and quickened; and shiverings, succeeded by heat, flushing, perspiration, and
other symptoms of slight febrile irritation, recurring
like the paroxysms of hectic, occasionally attend. In

---

* See a case related by Dolæus, in the Ephemer. Nat. Cur. dec. ii.
ann. iv. obs. 118, which occurred in a boy, " cujus omne corpus, absque
dolore, febre, aut lassitudine prægressâ, subito unà cum facie, labiis, et
lingua, ubi mane adsurgeret, numerosissimis maculis lividis et niger-
rimis obsitum fuit, &c. — Similar cases are described by Zwingerus, in
the Act. Nat. Cur. vol. ii. obs. 79. and by Werlhoff, in the Commerc.
Liter. Norimberg. ann. 1735, hebd. 7 & 2. In all these instances, the
eruption was discovered on rising in the morning, having taken place
during the night.

some patients, deep-seated pains have been felt
about the præcordia, and in the chest, loins, or
abdomen ; and in others a considerable cough has
accompanied the complaint, or a tumour and tension of the epigastrium and hypochondria, with
tenderness on pressure, and a constipated or irregular state of bowels. But in many cases, no febrile appearances have been noticed ; and the functions of the intestines are often natural. In a few
instances frequent syncope has occurred. When
the disease has continued for some time, the patient
becomes sallow, or of a dirty complexion, "the conjunctiva is tinged with bile ; there is often a fœtid
odour about the body," and he is much emaciated ;
and some degree of œdema appears in the lower
extremities, which afterwards extends to other
parts.

The disease is extremely uncertain in its duration : in some instances it has terminated in a
few days ; while in others it has continued not
only for many months, but even for years. Dr.
Duncan related a case to me, when I was preparing
my thesis on this subject, which occurred in a boy,
who was employed for several years by the players
at *golf* to carry their sticks, and whose skin was
constantly covered with petechiæ, and exhibited
vibices and purple blotches wherever he received
the slightest blow. Yet he was, in other respects,
in good health. At length a profuse hæmorrhage
took place from his lungs, which occasioned his
death. When the disease terminates fatally, it is

commonly from the copious discharge of blood, either suddenly effused from some important organ, or more slowly from several parts at the same time. A young medical friend of mine was instantaneously destroyed by pulmonary hæmorrhage, while affected with Purpura, in his convalescence from a fever, after he had gone into Lincolnshire to expedite his recovery * : and I have seen three instances of the latter mode of termination ; in all of which there was a constant oozing of blood from the mouth and nostrils, and at the same time considerable discharges of it from the bowels, and from the lungs by coughing ; and in one it was likewise ejected from the stomach by vomiting, for three or four days previous to death. † On the other hand, I lately saw a case of Purpura simplex, in which the petechiæ were confined to the legs, in a feeble woman, about forty years of age, who was suddenly relieved from the eruption and its attendant debility, after a severe catamenial flooding. ‡

The causes of this disease are by no means clearly ascertained, nor its pathology well understood.   It

---

* Several instances of sudden death, in this disease, from the occurrence of profuse hæmorrhage, are mentioned by respectable authors. See Lister, Exercit. de Scorbuto, p. 96, &c. — Greg. Horst. lib. v. obs. 17. Two examples (one from pulmonary and the other from uterine hæmorrhage) were communicated to me by my friend Mr. James Rumsey, of Amersham, one of which occurred in his own family.

† Two of these cases were described in my Report of the Diseases treated at the Dispensary, Carey Street, in the spring of 1810. See Edin. Med. and Surg. Journal, vol. vi. p. 374.

‡ See my Report for 1810, ibid. p. 124. — See also a case related by Wolff, in the Act. Acad. Natur. Curios. vol. iii. obs. 79.

occurs at every period of life, and in both sexes;
but most frequently in women, and in boys before
the age of puberty, particularly in those who are of
a delicate habit, who live in close and crowded
situations, and on poor diet, or are employed in
sedentary occupations, and subject to grief and
anxiety of mind, fatigue and watching. * It has
likewise attacked those who were left in a state of
debility by previous acute or chronic diseases. In
one of the fatal instances above mentioned, it came
on during a severe salivation, which had been accidentally induced by a few grains of Mercury,
given, as I was informed, in combination with
opium, for the cure of rheumatism. It has sometimes occurred as a sequela of smallpox, and of
measles; and sometimes in the third or fourth week
of puerperal confinement. † The disease, however,
appears occasionally, and in its severest and fatal
form, where none of these circumstances existed:
for instance, in young persons living in the country,
and previously enjoying good health, with all the
necessaries and comforts of life.

This circumstance tends greatly to obscure the
pathology of the disease. For it not only renders
the operation of these alleged causes extremely
questionable, but it seems to establish an essential
difference in the origin and nature of the disorder,

---

* See Dr. Willan's Reports on Dis. in London, p. 90.

† See Joerdens, in Act. Acad. N. Cur. vol. vii. obs. 110. — This is
the Purpura *Symptomatica* of Sauvages, class iii. gen. vi. spec. 3.

from that of *scurvy* *, to which the majority of
writers have contented themselves with referring it.
In scurvy, the tenderness of the superficial vessels
appears to originate from deficiency of nutriment;
and the disease is removed by resorting to wholesome and nutritious food, especially to fresh vegetables and to acids: while in many cases of Purpura,
the same diet and medicine have been taken abundantly, without the smallest alleviation of the complaint. In the instance of the boy mentioned by
Dr. Duncan, the remedies and regimen which would
have infallibly cured the scorbutus, were liberally
administered, without affording any relief; and in
other cases, above alluded to, where a residence in
the country, and the circumstances of the patients
necessarily placed them above all privation in
these respects, the disease appeared in its severest
degree.

On the other hand, the rapidity of the attack,
the acuteness of the pains in the internal cavities,
the actual inflammatory symptoms that sometimes
supervene, the occasional removal of the disease by
spontanous hæmorrhage, the frequent relief derived from artificial discharges of blood†, and from

* I mean the true *scurvy*, or rather *sea scurvy*, formerly prevalent
among seamen in long voyages, and among people in other situations,
when living upon putrid, salted, dried, or otherwise indigestible food,
yielding imperfect nutriment. See Lind, Trotter, &c. on the Scurvy,
and Vander Mye, de Morbis Bredanis. The symptoms are concisely
detailed by Boerhaave in his 1151st aphorism.

† See two cases of Purpura, related by an able and distinguished
physician, Dr. Parry of Bath, which were speedily cured by two bleed-

purging, all tend to excite a suspicion that some local visceral congestion or obstruction is the cause of the symptoms in different instances. This point can only be ascertained by a careful examination of the viscera, after death, in persons who have died with these symptoms. The ancient physicians directly referred some of them, especially the hæmorrhages from the nose, gums, and other parts, to morbid enlargement of the spleen. * In one case, in which an opportunity of dissection was afforded at the Public Dispensary, and which occurred in a boy under the inspection of my friend and colleague Dr. Laird, the spleen, which had been distinctly felt during life protruding itself downwards and forwards to near the spine of the ilium, was found enormously enlarged. In another instance, which occurred under my own care, in a boy thirteen years old, the abdominal viscera were found to be sound ; but a large morbid growth, consisting of a fleshy tumour, with a hard cartilaginous nucleus, weighing about half a pound, was found in the situation of the thymus gland, firmly attached to the sternum, clavicle, pericardium, and surrounding parts.† Cases not unfrequently occur, in which

---

ings from the arm. In both these cases, which occurred in a lady and an officer, the latter accustomed to free living, some degree of feverishness accompanied the symptoms of Purpura ; and the blood drawn exhibited a tenacious, contracted coagulum, covered with a thick coat of lymph. See Edin. Med. and Surg. Journal, vol. v. p. 7, for Jan. 1809.

* See Celsus de Med. lib. ii. cap. 7.

† This boy, though delicate, had enjoyed a moderate share of health, until ten or twelve days previous to his death, notwithstanding the di-

hepatic obstruction is connected with Purpura. A man, habituated to spirit-drinking, died in about a fortnight from the commencement of an eruption of petechiæ, which was soon followed by profuse and unceasing hæmorrhage from the mouth and nostrils; but I had no opportunity of examining the body. The jaundiced hue of the skin and eyes, however, with the pain in his side, dry cough, and quick wiry pulse, left no doubt of the existence of considerable hepatic congestion. And, lastly, I attended a young woman, about the same time, labouring under the third species of the disease (P. *urticans*), with a sallow complexion, a considerable pain in the abdomen, and constipation, without fever. While she was taking acids and purgatives, which had scarcely acted upon the bowels, the pain on a sudden became extremely acute, the pulse frequent and hard, and the skin hot, with other symptoms denoting inflammation in the bowels, which were immediately relieved by a copious bleeding from the arm, followed by purgatives; after which the sallowness of the skin was gone, and the purple spots soon disappeared.

These facts are not sufficient to afford any general inference, respecting the nature or requisite treatment of Purpura hæmorrhagica; on the contrary, they tend to prove, that the general conclusions which are usually deduced, and the simple indi-

---

minution of the cavity of the thorax, occasioned by this tumour. See the Edin. Journal, vol. vi. just referred to.

M

cations* which are commonly laid down, have been too hastily adopted, and that no rule of practice can be universally applicable in all cases of the disease.

In the slighter degrees of the Purpura, occurring in children who are ill fed and nursed, and who reside in close places, where they are little exercised, or in women shut up in similar situations, and debilitated by want of proper food, and by fatigue, watching, and anxiety, the use of tonics, with the mineral acids and wine, will doubtless be adequate to the cure of the disease, especially where exercise in the open air can be employed at the same time.† But when it occurs in adults, especially in those already enjoying the benefits of exercise in the air of the country, and who have suffered no privation in respect to diet; or when it appears in persons previously stout or even plethoric; when it is accompanied with a white and loaded tongue, a quick and somewhat sharp, though small, pulse, occasional chills and heats, and other symptoms of

---

* I am sorry to be under the necessity of differing from my respected friend and preceptor, on this subject; who would, perhaps, subsequently, have deemed the following statement, respecting the method of cure in the hæmorrhagic Purpura, too general. "The mode of treatment for this disease is simple, and may be comprised in a very few words. It is proper to recommend a generous diet, the use of wine, Peruvian Bark, and acids, along with moderate exercise in the open air, and whatever may tend to produce cheerfulness and serenity of mind." See Reports on the Dis. of London, p. 93, for May 1797.

† In enumerating the remedies, mentioned in the preceding note, Dr. Willan lays the most particular stress upon this point, and adds, that "without air, exercise, and an easy state of mind, the effect of medicines is very uncertain." On Cutan. Dis. p. 461.

feverishness, however moderate ; and if at the
same time there are fixed internal pains, a dry
cough, and an irregular state of the bowels ; —
symptoms which may be presumed to indicate the
existence of some local congestion ; — then the
administration of tonic medicines, particularly of
wine, Cinchona, and other warmer tonics, will be
found inefficacious, if not decidedly injurious. In
such cases, free and repeated evacuations of the
bowels, by medicines containing some portion of
the Submuriate of Mercury, will be found most
beneficial. The continuance or repetition of these
evacuants, must, of course, be regulated by their
effects on the symptoms of the complaint, or on
the general constitution, and by the appearance of
the excretions from the intestines. * If the pains
are severe and fixed, and if the marks of febrile
irritation are considerable, and the spontaneous
hæmorrhage not profuse, local or general blood-
letting may, doubtless, be employed with great
benefit, especially in robust adults. " When the

* While these sheets were in the press, I received a valuable communication from my friend Dr. Harty, of Dublin, detailing the result
of his experience in this obscure disease ; and it afforded me great satisfaction to learn, that, after having witnessed the death of a patient,
who was treated in the ordinary way, with nutritive diet and tonic medicines, he has been uniformly successful in the management of upwards of a dozen cases, since he relied solely upon the liberal administration of purgatives. He prescribed Calomel with Jalap, in active doses,
daily, which appeared to be equally beneficial in the hæmorrhagic, as in
the simple Purpura : the hæmorrhage ceased, and the purple extravasations disappeared, after a few doses had been taken.

This document being, in my estimation, too valuable to be lost, I
transmitted it to Edinburgh, and it was published in the Medical and
Surgical Journal, for April 1815.

disease arises from congestion, and languor of the absorbents, blood-letting may be useful by taking off the load which obstructs the action both of the blood-vessels and the absorbents. It is a well-known fact, that blood-letting promotes absorption; and if Purpura be blood effused into the substance of the cutis, the bleeding, both by promoting absorption and relieving a congestion which implicates the venous capillaries, must be useful in Purpura. But it must be employed with cautious reference to the state of strength of the patient, separated from the temporary debility occasioned by the disease.

"In the majority of cases, in which blood-letting has been requisite, the blood has exhibited the buffy coat: in general there is little or no serum separated.

"When no congestion exists, and the disease appears to be referrible to want of tone in the extreme vessels, Dr. Whitlock Nicol has proposed the use of Oil of Turpentine, and has detailed two cases in which it proved successful. * It has also been successfully given by Dr. Magee of Dublin, in doses of fʒss mixed with fʒss of Castor Oil, and some Cinnamon or Peppermint Water."

When the urgency of the hæmorrhagic tendency has been diminished by these means, the constitution rallies, though not rapidly, with the assistance of the mineral acids, and the Decoction of Cinchona, or of Cascarilla; or with the aid of some

* London Med. Repository, July 1811.

preparation of Iron, together with moderate exercise, and nutritious diet.

SPECIES 3. PURPURA *urticans*, NETTLE RASH SCURVY.

Syn. Porphyra simplex ; ε. *urticans* (*Good*).

This species (Plate XXIX. of BATEMAN ; Pl. 12. of THE ATLAS,) is distinguished by this peculiarity, that it commences in the form of rounded and reddish elevations of the cuticle, resembling wheals, but which are not accompanied, like the wheals of Urticaria, by any sensation of tingling or itching. These little tumours gradually dilate, but, within one or two days, they subside to the level of the surrounding cuticle, and at the same time their hue becomes darker, and at length livid. As these spots are not permanent, but appear in succession in different places, they are commonly seen of different hues; the fresh and elevated ones being of a brighter red, while the level spots exhibit different degrees of lividity, and become brown as they disappear. They are most common on the legs, where they are frequently mixed with petechiæ; but they sometimes appear also on the arms, thighs, breast, &c.

The duration of the complaint is various, from three to five weeks. It usually occurs in summer and autumn; and attacks those who are liable to fatigue, and live on poor diet : or, on the contrary, delicate young women, who live luxuriously, and take little exercise. Some œdema of the extremities usually accompanies it, and it is occasionally preceded by a stiffness and weight of the limbs.

" Bleeding and purging are more decidedly useful in this than in the preceding species ; but in general the same rules of treatment are applicable to all of them."

SPECIES 4. PURPURA *senilis*, SCURVY OF OLD AGE.

I give this appellation to a variety of the complaint (Plate XXX. of BATEMAN ; Pl. 12. of THE ATLAS,) of which I have seen a few cases, occurring only in elderly women. It appears principally along the outside of the fore-arm, in successive dark purple blotches, of an irregular form and various magnitude. Each of these continues from a week to ten or twelve days, when the extravasated blood is absorbed. A constant series of these ecchymoses had appeared in one case during ten years, and in others for a shorter period ; but in all, the skin of the arm was left of a brown colour. The health did not appear to suffer ; nor did purgatives, blood-letting (which was tried in one case, in consequence of the extraordinary hardness of the pulse), tonics, or any other expedient, appear to exert any influence over the eruption.

SPECIES 5. PURPURA *contagiosa*, CONTAGIOUS SCURVY.

Syn. Purpura maligna (*Sauv.*)

This species is introduced for the purpose of noticing the eruption of petechiæ, which occasionally accompanies typhoid fevers, where they occur in close situations : but as these are merely symptomatic, it would be superfluous to dilate upon the subject here. I may observe, in addition to the facts which I formerly communicated to Dr. Willan, respecting the occurrence of petechiæ in patients admitted into the Fever-House *, that such an efflorescence is very rarely seen in that establishment.

Works which may be consulted on Purpura.

EDINBURGH Med. and Surg. Journal.
EYSEL, Dis. de Febre purpurata, 1702.
LONDON Med. Repository.
MASSIE (Steph.) de Purpura, 8vo. 1762.
MENTZLER, de Venæsect. in Purpura abusu, &c. 1744.
NEUCRANTZ, de Purpura liber singularis, 1660.
PLUMBE on Diseases of the Skin, 2d edit. 1827.
RAYER, Traité des Maladies de la Peau, 1827.
STOKER's Pathological Observations, Part I. Dub. 1825.

GENUS VI. ERYTHEMA, INFLAMMATORY BLUSH.

Syn. Εϱυθημα *(G.)*: Erysipelas *(Celsus, Galen)*: Hieropyr *(Vog.)*: Dartre erythemoïde, Herpes erythemoïdes *(Alibert)*: Efflorescence cutanée, *(F.)*: die Hautröthe *(Germ.)*: *Inflammatory Blush.*

Def. A RED SMOOTH FULNESS OF THE INTEGUMENTS : ACCOMPANIED WITH BURNING PAIN ; TERMI-

---

* See his Treatise on Cutan. Dis. p. 468 and 469, *note.*

NATING GENERALLY IN SCALES; OCCASIONALLY, BUT
RARELY, IN GANGRENE: NOT CONTAGIOUS.

ERYTHEMA, like Roseola, is commonly symptomatic, and occurs with much variety in its form;
yet sometimes, like the same efflorescence, it is the
most prominent symptom, and is, therefore, in like
manner, liable to be mistaken for the idiopathic.
eruptive fevers. This term is often erroneously
applied to eruptions, which, together with redness,
exhibit distinct papular and vesicular elevations *;
as, for example, to the *Eczema* produced by the
irritation of mercury.

Dr. Willan has described six species of Erythema, which include all the ordinary forms of the
efflorescence; but there are, properly speaking,
seven species:

1. E. *fugax.*	5. E. *tuberculatum.*
2. E. *læve.*	6. E. *nodosum.*
3. E. *marginatum.*	7. E. *intertrigo.*
4. E. *papulatum.*	

* The word ερυθημα, as used every where by Hippocrates, signifies
simply *redness;* and is therefore correctly appropriated to this affection, which differs from Erysipelas, inasmuch as it is a mere rash or
efflorescence, and is not accompanied by any swelling, vesication,
or regular fever. — Modern authors have not agreed in their distinctions between these two terms. Dr. Cullen applies the word
Erythema, to a slight affection of the skin, appearing without fever, or
attended by a secondary fever of irritation; and *Erysipelas,* to an
affection of the skin, when it is the result, or is symptomatic of fever;
making no distinction as to the termination in bullæ, &c. See his
Nosol. Meth. gen. vii. spec. 2.; and First Lines, § 274. — Prof. Callisen
deems Erythema only a lesser degree of Erysipelas. See his Systema
Chirurg. Hodiern. § 483.

Mr. Travers considers Erythema and Erysipelas "modes of inflammation with inadequate power to carry them on to a termination.
Thus they are deficient in the adhesive state; they are incapable of a

In some of these, as appears from their titles, the surface is more or less elevated during the course of the disease, approximating to the papular or tubercular tumours : but these elevations are obscurely formed, and soon subside, leaving the redness undiminished.

SPECIES 1. ERYTHEMA *fugax*, FUGACIOUS INFLAMMATORY BLUSH.

Syn. L'Erythème symptomatique (*Rayer.*)

This species consists of red patches, of an irregular form, and short duration, resembling the redness produced from pressure. These patches appear successively on the arms, neck, breast, and face, in various febrile diseases, and in bilious diarrhœa, generally denoting, as Hippocrates and the ancients have observed, a tedious and dangerous disease. They sometimes occur in chronic affections, especially those in which the primæ viæ are deranged ; as in dyspepsia, hysteria, hemicrania, &c.

SPECIES 2. ERYTHEMA *læve*, SMOOTH INFLAMMATORY BLUSH.

Syn. Erythema œdematosum (*Good*): L'Erythème idiopathique (*Rayer*): Œdematous inflammation (*J. Hunter*).

This species exhibits an uniformly smooth,

---

healthy suppuration ; and their imperfect effusion or suppuration is at the expence of the life of the part." See his vol. on Constitutional Irritations, p. 220. However we might in part admit this reasoning in some of the species of Erysipelas, it certainly does not apply in Erythema. T.

shining surface, and chiefly appears on the lower extremities, in confluent patches, and is generally accompanied by anasarca. It affects young persons, who are sedentary, with slight fever, and terminates gradually, after an uncertain period, in extensive desquamation, as soon as the anasarca has disappeared. Exercise, with diuretics and corroborants, contributes to shorten its duration in this class of patients. It occurs also in elderly persons, labouring under Anasarca (especially in those accustomed to excessive drinking), and is liable to terminate in gangrenous ulcers. Indeed, under whatever circumstances Anasarca occurs, so as to stretch the skin greatly, this Erythema is liable to be produced : it is often chequered with patches and streaks of a dark red or purple hue. Relief is afforded by the horizontal posture of the limbs, by the internal use of diuretics and bark, and also by weak spirituous lotions, or those formed with Solution of Acetate of Ammonia and Camphor Mixture, or of diluted Acetate of Lead, applied to the surface.

This species of Erythema sometimes occurs, without œdema, when the bowels have been much disordered; and, occasionally, in women, at the menstrual periods.

SPECIES 3. ERYTHEMA *marginatum*, MARGINATED INFLAMMATORY BLUSH.

(Plate XXXII. fig. 2. of BATEMAN; Pl. 13. of THE ATLAS). The eruption in this species occurs in patches, which are bounded on one side by a hard, elevated, tortuous, red border, in some places obscurely papulated; but the redness has no regular boundary on the open side. The patches appear on the extremities and loins in old people, and remain for an uncertain time, without producing any irritation in the skin. They are connected with some internal disorder, and their occurrence is to be deemed unfavourable.

SPECIES 4. ERYTHEMA *papulatum*, PAPULATED INFLAMMATORY BLUSH.

(Plate XXXI. fig. 1. of BATEMAN; Pl. 13. of THE ATLAS.) This rash occurs chiefly on the arms, neck, and breast, in extensive irregular patches, "frequently slightly elevated above the unaffected skin," of a bright red hue, presenting not an inelegant painted appearance. For a day or two, before the colour becomes vivid, the surface is rough or imperfectly papulated. The redness afterwards continues for about a fortnight; and as the eruption declines, it assumes a blueish or pale purple hue, especially in the central parts of the patches. "It is generally attended, during the height of the eruption, with a sensation of tingling, which is much increased at night; and is sometimes followed, as the patches change in colour, by a sensation of soreness." I have seen this eruption attended with great disorder of the constitution; especially with a frequent small pulse, anorexia, watchfulness, and extreme depression of strength and spirits, and with acute pains and great tenderness of the limbs: but the general disorder is often trifling. * Light diet, with diaphoretics, and the mineral acids, and an attention to the state of the bowels, comprise all that is necessary in the treatment of this disorder. "To allay the uneasy tingling, and secure rest at night, combinations of Tartar emetic, or of James' powder and Opium, will be found useful."

SPECIES 5. ERYTHEMA *tuberculatum*, TUBERCULATED INFLAMMATORY BLUSH.

(Plate XXXI. fig. 2. of BATEMAN; Pl. 13. of THE ATLAS.) This species resembles the last in the large irregular patches of red efflorescence which it exhibits; but there are small, slightly-elevated tumours interspersed through the patches, subsiding in about a week and leaving the Erythema,. which becomes livid and disappears in about a week more. It commences with fever, and is accompanied with great languor, irritability, and restlessness, and succeeded by hectic. In the only three cases of this Erythema which had occurred to Dr. Willan, the medicines employed did not appear to alleviate the symptoms, or to prevent the subsequent hectic. I have not seen any instance of it.

SPECIES 6. ERYTHEMA *nodosum*, NODOSE INFLAMMATORY BLUSH.

* See Report of the Public Dispensary, Edin. Med. and Surg. Journ. for Jan. 1812.

(Plate XXXII. fig. 1. of Bateman; Pl. 13. of The Atlas). This species is a more common and milder complaint : it seems to affect females chiefly ; "but Dr. Merriman says, that he has 'frequently witness- ed it in children of both sexes * :' and Mr. Plumbe has also seen it in children. † I have seen it several times in girls under ten years of age, and once only in a boy:" it occurs on the fore part of the legs. It is preceded by slight febrile symp- toms for a week or more, which generally abate when the Erythema appears. It shows itself in large oval patches, the long diameter of which is parallel with the tibia, and which slowly rise into hard and painful protuberances, and as re- gularly soften and subside, in the course of nine or ten days; the red colour turning blueish on the eighth or ninth day, as if the leg had been bruised. It has always gone through its course mildly, un- der the use of small doses of Calomel and mild laxatives, followed by the mineral acids, Decoction of Cinchona Bark, and other tonics. When the pain is severe, an opiate, combined with James' powder and Calomel, is necessary. The best local appli- cation is a lotion compounded of f3x of Alcohol, and f3v of Rose Water.

SPECIES 7. ERYTHEMA *intertrigo*, FRET OR ERO- SION OF THE SKIN.

Syn. Erythema intertrigo (*Sauv.*) : Intertrigo (*Linn. Vog.*) : Erythema ab acri inquilino (*Cull.*) :

---

* Underwood on the Diseases of Children, 8th edit. p. 176.
† Plumbe on Diseases of the Skin, 2d edit. p. 449.

Maculæ volaticæ (*Auct. var.*): Kereh (*Arab.*): Erat (*German*): Ecorchure, Rougeurs des nouveau nés (*F.*) *Fret.*

Under the head of Erythema, Dr. Willan has made mention of that form of *Intertrigo* which is produced in some persons, especially those of sanguine temperament and corpulent habit, by the attrition of contiguous surfaces. * It most frequently occurs beneath the breasts, round the axillæ, in the groin, and at the upper part of the thighs. "This species of Intertrigo is very common in fat children, occurring in all the folds of the skin, and causing an acrimonious discharge, which excoriates the surface beyond the affected parts, if attention to cleanliness be neglected." Sometimes it is accompanied by a glairy fetid secretion; and sometimes the surface is dry, and the redness terminates in a scurfy or scaly exfoliation. An erythematous appearance, analogous to the Intertrigo, is occasioned by acrimonious discharges, as by those of fluor albus, dysentery, gonorrhœa, &c. and by the irritation of the urine and alvine discharges, in infants, when a sufficient attention is not paid to the proper changes of their linen.

The heat and uneasiness attendant on this complaint are allayed by frequent tepid ablution, which removes the acrid secretion, where it occurs, and

---

* Sauvages includes this variety of Intertrigo, and the chafing and inflammation produced by riding on horseback, tight shoes, the use of tools, and even that of bedridden persons, under Erythema, denominating the former Erythema *intertrigo* (spec. 5), and the latter E. *paratrimma* (spec. 6.)

tends to prevent excoriation. If this take place, any simple ointment, or, which is preferable, some mild absorbent powder, such as that of Calamine or of Cerussa, will be applied with relief. " When the discharge is fœtid, the odour is almost immediately destroyed, and the inflammation rapidly allayed, by frequently bathing the affected parts with a lotion composed of six fluid drachms or a fluid ounce of the Chloro-sodaic solution and five fluid ounces of Water." When there is much irritability, a lotion composed of ten grains of Oxymuriate of Mercury, and six fluid ounces of Lime Water, will be found serviceable.

Books which may be consulted on Erythema.

ALIBERT, sur les Maladies de la Peau.
LECOURT-CHANTILLY, sur l'Erythème et l'Erysipile, 4to. 1804.
PLUMBE on Diseases of the Skin, 2d edit. 1827.
RAYER, Traité des Maladies de la Peau, 1826.

GENUS VII. ERYSIPELAS.*

Syn. Febris erysipelatosa (*Sydenham*): Febris erysipelacea (*Hoffm. Vog.*): Emphlysis Erysipelas, (*Good*): Rosa, Ignis Sancti Anthonii (*Auct. var.*):

*.In the former editions of this work, Erysipelas is ranked among Bullæ. It may, in my opinion, with more propriety be regarded as one of the Exanthemata; I have therefore removed it to this place. Vesications certainly occur in severe and aggravated cases of the disease; but, in the great majority of instances, this symptom is absent: and unless it be an invariable attendant of the disease, there is more propriety in placing Erysipelas in its present situation, than where it formerly stood in this work. T.

Erésipèle (*F.*): Rothlauf (*Germ.*): Hemnet (*Arab.*): Akki (*Tam. Tel.*): Shirjah (*Duk.*): Pittā vichārchika (*Sans.*): Soorkh (*Pers.*): Kaszalapani (*Malayalie*): *The Rose.*

Def. A FEBRILE DISEASE, IN WHICH SOME PART OF THE BODY IS AFFECTED EXTERNALLY WITH HEAT, REDNESS, SWELLING, AND SOMETIMES VESICATIONS.

The tumour in this affection is soft, diffuse, and irregularly circumscribed, and not accompanied by throbbing or acute pain, nor terminating in true suppuration.

The last-mentioned circumstances distinguish the tumour of Erysipelas from that of Phlegmon [*] ; and the presence of tumour, together with vesication, distinguishes the disease from Erythema. The disappearing of the redness on pressure, and its immediate return when the pressure is removed, are commonly mentioned among the characteristics of Erysipelas, by medical writers, from Galen downwards.[†] This phænomenon, however, belongs to Erysipelas in common with several of the Exanthemata ; as with the efflorescence in Scarlatina, in some varieties of Roseola, and in Erythema. Erysipelas is often a contagious disease. It more frequently attacks women than men.

---

[*] See Galen Meth. Med. cap. xiv. and Comment. in aph. 20., lib. iv. also Aëtius, tetrab. iv. serm. ii. cap. 59.

[†] Galen speaks of Erysipelas *phlegmonodes*, and *œdematodes*, in which he has been followed by Forest, Obs. Chirurg. lib. ii. 1. 3. & 4.; by Plater, De Superfic. Corp. Dolore, cap. 17.; and Frank, De Curand. Hom. Morbis, lib. iii. — Mr. Pearson divides Erysipelas into three species, adding the *gangrenous* to the two just mentioned. See his Principles of Surgery, chap. x.

" Mr. Lawrence, in a paper on Erysipelas *, conceives that this disease in every instance is a modification of inflammation, and that its various forms depend upon accidental circumstances. This doctrine appears to be evidently erroneous. It is indeed highly probable that Erysipelas arising from wounds or. other injuries is simple inflammation, modified by the structure which it has attacked ; but that there is a distinct febrile affection, of which the eruption termed Erysipelas is a characteristic symptom, as much as the eruption in Scarlatina, or in any other of the Exanthemata, is undoubted. The eruption being preceded by the fever, the disease running a tolerably regular course, its being occasionally contagious, and never by any treatment being cut short, are very strong evidences in favour of this opinion."

There are four species of Erysipelas :

1. E. *phlegmonodes.* 3. E. *gangrænosum.*
2. E. *ædematodes.* 4. E. *erraticum.*

SPECIES 1. ERYSIPELAS *phlegmonodes*, PHLEGMONOUS ERYSIPELAS. †

It is scarcely necessary to enter into a minute description of the well-known appearance of acute Erysipelas. ‡ This form of it most frequently occurs in the face, the head, the neck, and some-

* Med. Chirurg. Trans. vol xiv.

† Mr. Arnot (Med. & Phys. Journ. vol. 57. p. 210.) objects to this name, as being "unnecessary, inaccurate, and applied to dissimilar morbid conditions." See Mr. Earle's paper in the same volume.

‡ Dr. Cullen has given an excellent history of the disease. First Lines, § 1696.

times the chest, affecting usually one side of it only;
sometimes it seizes one of the extremities ; and in
both cases it is ushered in by a smart feverish
attack, " with great irritability of the stomach, often
with delirium, and a tendency to coma.　The colour of the eruption is more of scarlet than of the
tint of the rose, as in the other species; and the
burning heat and tingling in the part are exceedingly distressing.　The swelling generally appears
on the second night, or the third day of the fever,
" and extends to the cranium from the face :
the cutis only, however, is affected, and in the
line of its progress is elevated, and shows a well-
defined edge, the diseased parts appearing upon
the healthy almost as embossed work."　The vesications, when they arise, appear on the fourth and
fifth, and break or subside on the fifth or sixth day,
when the redness changes to a yellowish hue, and
the swelling and fever begin to diminish ; — and on
the eighth day both disappear : on the tenth, the
new cuticle is commonly left exposed, the old one
having cracked and separated : the brownish or
dark scab, which had formed where the fluid of the
vesications had been discharged, having fallen off. —
The progress of the disease, however, is more rapid,
and its duration shorter, in young and sanguine
habits, than in those more advanced in life* : in the
former, the tumefaction is sometimes fully formed
on the second day, and the whole terminates on the

---

* Quo vehementius malum, eo etiam gravius est, sed brevius.　Lorry
de Morb. Cutan. 4to. p. 192.

sixth or seventh; while in the latter, it may be protracted to the tenth or twelfth, and the desquamation may not be completed before the fourteenth
day. The vesications, in the latter instances, are
often succeeded by a profuse discharge of acrimonious lymph for several days, so that scabs do not
form. Suppuration very rarely occurs in this
species of Erysipelas, especially when it affects the
face. It rarely terminates in death.

SPECIES 2. ERYSIPELAS *œdematodes*, EDEMATOSE
ERYSIPELAS.

In this species, which is less severe in its attack,
the tumour is more gradual in its rise and extension, is of a paler red, or of a yellowish
brown colour, and is accompanied by less heat and
local distress; its surface is smooth and shining;
and if it be strongly pressed with the finger, a
slight pit remains for a short time. * Vesications,
which are smaller, less elevated, and more numerous
than those which occasionally appear in the former
species, rise on the third or fourth day from the
commencement of the swelling; and are succeeded, in two or three days, by thin, dark-coloured scabs, giving an appearance not unlike
the confluent smallpox, from the edges of which
a clear lymph exudes. The whole face is much

---

* Mr. Pearson observes, that " the part affected is almost wholly free
from tension, and gives the sensation of an *œdematose* or *emphysematose*
state, except that there is no crepitation." He compares the sensation,
on pressing a part in which a considerable formation of pus has taken
place in Erysipelas, " to that which is excited by a quagmire or morass."
Loc. cit.

enlarged, so that the form of the features is scarcely recognised, and the appearance is not unaptly compared by Dr. Willan to that of a bladder distended with water. " This species is often accompanied with an affection of the throat, evidently erysipelatous. The symptoms are a red blush over the velum palatum and uvula, slight tumefaction, and considerable pain on deglutition. After a few days, excoriation and superficial ulceration sometimes extends to the larynx, affecting speech and respiration ; sometimes to the pharynx and œsophagus."

Edematose Erysipelas is attended with considerable danger when it affects the face, as above described ; for the disorder of the functions increases with the advancement of the external disease. Vomiting, rigors, and delirium, followed by coma, take place about the height of the disorder, and often terminate fatally on the seventh or eighth day : " there is great depression of the muscular strength ; the pulse is feeble and quick, and the tongue dry with a brown streak in the centre :" while in other cases, the symptoms continue undiminished, and death occurs at a later period ; or a slow and tedious convalescence ensues.

This form of Erysipelas most commonly affects persons of debilitated constitution, dropsical patients, and those who have long been subject to other chronic maladies, or live in habitual intemperance. It is not attended with danger, however, when it affects one of the extremities ; unless symptomatic of a punctured wound in a bad state of the habit. In some unfavourable cases matter is formed, which is apt to make its way through the cellular substance, producing irregular sinuses between the muscles, which it often materially injures, and prolonging the sufferings of the patient for many weeks.

SPECIES 3. ERYSIPELAS *gangrænosum*, GANGRENOUS ERYSIPELAS.

This species commences sometimes like the one, and sometimes like the other of the foregoing species; and most commonly occurs in the face, neck, or shoulders. "It is not improbable that it is merely an increased degree of the first species." It is accompanied with symptoms of low fever, and with delirium, which is soon followed by coma, which remains through the subsequent course of the disease. The colour of the affected part is a dark red; and scattered phlyctænæ, with a livid base, appear upon the surface, and frequently run into gangrenous ulcerations. Even when it terminates favourably, suppuration and gangrene of the muscles, tendons, and cellular substance often take place, producing little caverns and sinuses, which contain an ill-conditioned pus, together with sloughs of the mortified parts, which are ultimately evacuated from the ulcers. It is always a tedious and precarious disease, and irregular in the period of its termination.

A peculiar variety of gangrenous Erysipelas oc-

N 3

casionally occurs in infants, a few days after birth,
especially in lying-in hospitals*, and is often fatal.
Sometimes, indeed, infants have been born with
livid patches, vesications, and even gangrene already advanced.†   It most frequently commences
about the umbilicus or the genitals, and extends
upwards, or downwards, affecting the parts which
it reaches with moderate swelling, and slight hardness ‡; the skin puts on a dark-red colour, and vesications with livid bases break out, terminating in
sphacelus, which, if the child be not speedily cut
off, nearly destroys some of the fingers or toes, or
even the genitals.   In the milder cases, when the
extremities alone are affected, suppurations take
place rapidly about the joints of the hands and feet.
The complaint, however, often terminates favourably in ten or twelve days.

SPECIES 4. ERYSIPELAS *erraticum*, WANDERING
ERYSIPELAS.

In this species the morbid patches appear, one
after another, on different parts of the body; in
some cases, those which appeared first remain till
the whole eruption be completed; in others, the
first patches decline as fresh ones appear.   Sometimes the disease thus travels progressively from

---

* See Underwood on the Diseases of Children, vol. i. p. 31. (5th edit.)
—and an ample account of it by Dr. Garthshore, in the Med. Communications, vol. ii. art. v. (1790)— with some references.

† See a case related by Dr. Bromfield, in the same vol. art. iv.

‡ Umbilicalem regionem in infantibus frequentius infestat, ac inde
per abdomen spargitur, cum pathematibus, funesto ut plurimum eventu.
— Hoff. de Morb Infantum, cap. 13.   T.

the face downwards to the extremities.* Sometimes it suddenly leaves one part, and appears at
another. It commonly terminates favourably, however, in a week or ten days. †

The exciting causes of Erysipelas are not always
obvious : but it is commonly attributed to the action
of cold or damp air, after being heated ‡, or to
exposure to a strong heat, whether from the direct
rays of the sun or from a fire ; to intemperance,
or to violent emotions of the mind, especially
anger and grief. " Some practitioners refer it, in
the majority of cases, to a superabundant acid in
the blood, arising from acid or acidifiable diet, such
as raw vegetables, too much fruit, sweets, &c. ; and
it has even been stated that the serum in the vesicles is of an acid nature, which can be detected
by tests." Erysipelas is likewise symptomatic of
wounds and punctures, the local application of

* Mr. Pearson mentions this progression of the disease as belonging
to the Erysipelas œdematodes ; and adds, that each renewed accession
of the complaint was less and less severe, as it receded to a greater distance from the part first affected. § 308. See also Frank, lib. iii. § 281.
    Ita à facie in genitalia sæpe ruit erysipelas, quod jam intellexerat
Hippocrates, ab aurium posticâ parte ad articulas fluxisse vidi, ab his in
oculos. Lorry de Morb. Cutan. 4to. p. 195. T.
    † ' It has been reasonably suggested by Mr. Arnott, that the term
Erysipelas is improperly applied to aponeurotic inflammation, in which
the skin is raised and becomes puffy, and often ends in suppuration.
Many cases of what is regarded as Erysipelas Phlegmonodes are of this
description.' T.
    ‡ Virum novi militarem qui nunquam aëris uvidi humiditati exponi-
tur per horam unam aut alteram, quin illicò corripiatur erysipelate.
Lorry de Morb. Cutan. 4to. p. 196. T.

poisons, the stings of insects, &c. * " This is particularly the case in slight injuries of the scalp ; and not unfrequently terminates fatally," especially when the periosteum is injured. " It is more prevalent in spring and autumn, but rarely appears in winter."

It has been the subject of some discussion, whether Erysipelas be not sometimes propagated by contagion and infection. The disease has been noticed, in several hospitals, to prevail in certain wards, among patients admitted with different complaints ; but has seldom been known to spread in private houses. Dr. Wells, indeed, has collected several examples of the apparent communication of Erysipelas by contagion, which occurred in private families. † But such cases are, at all events, extremely rare, and perhaps never happened in well-ventilated and cleanly houses. From the Royal Infirmary, at Edinburgh, this disease, like the puerperal fever, was banished by ventilation, whitewashing, and other means of purification ; and it has not occurred in any hospital of late years, since a better system has been adopted in these respects. Other diseases, not infectious in themselves, appear to become united with typhus, or contagious fever, under similar circumstances, and thus to be propagated

---

* An erysipelatous affection, which has even proved fatal, has occasionally come on two or three days after inoculation, both variolous and vaccine, in children of irritable habits. See some cases in the Med. and Phys. Journal for 1801.

† See Transact. of a Soc. for the Improvement of Med. and Chirurg. Knowledge, vol. ii. art. xvii. (1800.)

in their double form; the dysentery*, for example, the peritonitis of women in childbed, ulcerated sore-throat, &c. †   The simple phlegmonous Erysipelas, at all events, was never seen to spread like an infectious disease.   " Persons who have once had the disease are very liable to a repetition of it. What, it may be asked, is the temperament which predisposes to it?   Is it simple increased irritability?   The solution of this question would throw great light upon the pathology of the disease."

The method of treatment must necessarily be widely different in the phlegmonous, from that which the other forms of the disease require.   In the ordinary cases of this species of Erysipelas, the principal plan of cure consists in the administration of moderate purgatives, with a light vegetable diet, and in enjoying repose of body and mind, and a cool apartment.   " M. Reil and M. Retz strongly recommend emetics in the commencement of Erysipelas.   Calomel, in full doses, is always beneficial in the early stage of the disease.   Saline and other diaphoretic medicines may be employed, as auxiliaries of secondary importance; as, for instance, the Liquor Ammoniæ Acetatis, Tartarised Antimony, and similar sudorifics.   Colchicum has been advantageously used in the two first species of the

---

* See Dr. Harty's Observations on Dysentery.

† In the case of Mr. Newly, who died of a disease closely resembling Erysipelas œdematodes, caused by a wound received in dissection, Mr. Travers states, that besides the nurse, who took the disease and died, another woman, who merely assisted in the room, was attacked, but recovered. Travers on Constitutional Irritation, p. 289. T.

disease." Blood-letting, which has been much recommended as the principal remedy for the acute Erysipelas, is seldom requisite; and, unless there is considerable tendency to delirium or coma, cannot be repeated with advantage, at least in London, and other large towns.* Local bleeding and blistering may be substituted in such cases. It is usual to forbid leeches to be applied upon, or very near the diseased surface; "but although the bites of leeches are, in some states of the habit, followed by Erysipelas, yet they do no harm when applied to the inflamed surface in this disease." The administration of Cinchona, Sulphate of Quinia, and Opium, in this form of the complaint, is certainly unnecessary, and appears to be of very equivocal safety, notwith-standing the authority upon which it has been ·recommended. "In general, however, some form of tonic is requisite after purging: the best is a light Infusion of Cascarilla Bark, so combined with Carbonate of Soda as to be taken in a state of effervescence. When spirits have been indulged in, they should be allowed, under due restraint.† Under the impression of a prevailing acidity, Car-bonate of Ammonia has been extolled as a remedy in this affection. It is probable that the benefit which results from it, depends more upon its power

---

* See Pearson's Principles of Surgery, § 320. — Bromfield's Chir. Obs. vol. i. p. 108;— also Prof. Callisen, Syst. Hodiern. § 491.

† See Sir A. Cooper's Surgical Lectures, vol. i. p. 249.

over the nervous system, than in its chemical union with the acid of the stomach."

In the Erysipelas *œdematodes*, and *erraticum*, the two last-mentioned remedies are highly useful, in accelerating the decline of the disease, and relieving irritation, when the active symptoms of the first three or four days have been subdued by purgatives and diaphoretics ; or, if the functions of the sensorium were considerably disordered, by a blister between the shoulders, or a topical bleeding in the same part. The strength should be supported, during the decline of the complaint, by a more cordial regimen, with a view to obviate the tendency to gangrene.

In the Erysipelas *gangrænosum* *, the Cinchona Bark is necessary, in considerable doses ; " but Sulphate of Quinia is preferable. It may be given to adults in two grain doses every three hours ; and in Erysipelas *infantum*, which is a variety of this species, it is the medicine chiefly to be relied upon." Opium also, Camphor, the mineral acids, Wine, and the general regimen adapted to gangrenous affections occurring under other circumstances, must be freely employed. The formation of sinuses, the separation of sphacelated parts, &c. will require surgical attention for some time.

With respect to external applications in the early stages of Erysipelas, experience seems to have de-

* " In tenellis infantibus observatum fuit Erysipelas à causa abscondita, sæpissime lethali, nisi corticis usu occurratur malo." Callisen, p. 493.—See also Underwood, and Garthshore, before quoted.

cided that they are generally unnecessary, if not prejudicial. *   " Puncturing or scarifying the skin with the point or the shoulder of a lancet has been found highly beneficial. In E. *phlegmonoides,* these incisions should be about an inch in length, and carried completely through the cutis vera; after which, fomentations should be applied over the incisions. This practice, however, is less frequently necessary than some modern surgeons would lead us to believe. It is useful in that state of the disease in which the inflammation runs so high as to threaten destruction to the subcutaneous structure. It requires, however, to be done with caution, as fatal hæmorrhages have followed these incisions." The application of powdery substances has commonly, according to my own observation, augmented the heat and irritation in the commencement; and afterwards, when the fluid of the vesications oozes out, such substances produce additional irritation, by forming, with the concreting fluid, hard crusts upon the tender surface. †   In order to allay the irritation produced by the acrid discharge from the broken vesications, Dr. Willan recommends us to foment or wash the parts affected, from time to time, with milk, bran and water, thin gruel, or a decoction of elder flowers and poppy heads. In the early state of the inflammation,

---

* Mr. Pearson, § 331.

† " Externa remediare solventia, emollientia, adstringentia, vel calida, vel frigida,—uti quoque pulveres varii, parum vel nihil in erysipelate prosunt; nec omnis noxæ suspicionem, experientiâ teste, effugiunt."— Callisen.

when the local heat and redness are great, moderate tepid washing, or the application of a cool but slightly-stimulant lotion, such as the diluted Liquor Ammoniæ Acetatis, has appeared to me to afford considerable relief. " Compresses dipped in Camphorated Spirits of Wine in the first stages are beneficial. The following lotion has generally proved useful:

R Plumbi Acetatis gr. xij,
   Aquæ Rosæ f3v,
   Aceti Distillati f3iij,
   Spiritus Vini rectificati f3v. M.

Dr. Merriman recommends fomentations made of extract of Poppies diffused in warm water, and poultices, made of crum of bread and the same fluid. * When gangrene supervenes, Port wine poultices or the Nitrous acid lotion, in the proportion of f3j of the acid to Oij of water, are the best applications: or the Chloro-Sodaic Solution of Labarraque, diluted with five parts of water. As a local application, in ordinary cases, Mr. Higginbottom, on his own experience, recommends the lunar caustic. He desires that the part be well washed with warm soap and water, and then a long stick of caustic applied to the inflamed surface: but not sufficiently strong to abrade the surface.

" No disease is so liable to return as Erysipelas. Tissot recommends the following as the best pro-

---

* See Merriman's edit. of Underwood, 8vo. p. 127.

phylactic plan : The patient must carefully avoid the use of milk, cream, all rich and viscid food, baked and strong meats, aromatics, strong wines, a sedentary life, mental irritations : and live on light, cooling, vegetable food; and drink water with a little weak wine."

The *zona*, *zoster*, or *shingles*, is considered as a variety of Erysipelas by the nosologists, as well as by several practical writers : but it is invariably an eruption of vesicles, and possesses all the other characteristics of Herpes.   See ord. vi. gen. 3.

Sauvages under the head of Erysipelas *pestilens* (spec. 5.) arranges the fatal epidemic disease, which prevailed extensively in the early and dark ages, as the sequel of war and famine, and which has received a variety of denominations; such as ignis sacer, ignis S^{ti} Anthonii, mal des ardens, ergot, Kriebel krankheit, die Feverflecke, &c. &c. according to its various modifications and degrees of severity, or according to the supposed cause of it.*
The erysipelatous redness, however, followed by the dry gangrene, which often destroyed the limbs

* Sagar has included the varieties of this disease under the genus *Necrosis*, of which he thus details the symptoms: " Est partis mors lenta, sine prævio tumore, mollitie, et dissolutione fœtidâ, cum dolore ardente ordinario et stupore, quæ sequitur exsiccatio partis, induratio, nigredo, et mumia: differt à gangrenâ in eo, quod lentius procedat, cum dolore rodente et stupore, et in mumiam abeat; gangrena contra mollescat, phlyctænas elevet, putrescat, fœteat, atque cito decurrat." Syst. Morbor. cl. iii. ord. vii. gen. 42.   He describes five species; and of the fourth, *epidemica*, he says, " Apud Flandros regnavit hæc Necrosis 1749-50. spasmi artuum cum doloribus vagis; post 2 vel 3 septimanas stupor, fremitus obscurus, artus cum frigore glaciali, contracturis, et anæsthesiâ; tandem livor partis, nigredo, flavedo, phlyctænæ, et siccissima mumia."

joint by joint, was only one of the forms or stages of that disease ; as the contracted and palsied state of the limbs, to which the ancients gave the name of *scelotyrbe* *, constituted another. Instead of originating from eating rye affected with the *ergot*, as was supposed in France † ; or barley with which the *raphanus* was mixed, as was imagined in Sweden ‡ ; the disease was, doubtless, the result of deficient nourishment, — a severe land-scurvy, which was a great scourge of the ancient world, and often denominated *pestilence*. § — The name of St. Anthony seems to have been first associated with an epidemic disease of this kind, which prevailed in Dauphiné about the end of the twelfth century. An abbey, dedicated to that saint, had recently been founded at Vienne, in that province, where his bones were deposited ; and it was a popular opinion, in that and the succeeding century, that all the patients who were conveyed to this abbey were cured in a space of seven or nine days ‖ ;

* See Plin. Nat. Hist. lib. xxv. cap. 3.

† See an able history of the Ergot, in the Mém. de la Soc. Roy. de Médecine de Paris, tom. i. p. 260. by MM. Jussieu, Paulet, Saillant, and the Abbé Tessier. — See also the Philos. Trans. vol. lv. p. 118. An interesting account of the Kriebel krankheit, which was endemic in Hessia and Westphalia during a season of dearth in 1597, is preserved by Greg. Horst. in Oper. lib. viii. obs. 22. tom. ii.

‡ See Linnæus, Amœnit. Academ. vol. v.

§ Several instances of pestilence mentioned by Livy appear to have been of this kind. Indeed the learned Heyne observes : " Nobis manifestum videtur, ne ullam quidem inter Romanos pestilentiam memorari, quæ pro *pestilentiâ propriè dictâ* haberi possit," &c. (Opusc. Academ. iii. p. 113.)

‖ Mezeray, Abrégé Chronologique. See the articles Ergot, and Ignis Sacer, in Dr. Rees's Cyclopædia.

a circumstance which the ample supply of food in those religious houses may probably satisfactorily explain. It would be foreign to my purpose to pursue the subject here.

Works which may be consulted on Erysipelas.

AERTS (Jos. Joan.) de Erysipelate Diss. Inaug. Paris, 1782.

BUREAU, James, on the Erysipelas, 12mo. Lond. 1777.

BROMFIELD's Cases, Medical Communications, vol. ii. p. 322. 1790,

EDINBURGH Med. and Surg. Journ. vol. viii—xvii.

ENGELHART, Diss. de Erysipelate, 1797.

GARTHSHORE, Med. Communications, vol. ii. p. 326.

HADEN, Pract. Obs. on Colchicum Autumnalis, 8vo. 1821.

HUTCHISON, Surgical Observations, 8vo. 1816.

JAMES, Jacksonian Prize Essay for 1818. 8vo.

LONDON Med. Repos. vol. iv.

MEDICAL and Phys. Journ. January, vol. 57.

MEDICO-CHIRURG. Trans. vol. v. and xiv.

PAULUS ÆGINETUS, l. iv. c. 21.

PLUMBE on Diseases of the Skin, 2d edit. 1827.

RAYER, Traité sur les Maladies de la Peau, 1826.

RENAUD, Diss. sur l'Erysipèle, 1802.

SYDENHAM Opusc. p. 135.

WEATHERHEAD, Diagnosis between Erysipelas, Phlegmon, &c. 8vo. 1819.

WILSON on Febrile Diseases, vol. ii. & iii.

Order IV.

BULLÆ.

BLEBS.

SYN. Phlyctænæ (*Auct. vet.*): Ecphlysis (*Good*): Inflammations Bulleuses, Bulles (*F.*): Wasserblattern (*Germ.*).

Def. A PORTION OF THE CUTICLE DETACHED FROM THE SKIN BY THE INTERPOSITION OF A TRANSPARENT WATERY FLUID.

In the original sketch of his arrangement, Dr. Willan conjoined in one Order the three following genera, ERYSIPELAS, PEMPHIGUS, and POMPHOLYX, and those which now constitute the Order of VESICLES: but he was led to separate them in consequence of a just criticism of Prof. Tilesius, of Leipsic.* The large and often irregular vesications, which are

---

* This criticism was contained in a paper on herpetic eruptions, " Uber die flechtenartigen Ausschläge," published in a German periodical work, the Paradoxien of Dr. Martens, at Leipsic, 1802, ii band, i heft. Dr. Tilesius pointed out the improper application of Dr. Willan's definition of Bulla, " of a large size, and irregularly circumscribed," to the small, regular, and clustered vesicles of Herpes; and he mentioned also the common inflamed base, upon which the herpetic clusters are seated, the scabby crust which invariably forms upon them, &c. as further grounds of separation. See p. 18, et seq. of the Paradoxien.—The substance of the descriptive part of this paper was inserted by myself in the Medical and Physical Journal, for March 1804, vol. xi. p. 250, with an engraving of the Herpes zoster.

termed *Bullæ,* discharge a watery fluid when they break ; and the excoriated surface sometimes becomes covered with a flat, yellowish or blackish scab, which remains till a new cuticle is formed underneath ; and sometimes is converted into an ulcer, that does not readily heal.

For the reasons previously stated, Erysipelas has been removed from this order into that of the Exanthemata.

The genera of Bullæ are

1. *Pemphigus.*
2. *Pompholyx.*

———

Genus 1. PEMPHIGUS.

Syn. Pemphigus (*Auct. var.*) : Pemphigus major (*Sauv.*) : Morta (*Lin.*) : Febris bullosa (*Vog. Selliger*) : Typhus vesicularis (*Young*) : der Blasenausschlag (*German*) : Dartre phlycténoide, Fièvre vesiculaire ou bulleuse (*Fr.*) *Vesicular Fever.*

Def. AN ERUPTION OF TRANSPARENT VESICLES, ABOUT THE SIZE OF A FILBERT, WITH A RED, INFLAMED EDGE, BUT WITHOUT SURROUNDING BLUSH OR TUMEFACTION, CONTAINING A PELLUCID FLUID ; ON BREAKING DISPOSED TO ULCERATE.

There is probably no such fever as that which has been described by a few continental physicians, under the titles of *Febris vesicularis, ampullosa,* or *bullosa,* and to which Sauvages applied the term

Pemphigus.* Subsequent nosologists have given definitions of the disease, upon the same authority, as an idiopathic, contagious, and malignant fever, in the course of which phlyctænæ or vesications, of the size of a filbert, with an inflamed base, appear in succession on different parts of the surface of the body, and sometimes in the mouth.† But Dr. Cullen justly expressed his doubts of the accuracy of the original writers. The case related by Seliger ‡, on which Sauvages founds his first species, Pemphigus major, is worthy of little attention, and was perhaps, as Dr. Willan suggests, a case of Erysipelas, with some incidental variation. The account of the epidemic at Prague, mentioned by Thierry §, which is the prototype of the Pemphigus castrensis (spec. 2.) of Sauvages, is not entitled to credit, as Dr. Cullen remarks, in some of its circumstances: the bullæ are supposed by Dr. Willan to have been symptomatic of severe typhus, or of pestilential fever, in the same manner as Dr. Hodges described those appearances in the plague of 1666, and as they are occasionally seen, inter-

---

* From πεμφιξ, bulla, phlyctæna. See his Nosol. Method. class iii. gen. 3.

† Dr. Cullen defines Pemphigus, " Typhus contagiosa; primo, secundo, vel tertio morbi die, in variis partibus vesiculæ, avellanæ magnitudine, per plures dies manentes, tandem ichorem tenuem fundentes." Nosol. Meth. gen. xxxiv. — Linnæus, who has designated the disease by the barbarous term Morta, characterizes it as " Febris diaria, malignissima, funestissima." Gen. Morbor. class. i. gen. 1.

‡ See Ephem. Acad. Nat. Cur. dec. i. ann. viii. obs. 56.—Also Delius, Amœnit. Medicæ, referred to by Sauvages.

§ See his Médecine Expérimentale, p. 134. Par. 1755.

mixed with petechiæ and vibices, or with patches,
of Erythema *fugax* in typhoid fevers.   Again, as
to the Pemphigus Helveticus (spec. 3.) of Sauvages, which is borrowed from the description of
Dr. Langhans *, Dr. Cullen is of opinion that the
disease was the Cynanche maligna; and Dr. Frank
viewed it in the same light, referring it to Scarlatina
anginosa.†   Dr. Willan, who points out the unsatisfactory nature of the history given by Langhans,
independently of the contradictions which it contains, proposes a query, whether the disease was
not rather *endemic*, than epidemic or contagious,
and referable to some local cause, like the *Ergot*,
Mal des Ardens, &c. before alluded to?

In a word, this conclusion seems to be deducible
from an examination of these slight and imperfect
histories of the subject, that the notion of an idiopathic contagious fever, terminating in a critical
eruption of bullæ, has been founded in error.   All
the cases of phlyctænæ, which have been related by
authors, are therefore referable either to typhoid
fevers, malignant dysentery, &c. in which they are

---

* In the Acta Helvetica, vol. ii. p. 260.

† " Quem *Helveticum* alii dixerunt Pemphigum, hic ad *Scarlatinæ* speciem *ulcerosæ* pertinere videtur." Lib. iii. p. 263.   Dr. Frank himself,
however, is the author of a singular confusion in regard to the genus
Pemphigus. He divides it into two species; the first of which, P. *am-
plior*, includes the eruptions of bullæ, which he deems in all cases *symptomatic* of gastric or nervous fevers, or of a chronic nature, without any
fever : and the second, P. *variolodes*, which is the chicken-pox; and
which he again subdivides into *vesicularis* (the true chicken or swine-
pox), and *solidescens* (the acuminated, warty, dry hornpock), which is,
in fact, smallpox.

accidental and symptomatic * ; or to the following genus, Pompholyx, in which they are unconnected with fever. " Notwithstanding the authorities which Dr. Bateman has brought forward to negative the existence of *Pemphigus*, I cannot help agreeing with those who take the opposite side of the question, having some years since been fortunate enough to meet with a case of it in a boy of fourteen years of age. The eruption appeared in successive crops, and was accompanied with fever not of a typhoid type. None of the vesicles exceeded the size of a filbert."

Dr. Willan mentions a Pemphigus *infantilis*, of which he had seen a few cases in infants, generally soon after birth, and which he considered as analogous to the Erysipelas, which occurs at the same period, and as originating from the same causes. It commonly affected weak and emaciated infants, with a dry shriveled skin, and proved fatal in a few days, from the complicated distress arising from pain, loss of sleep, and violent fever. The vesications, which were at first small and transparent, became large, oblong, and of a purplish hue, and finally turbid, and were surrounded by a livid red border. After breaking, they left ulcerations, which spread beyond their original limits, and became extremely painful.† " Gentle purga-

* Such was the Pemphigus Indicus (spec. 4.) of Sauvages, taken from a single case mentioned by Bontius. — The swine-pox, however, seems to have been described by mistake under the title of Pemphigus, by Mr. R. B. Blagden, in the Med. Facts and Observations, vol. i. p. 205.

† Consistently with the opinion that all these bullæ are symptomatic,

tives, with Bark, are the remedies which have been
found most beneficial in this affection."

Books which may be consulted on Pemphigus.

Braune, Versuch über den Pemphigus und das Blasen fieber, 1795.
Bunnel, Dissertation sur le Pemphigus, 4to. Paris, 1811.
Dickson, Trans. of the Roy. Irish Academy, 1787.
Gaitskell, Mem. of the Med. Society of London, vol. iv.
Giljbert, Monographie du Pemphigus, 8vo. Paris, 1813.
Hall, Duncan's Annals of Medicine, 1799.
Rayer, des Maladies de la Peau, Paris, 1827.
Wichmann, Boitrag zur kenntniss des Pemphigus, Erfurt, 1791.
Wilson on Febrile Diseases, vol. ii. 8vo. 1800.

Genus II. POMPHOLYX.

Syn. Πομφολυξ (*Auct. Græc.*): Pemphigus sine
pyrexia (*Sauv.*): Pemphigus apyretus (*Plenck.*):
Dartre phlyctenoïde confluente—Herpes phlycte-
noïdes confluens (*Alibert*): Ecphlysis Pompholyx (*Good*): Wassenblasen (*G.*): Ahenje (*Arab.*)
Water blebs.

Def. An eruption of bullæ, or blebs, "without any inflammation round them, and without
fever," breaking and healing without scale
or crust.

---

and that the existence of a peculiar eruptive fever, characterized by such
vesications, is imaginary, this infantile disease should, I conceive, have
been referred to Pompholyx, since it appears to differ from the Pompholyx benignus of infants, only in being connected with a severe and
fatal marasmus, instead of the irritation of dentition.

Dr. Willan has described three species of Pompholyx * :

1. P. *benignus.*   2. P. *diutinus.*
3. P. *solitarius.*

SPECIES 1. POMPHOLYX *benignus*, MILD WATER BLEBS.

This species exhibits a succession of transparent bullæ, about the size of a pea, or sometimes of a hazel-nut, which break in three or four days, discharge their lymph, and soon heal. They appear chiefly on the face, neck, and extremities; and occur in boys in hot weather, in infants during dentition, and in young persons of irritable habit from eating acrid vegetable substances, or from swallowing a few grains of mercury. " This appears to be the disease which Dr. Underwood has described under the title Phlyctænæ. He says it occurs during dentition, and sometimes in new-born infants, and always appears to be beneficial: ' it consists of vesications or blisters, of different sizes, resembling little scalds or burns, and continues for several days. They come out in different parts, but chiefly on the belly, ribs, and thighs; and contain a sharp lymph, which it may be pru-

* Foësius observes (Œconon. Hippoc. ad voc. πομφοι) that Hippocrates uses that word to denote wheals, or those eminences which resemble the eruption produced by nettles (lib. ii. Περι Παθων), and that πομφολυγες are bubbles of air, which appear upon water: but that Galen explains the *pomphi*, as eminences of the cuticle, containing a fluid; in Exegesi, lib. ii. de Mulier. — See also Gorræus, Def. Med.

dent to let out by a puncture.' No medicine is necessary but such as the particular state of the bowels may call for."

SPECIES 2. POMPHOLYX. *diutinus*, LINGERING or CHRONIC WATER BLEBS.

Syn. Le Pemphigus chronique (*Rayer*).

(Plate XXXIII. of BATEMAN; Pl. 14. of THE ATLAS). This is a tedious and painful disorder, and is usually preceded for some weeks by languor and lassitude, headach, sickness, and pains in the limbs. Numerous, red, pimple-like elevations of the cuticle appear, with a sensation of tingling. These are presently raised into transparent vesications, that become as large as a pea within twenty-four hours, and, if not broken, afterwards attain the size of a walnut. If they are rubbed off prematurely, the excoriated surface is sore and inflamed, and does not readily heal. The bullæ continue to arise in succession on different parts of the body, and even re-appear on the parts first affected, in some cases for several weeks, so that the whole number of bullæ is very great; and when the excoriations are thus multiplied, a slight febrile paroxysm occurs every night, and the patient suffers much from the irritation, and from want of sleep.

This disease chiefly affects persons of debilitated habits, and is very severe in the aged. It seems to originate under different conditions of the body, but often after continued fatigue and anxiety, with low diet; sometimes from intemperance; and not unfrequently it is connected with anasarca, or general dropsy, scurvy, Purpura, and other states of the constitution, in which the powers of the cutaneous circulation are feeble. It has, in some instances, appeared after profuse sweating, during which cold liquors were copiously swallowed, in common with several other forms of chronic cutaneous disease. In the fevers in which it has been observed, it was obviously symptomatic; for it has not only occurred at various periods, and varied much in its duration, but has accompanied fevers of the continued, remittent, and intermittent type, as well as arthritic, and other secondary fevers. *

It is sufficiently clear, from the statements of the writers just referred to, that the Pompholyx is never communicated by contagion—" indeed, when lymph was taken from a vesicle, and introduced by inoculation into the system of another individual, no disease followed. The fluid contained in the vesicles is not ichorous, but a bland

* Many cases illustrative of these observations are on record; especially those related, under the appellation of Pemphigus, by Mr. Gaitskell, and Mr. Upton, in the Memoirs of the Medical Society of London, vol. iv. art. i. and vol. iii. appendix; by Mr. Christie, in the Lond. Med. Journal, vol. x. p. 385 (for 1789); by Dr. Stewart, in the Edin. Med. Commentaries, vol. vi. art. 3. p. 79; by Dr. Hall, in the Annals of Med. vol. iii. art. ix.; by Mr. Ring, in the Lond. Med. Journ. xi. p. 235; by Dr. Dickson, in the Trans. of the Royal Irish Academy for 1787, and Lond. Med. J. vol. ix. p. 309; and by Bang, in the Acta Reg. Soc. Med. Hauniensis, vol. i. p. 8, &c. See also Frank, de Curand. Hom. Morbis, lib. iii. p. 263. Sennert. de Scorbuto, cap. v. § 59.

lymph *, resembling that which is poured into the ventricles of the brain in hydrocephalus. In several of the persons, whose cases are recorded, the disease occurred more than once. The Pompholyx is most troublesome and obstinate in old persons, in whom the transparent bullæ sometimes equal the size of a turkey's egg, while others of a smaller size are intermixed with them, which appear dark and livid. When broken, they leave a black excoriated surface, which sometimes ulcerates. "The first-mentioned form of this disease is seldom severe, and never fatal, unless complicated with some internal inflammation: but the second, the *diutinus*, is often followed by severe ulcerations, which, in the aged, are not devoid of danger."

The warm bath, used every second day, was considered by Dr. Willan as the most active palliative, and the best remedy. I think I have seen the decoction of Cinchona, with cordials and diuretics, of considerable advantage in these cases, especially when the eruption was combined with anasarca. In young persons, in whom the Pompholyx is seldom severe, these remedies are affirmed by Dr. Willan to be successful within two or three weeks; but the warm bath seems to increase both the tingling in the skin, and the number of the vesications, in these patients.† "In the benign form

* Mr. Gaitskell not only proved this by analysis; but also ascertained the uncontagious nature of the fluid, by inoculating himself with it with perfect impunity.

† The warm bath sometimes aggravates the disease, even in the aged;

of the disease little is required from the physician: diluents, or vegetable cooling diet and mild purgatives, constitute the whole of the treatment. When accompanied with inflammation of the mucous membrane, the necessary remedies to relieve this are to be prescribed without any reference to the cutaneous eruption. The excoriations which follow the rupture of the vesicles are to be dressed with any mild ointment, and if troublesome, to be touched with the nitrate of silver. In the more severe form of the disease, the warm bath proves often highly beneficial; but it must not be too long continued; never to produce fainting. If there is internal inflammation, the antiphlogistic treatment is to be pushed to its utmost length. Narcotics are also useful; but the preparations of these ought not to contain either wine or alcohol. In old persons, and those of a delicate habit, acidulated decoction of Cinchona Bark, or the Sulphate of Quinia, if not forbidden by intestinal irritation, are necessary for maintaining the tone of the habit. Purgatives are always injurious in the chronic form of Pompholyx."

SPECIES 3. The POMPHOLYX *solitarius* is a rare form of the disease, which seems to affect only

---

as I lately had an opportunity of witnessing in an old lady of 80. In this case, however, the *bullæ*, of which eight or ten arose daily for several months, were surrounded by an extensive erythematous inflammation, and there was a considerable tendency to the febrile state. A single immersion in the warm bath excited a violent fever; and Bark, Sarsaparilla, and other tonics, produced a similar effect. She ultimately recovered, under a light and refrigerant diet and regimen.

women. One large vesication usually appears in
the night, after a sensation of tingling in the skin,
and rapidly distends itself so as to contain sometimes a tea-cupful of lymph, " and closely resembles the effect produced by a blistering plaster."
Within forty-eight hours it breaks, discharging its
fluid, and leaving a superficial ulceration. Near
this another bulla arises in a day or two, and goes
through the same course; and it is sometimes followed, in like manner, by two or three others in
succession; so that the whole duration shall be
eight or ten days. Cinchona, with the diluted
Sulphuric Acid, internally, and linseed poultices,
followed by light dressings to the sores externally,
were employed with advantage in three cases seen
by Dr. Willan.

*Books which may be consulted on Pompholyx.**

ACTA Reg. Soc. Med. Hauniensis, vol. i.
ANNALS of Medicine, vol. iii.
BUNEL, Dissertation sur le Pemphigus, 4to. 1811.
EDIN. Med. Commentaries, vol. vi.
FRANK de Curand. Hom. Morb. lib. iii.
GILIBERT, Monographie du Pemphigus, 8vo. 1813.
LONDON Med. Journ. vol. ix. x. xi.
LONDON Med. Repository, vol. ii. vi.
MEM. of the Med. Society of London, vol. iii. iv.
PLUMBE's Practical Treatise on Diseases of the Skin, 2d edit. 1827.
RAYER, Traité des Maladies de la Peau, 8vo. 1826.
TRANS. of the Roy. Irish Acad. 1787.
WICHMANN, Boitrag zur kenntnis des Pemphigus, 1791.
WILLAN on Cutaneous Diseases.

* In most of the works referred to, the disease is termed Pemphigus.

Order V.

PUSTULÆ.

PUSTULES.

SYN. Φλυκταιναι (*Auct. Græc.*): Pustulæ (*Linn. Sag.*): Pustules, Boutons (*F.*): die Eiterblattern (*German*).

Def. (PUSTULE): AN·ELEVATION OF THE CU-TICLE, WITH AN INFLAMED BASE CONTAINING PUS.

There are four varieties of pustules.

a. Phlyzacium; a·pustule commonly of a large size, raised on a·hard circular base, of a vivid red colour, and succeeded by a thick, hard, dark-coloured scab. *

b. Psydracium; a small pustule, often irregularly circumscribed, producing but a slight elevation of the cuticle, and terminating in a laminated scab. †

---

* The derivation of this term, " απο του φλυω, φλυζω, sive φλυσσω, quod *fervere* significat, et *ebullire*," (Gorræi Def. Med.) would render it sufficiently appropriate to elevated and inflamed pustules, if we had not possessed also the interpretation left by Celsus : " φλυζακιον autem paulo durior pustula est, subalbida, acuta; ex qua quod exprimitur, humidum est. Ex pustulis vero nonnunquam etiam ulcuscula fiunt, aut aridiora, aut humidiora : et modo tantum cum prurigine, modo etiam cum in-flammatione aut dolore; exitque aut pus, aut sanies, aut utrumque. Maximeque id evenit in ætate puerili : raro in medio corpore; sæpe in eminentibus partibus." (De Medicina, lib. v. cap. 28. § 15.)

† As the *Phlyzacia* were denominated from the heat of the eruption, so the *Psydracia* received their appellation from the opposite quality, " quasi ψυκρα υδρακια, id est, *frigidæ* seu frigefactæ *guttulæ*," says Gor-ræus. — The psydracia are enumerated among the eruptions peculiar to

Many of the psydracia usually appear together, and become confluent; and, after the discharge of pus, they pour out a thin watery humour, which frequently forms an irregular incrustation.

c. Achor; and

d. Favus. These two pustules are considered by the majority of writers from the Greeks downwards, as varieties of the same genus, differing chiefly in magnitude.* The *Achor* may be defined, a small acuminated pustule, containing a straw-coloured matter, which has the appearance and nearly the consistence of strained honey, and succeeded by a thin brown or yellowish scab. The *Favus,* or κηριον, is larger than the *achor,* flatter, and not acuminated, and contains a more viscid matter; its base, which is often irregular, is slightly inflamed; and it is succeeded by a yellow, semitransparent, and sometimes cellular scab, like a honeycomb; whence it has obtained its name.

Pustules† originate from an inflammation of the skin, and the consequent partial effusion of puru-

---

the head by Alexander and Paul, and some other Greek writers; but Galen and others mention them as common to other parts of the body (See Alex. Trall. Op. lib. i. cap. 5. Paul. Ægin. lib. iii. cap. 1. Actuarius, lib. vi. cap. 2.) See also Impetigo, below, p. 145.

* See Aëtius, tetrab. ii. serm. ii. cap. 68. — Alex. Trall. lib. i. cap. 8 & 9. — Paul Ægin. de Re Med. lib. iii. cap. 3. — Oribas. de Loc. Affect. lib. iv. cap. 12.

† Although it seems obvious, that the origin of this term was deduced from the *purulent* contents of the eruption (quasi, *pus tulit*); yet the best ancient authority sanctions the common indefinite and unlimited use of it. For Celsus applies it to every *elevation* of the cuticle, including

lent matter under the cuticle, by which the latter is elevated into small circumscribed tumours. Sometimes several of these elevations arise upon a common inflamed surface; but most frequently the inflammation of the base of each is distinct and circumscribed. The fluid contained in them desiccates, and often terminates in a scabby incrustation, varying in hardness according to the various tenacity of the contained fluid: sometimes in superficial ulceration. " Rayer justly remarks, that the number, form, and aspect of the pustulous ulcerations, of the tubercles which succeed them, and even of the cicatrices, should be attentively studied, as they are often characteristic of the genera." The five genera of pustular diseases, comprehended in this order, have nothing in common in their character, except the appearance of pustules in some state of their progress; for some are contagious, and others not; some are acute, and others chronic. These genera are,

1. Impetigo.   4. Variola.

2. Porrigo.   5. Scabies.

3. Ecthyma.

---

even wheals and papulæ, "quæ ex urtica, vel ex sudore nascuntur;" and he deems it synonymous with εξανθημα of the Greeks, which was in fact the general term for every species of *eruption*. (Celsus de Med. lib. v. cap. 28. § 15.) — The Greek physicians appear to have comprehended both pustules and vesicles under the term φλυκταιναι, which their translators have rendered by the word *pustulæ*; and in this double sense the latter has also been generally used. Some discriminating writers, however, have correctly appropriated it to suppurating eruptions. "Pustularum nimirum conditio," says Prof. Arnemann, "exigit, ut in apice *suppurentur* vel in *pus* abeant." Commentar. de Aphthis, Gött. 1787. § 2. See also Linn. Gen. Morb. class xi. ord. 4. — Sagar, class i. ord. 2.

Genus I. IMPETIGO.

Syn. Lepra Squammosa(*Auctorum*): Ecpyesis Impetigo (*Good*) : Phlysis Impetigo (*Young*): Herez (*Arab.*): Courap (*Hindos.*): der Kleienausatz (*G.*): Dartre crustacée, Lepre humide (*F.*): *Humid* or *Running Tetter*, or *Scall.*

Def. An eruption of yellow, itching pustules appearing in clusters ; and terminating in a yellow, thin, scaly crust.

This eruption is characterised by the appearance of the small pustules, denominated *Psydracia.* It is not accompanied by fever, is not contagious, nor communicable by inoculation. It chiefly occurs on the extremities, although sometimes on the face. It appears under the five following forms* :

1. I. *figurata.*   4. I. *scabida.*
2. I. *sparsa.*   5. I. *rodens.*
3. I. *erysipelatodes.*

Species 1. Impetigo *figurata*, Figured or Herpetic Scall.

Syn. Ecpyesis Herpetica (*Good*): Herpes (*Cullen*): Phlyctæna (*Vog.*).

This species (Plate XXXIV. of Bateman ; Pl. 15. of The Atlas,) is the most common variety of the moist tetter. " It generally attacks the young,

---

* Celsus has described four species of Impetigo, the first of which is a pustular disease, terminating in excoriation, and corresponds with the affection described in the text. His other varieties seem to include some of the more violent forms of Psoriasis, or Lepra. See the 28th chapter of his 5th book, § 17.

The ulcerated Psora (ψωρα ἑλκωδης) of the Greeks was apparently the same affection with the Impetigo of Celsus.

and those of what is termed a lymphatic temperament; but is rarely preceded by symptoms of fever, or general derangement of the habit. It is more commonly situated on the face, as the cheeks, the upper lip, the sides of the nostrils, than on other parts of the body: but it occasionally occurs on the extremities." It appears in circumscribed patches, of various figure and magnitude, which are usually small and circular on the upper, and large, oval, and irregular on the lower extremities. The patches consist at first of clusters of the yellow psydracious pustules, set close together, and surrounded by a slight inflammatory border; the whole being somewhat raised, but the pustules not very prominent nor acuminated. In a few days the pustules break, and discharge their fluid; the surface becomes red and excoriated, shining as if it were stretched, but exhibiting numerous minute pores, from which a considerable ichorous discharge is poured out, accompanied with much troublesome itching, heat, and smarting. The discharge soon concretes partially into thin yellowish or greenish scabs; but it still continues to ooze from under the scab, which it forms. In the course of three or four weeks, as the quantity of the discharge diminishes, the scabs dry and fall off, leaving the surface of the cuticle red, rough, and somewhat thickened, and at the same time extremely brittle, and liable to crack and to be excoriated; so that the ichorous discharge and scabbing are easily reproduced, and the disease is

P

often thus much prolonged in its duration. Occasionally fresh crops of the psydracious pustules re-appear, as at the commencement; and the whole course of the eruption is repeated.

When the Impetigo figurata is beginning to heal, the patches undergo a process somewhat similar to that which takes place in the Lepra vulgaris. The amendment commences at the centre of the patch, which first subsides, leaving the border elevated: at length this also disappears; but the cuticle, which was the seat of the patch, remains for some weeks red, shining, and tender.

But though this is the most usual and regular, it is by no means the uniform progress of Impetigo. For this eruption, like Scabies and Eczema, varies so much in its phænomena, as almost to bid defiance to arrangement. Sometimes the patches enlarge by the formation of successive pustular margins; an exterior circle of pustules arising, while the preceding border is drying, to be followed by others which go through the same course, until the patch attains a considerable extent. The area, in the mean time, becomes dry and rough, with a scaly or scabby incrustation in its centre.* Sometimes

---

* This impetiginous *ring-worm* bears a considerable resemblance to the Herpes circinatus, which spreads by a succession of *vesicular* borders. A severe form of this tetter occurs in hot climates, according to the testimony of physicians who have practised there. See Hilary on the Diseases of Barbadoes, p. 352. (2d edit.)—Towne on the same, chap. 8.—Winterbottom's Account of Sierra Leone, vol. ii. chap. 9.— Probably it is this form of Impetigo, which Bontius mentions, as a most distressing disease in India, where it is called by the natives *Courap.* (De Med. Indorum, cap. 17.)

the papulæ of the Lichen agrius become pustular, or are intermixed with psydracia, as before mentioned, and the disease assumes all the characters of Impetigo.

But the affinity of Impetigo with the vesicular diseases is manifested by a common variety of it, in the upper extremities, in which the psydracious pustules are intermixed with transparent vesicles, resembling the pustules in size and form. Where this intermixture occurs, the disease is much more troublesome, from the extreme irritation, itching, smarting, and heat, which accompany it; and much more tedious and difficult of cure. It takes place chiefly on the hand, about the knuckles and sides of the fingers, or on the wrist; and the space between the metacarpal bones of the fore-finger and thumb is usually the seat of one of the blotches. The vesicles are slower in their progress than the psydracia: they remain many days transparent, but not much elevated, the cuticle over them being thick in that situation. — When they break, an acrid ichor is discharged, which produces inflamed points where it touches the cuticle, and these become vesicles or psydracia. Each vesicle, thus broken, is not disposed to heal; but the cuticle round its base now becomes inflamed and raised, and discharges a thin ichor, when in any degree irritated. The vesicles appear, in slow succession, at a little distance from each other and from the pustules; and at length an irregular blotch is produced, of a red, chopped, and thickened cuticle, interspersed with the rising eruptions, little humid ulcers, and chops or fissures. * The sense of burning and intense itching, accompanying especially the first rise of the vesicles, is extremely distressing, and is much aggravated by the irritation of almost every application that is resorted to.

SPECIES 2. IMPETIGO *sparsa*, SCATTERED RUNNING SCALL.

Syn. Ecphyesis sparsa (*Good*).

This species (Plate XXXV. of BATEMAN; Pl. 15. of THE ATLAS,) differs from the preceding rather in the *form*, than in the nature and progress of the eruption: for, with the exception of the indeterminate distribution of the pustules, which are not congregated in circumscribed clusters, but dis-

---

* This mixed form of the disease has misled the generality of writers to confound it with Herpes, under which term it is commonly described. Such is the Herpes of Dr. Cullen. " Phlyctænæ, vel ulcuscula plurima, gregalia, serpentia, dysepuleta." Nosol. gen. 147. And Prof. Callisen's brief description of Herpes, in one of its varieties, is an accurate delineation of this Impetigo. " Herpes *pustulosus, crustosus, serpigo*, quem constituunt papulæ pejores corrosivæ, quæ congestæ aream circularem constituunt, acutè pungentem, valdè pruriginosam, deinde pars illa tegitur crusta cuti firmiter adglutinata, à transudatione humoris tenuis et acris è cute porosa; ichor, si' tangit alias partes, istas simili malo defædat, unde late serpere solet hoc malum, tamen absque exulceratione." (Chirurg. Hodiern. § 612.) See also Wiseman's Chirurg. Treatises, i. chap. 17. on Herpes. Turner on the Dis. of the Skin, chap. v. where Herpes and Tetter are used as synonymous terms.— But it is to be recollected, that, in this arrangement, Herpes is appropriated to a purely vesicular disease, which has a short and nearly uniform course of ten or twelve days, the vesicles of each patch becoming confluent, and at length covered with a dry crust. Of this genus, the shingles afford the most characteristic example.

persed without any regular order along the extremities, and sometimes about the neck and shoulders, and even on the face, ears, and scalp, the foregoing description is applicable to both species of the disorder. The Impetigo sparsa more frequently occurs in the lower extremities, than the former; and is, in that situation, more troublesome and obstinate. In elderly people, especially of debilitated habits, the excoriations are liable to pass into deep, irregular ulcers, surrounded by a purplish colour, and often accompanied with œdema.

These two forms of Impetigo are not always traced to any obvious exciting cause: but they are frequently preceded by some derangement of the digestive organs, languor, and headach. A predisposition to the disease appears to be connected with the sanguine temperament, with a thin soft skin, and a relaxed and bloated habit of body; or with the sanguineo-melancholic temperament, a spare form, and a thin but harsh skin. Certain seasons appear to have great influence on the disease, in those who are predisposed to it. " Certain kinds of diet also, as salt and especially tainted food." The I. sparsa, especially on the lower extremities, is apt to return with regularity at the latter end of autumn, and to harass the patient during the whole of the winter, but disappears in the warm weather: while the I. figurata, affecting the upper extremities, is liable to recur in the spring; of both

which I have witnessed several examples.* The
accession of the eruption has, in other instances,
been ascribed to violent exercise, intemperance,
cold, and sudden depressing passions, especially
fear and grief. †

The I. sparsa is not unfrequent in young children, in whom it appears to be a sequela of the
Porrigo larvalis; if indeed it be not the same
disease, as I have above hinted. The disease in
these young subjects, fixes itself particularly in the
flexures of the large joints, and is accompanied
with intense itching, which greatly disturbs the
rest. It recurs frequently under every irritation,
as from dentition, &c., sometimes, even till after the
second dentition is completed, or till near the
period of puberty; after which the predisposition
to its attacks ceases.

---

* In this and some of the preceding circumstances, the accuracy of
the brief description of Celsus is manifest. The first form of Impetigo
is that, " quæ similitudine scabiem repræsentat; nam et rubet, et durior est, et exulcerata est, et rodit. Distat autem ab ea, quæ magis exulcerata est, et varis similes pustulas habet, videnturque esse in ea quasi
bullulæ quædam, ex quibus interpositio tempore quasi squamulæ
solvuntur; certioribusque hæc temporibus revertitur."

† In two gentlemen, whom I lately had occasion to see, affected with
Impetigo, the eruption was imputed to great alarm and agitation of
mind. Some of the scaly eruptions also are now and then referred to
fear and grief, as well as the tubercular Elephantiasis. See Dr. Tho.
Heberden's remarks on the Elephantiasis in Madeira (Med. Trans. vol. i.
art. 2.); and those of Dr. Joannis on that of Martigues (Med. Obs. and
Inquir. vol. i. art. 19.) Some time ago we witnessed the extraordinary
influence of mental alarm on the cutaneous circulation, in a poor woman, who became a patient of the Public Dispensary. A sudden universal anasarca followed, in one night, the shock occasioned by the loss
of a small sum of money, which was all she possessed. (See Edinb.
Med. and Surg. Journal, vol. v. p. 127.

Local Tetters are produced by the action of particular irritants on the cuticle, which soon disappear, when the source of irritation is withdrawn. The affection of the hands and fingers, in those who work among sugar, which is called the *grocer's itch*, is of this nature; and similar eruptions are produced on the hands of bricklayers, by the acrid stimulus of lime. It is worthy of remark, that both the grocer's and the *bricklayer's itch* is, in some individuals, a pustular, and in others a vesicular eruption, referable to the Eczema; but in neither case contagious, as the popular appellation might lead us to suppose.

Local pustular patches are also the result of the application of the Tartrate of Antimony to the skin by friction, and in some cases of the application of blisters, and other stimulating plasters. These pustules are liable to extend considerably beyond the blistered or stimulated part, and sometimes continue to arise in succession for a fortnight or more; and many of them often assume the form of Phlyzacia (Def. 5. *a*), or of large, protuberant pustules, with a hard, elevated, and inflamed base. Some of these even acquire the size of small boils, and suppurate deeply and slowly, with great pain, and considerable restlessness and feverish heat in the night.

The Impetigo figurata and sparsa are sometimes confounded with two contagious diseases, of the pustular order, Porrigo and Scabies. The appellation of *ring-worm*, which is popularly given to the oval or circular patches of the first, has partly contributed to occasion this mistake. They differ, however, from the contagious circles of Porrigo, inasmuch as the I. figurata seldom affects children, — occurs principally on the extremities, — and they do not continue to discharge a purulent and glutinous, but, after the first eruption, an ichorous humour, — nor do they form the thick, soft, and copious scabs of Porrigo: not to mention the absence of contagion.

The prevalence of transparent vesicles in the patches of Impetigo, may mislead an incautious or inexperienced observer into a suspicion that the disease is Scabies: but the distribution of the eruption in patches, — the copious exudation of ichor, — the rough, reddened, and fissured cuticle, — the magnitude and slow progress of the vesicles, and the heat and smarting, which accompany the itching in Impetigo, will serve in general to determine the diagnosis. In the strictly purulent form of Scabies, the pustules about the hands arise to a much greater magnitude and elevation, than the psydracia; they are filled with a thick yellow pus, and are more considerably inflamed round their base.

The Impetigo in its advanced stage is, however, more liable to be mistaken by common observers, and is, in fact, daily mistaken for Psoriasis or Lepra; as a sufficient discrimination is not made between the laminated and scale-like concretions of the ichorous matter, and the exfoliations of morbid cuticle, which constitute the true *scab*. But the scaly diseases emit no fluid, and the very existence of a discharge, however slight, is sufficient to determine the diagnosis of the eruption.

In the incipient state of these two forms of Impetigo, it is useful to administer Sulphur internally, in such quantities as not to induce purging; and, if there is much irritability or inflammation of the cuticle, a portion of Soda, Nitre, or Crystals of Tartar, with which Conium, and Acids, as that of Lemons, Limes, or Barberries, may be advantageously combined. The Impetigo sparsa commonly yields to these medicines, particularly if diligent ablution with tepid water be at the same time employed. But when the disease is of long standing, it requires a treatment somewhat similar to that recommended for inveterate Psoriasis; namely, the diet drinks, decoctions of Sarsaparilla and Cinchona, with the fixed Alkalies and Antimonials. The mercurial alteratives, however, in this affection are of essential assistance to this plan of cure; such as small doses of Cinnabar, the Hydrargyrus cum Creta, or the pill of Dr. Plummer. "In those cases which have come under my care, I have seen more benefit from the occasional administration of from gr. v to gr. viij of Submuriate of Mercury, at bedtime, and a brisk cathartic on the following morning, than from a continued course of alteratives."

The external applications adapted to these forms of Impetigo, especially to the figured species, are the mild desiccative ointments; for, in the majority of cases, the irritable surface of the tetter will not bear stimulants with impunity. When the discharge is considerable, the ointments prepared with the Oxide of Zinc, alone, or united with Saturnine Ointment, or with the white precipitated Oxide of Mercury, are the most efficacious, in allaying the inflammatory condition of the excoriated surface, and in reducing the quantity of the discharge. When there is less of this irritability and exudation, the Tar Ointment most effectually relieves the itching; the ointment of the Nitrate of Mercury, diluted with five or six parts of simple ointment, will also be beneficial. From the too active employment of this ointment, and still more of that of the Nitric Oxide of Mercury, and various other stimulant lotions and applications, by practitioners unacquainted with the character of the disorder, a great aggravation of the eruption and of the sufferings of the patient is sometimes occasioned. *

In some instances, indeed, the skin, under this impetiginous affection, is peculiarly sensible to the stimulus of Mercury, whether employed internally or externally. I think I have observed this circumstance most frequently in a few cases which were the sequelæ of Lichen. But the most irritable of all the varieties of Impetigo are those in which vesicles abound; in some of which the Zinc, and saturnine applications, and even simple lard, occasion an aggravation of the symptoms. In these

---

* Formerly a lotion made by macerating the root of the Water Dock (Lapathum) in vinegar was much employed. T.

cases, it is particularly necessary to keep the parts
covered, with a view to avoid the effects of friction
from the clothes, as well as of heat, and of cold;
to wash the surface daily with some emollient fluid,
such as milk and water, or an infusion of bran; to
interdict the use of soap; and to besmear the parts
with cream, or an emulsion of almonds. A lotion
prepared by boiling Mallow, Digitalis, and Poppy-
heads has been found serviceable, where the parts
are very painful. In many cases, however, the
stiffness, which ensues upon the speedy drying of
these lotions, renders it impossible to use them,
and it is necessary to cover the part lightly with
dry lint only, or to interpose between it and the
diseased surface a sprinkling of the Oxide of Zinc:
sometimes, however, the application of linen dipped
in melted suet affords relief, when no other greasy
substance can be used. "The editor was induced,
some years since, to apply the Hydrocyanic Acid in
the form of lotion in Impetigo, and found that it
allayed the irritation more effectually than any
other means. It has since been very generally
employed for this purpose. The following is the
formula which he originally used:

R. Acidi Hydrocyanici f℥iv,
    Aquæ distillatæ f℥vij,
    Alcoholis f℥iv;
Misce ut fiat lotio.

"He has, however, lately found, that the efficacy
of this application is greatly increased by the
addition of sixteen grains of the Acetate of Lead.
This lotion not only soothes the irritability of the

part, but also disposes the skin to take on its healthy action. Mr. Plumbe cautions against the external employment of Hydrocyanic Acid, and mentions that in two cases, of both legs, in which the eruption extended from the ancle to the knee, where it was employed, a considerable intermission of the pulse took place, which ceased on its being discontinued. In my experience of the external use of Hydrocyanic Acid, I have seen no bad effects result from it."

In the drier and less irritable forms of the Impetigo, the use of the waters of Harrowgate is the most effectual remedy, and likewise the best preventive of its returns : under the same circumstances, the warm sea-water bath, followed by a course of bathing in the open sea, is productive of great benefit. But during the existence of any actual inflammation, the irritation of salt-water is decidedly injurious. " Nothing in the form of bath is so successful as the Sulphur Vapour Bath."

SPECIES 3. IMPETIGO *erysipelatodes*. ERYSIPELA-TOUS RUNNING SCALL.

Syn. Ecpyesis Erythematica (*Good.*)

This form of the disease, in its commencement, presents nearly the ordinary appearances of Erysipelas ; namely, a redness and puffy swelling of the upper part of the face, with œdema of the eyelids ; and is accompanied with slight febrile symptoms for the space of two or three days. But on a minute examination, the surface, instead of the smooth polish of Erysipelas, is found to exhibit a slight inequality, as if it were obscurely papulated; and, in a day or two, the true character of the disease is manifested, by the eruption of numerous psydracious pustules, over the inflamed and tumid skin, instead of the large irregular bullæ of Erysipelas. These pustules first appear below the eyes, but soon cover the greater part of the face, and sometimes extend to the neck and breast : they are accompanied with a distressing sense of heat, smarting, and itching. When they break, they discharge a hot and acrid fluid, which adds to the irritation and excoriation of the surface. In this painful condition the face remains for ten days or a fortnight, when the discharge begins to diminish, and to concrete into thin yellowish scabs. But on the interstices between the scabs, fresh pustules arise at intervals, with renewed heat and pain, and subsequently discharge, ulcerate, and form scabs like the former. The disease continues thus severe and troublesome for an uncertain period, from one to two or three months; and ultimately leaves the cuticle in the same dry, red, and brittle state, which remains after the other forms of Impetigo. The constitution is scarcely disturbed during the progress of this disease, and is much less disordered in the outset than in Erysipelas. Its affinity with Impetigo has been further evinced, in some cases which I have seen, by the occurrence of the other forms of the eruption on the extremities, during its course : occasionally, indeed, extending over the whole surface, a capite ad calcem.

In the commencement of the disease, purgative medicines, with the antiphlogistic regimen, afford great alleviation to the symptoms; but when the copious exudation and scabbing take place, the Cinchona in considerable doses, alone or with the Sarsaparilla, or the mineral acids, is administered with the greatest benefit. The same local treatment is requisite as in the other forms of the eruption; viz. tepid ablution, with emollient liquids; the application of the mildest ointments; and the use of sea-bathing, or of the sulphureous waters, in its decline.

SPECIES 4. IMPETIGO *scabida*, CRUSTED RUNNING SCALL.

Syn. Lepra Herpetica (*Sauvages*): Ecpyesis laminosa (*Good*).

In this more rare and severe form of the disease, (Plate XXXVI. OF BATEMAN; Plate 15. OF THE ATLAS,) one or more of the limbs becomes encased in a thick, yellowish, scabby crust, not unlike the bark of a tree, which is accompanied with a disagreeable heat and itching, and renders the motion of the affected limbs difficult and painful. This crust is the result of the concretion of an acrimonious humour, which is discharged in great abundance from numerous psydracious pustules, as they successively form, break, and ulcerate over the surface of the limb. The concretion commences about the third or fourth week, when the discharge begins to abate, and invests the whole of the arm from the elbow to the wrist, or the leg from the knee to the ancle.* After some time longer, the scabby coating is divided by large cracks or fissures, from which a thin ichor exudes, and concretes into additional layers of scabs. If any portion of the scab be removed, the excoriated surface pours out its fluid again, and fills up the space with a new concretion. In the lower extremities the disease is most severe and obstinate, is ultimately conjoined with Anasarca, and often produces severe ulceration. The incrustation sometimes extends to the fingers and toes, and destroys the nails; and, as in other similar instances, the new ones are thick, notched, and irregular.†

The I. scabida requires the same internal medicines which have been recommended for the inveterate forms of the preceding varieties, especially the sulphureous waters. The chief peculiarity of its treatment consists in clearing the surface of its incrustation, and correcting the morbid action of the superficial vessels. The thick scab can only be softened and gradually removed, by perseverance in the application of the steam of warm water to it, for a short time, daily ; or mild poultices. Those parts of the surface which are thus cleared must

* Sauvages observes that this affection is called *Dartres encroutées* by the French; but he describes it under the appellation of *Lepra* herpetica. " Cognoscitur ex herpetibus crustaceis, squamosis, albis, hyeme majoribus, et suppurantibus; noctu intolerabiliter prurientibus: brachia ambo usque ad carpum, ambo femora tibiasque usque ad pedes, quandoque tegentibus; scalptu cruentatur hæc lepra; poplites et cubiti vix flecti possunt: præcesserunt non raro tineæ malignæ." Class. x. gen. xxvii. spec. 7.

† See Lepra, above, p. 27.

be covered with soft linen, after tepid ablution, twice a day; and some of the Unguentum Zinci, or a much-diluted ointment of Nitrate of Mercury, with common cerate (containing, for example, a fourth or fifth part of the mercurial), or simply the Oxide of Zinc, or Calamine in powder, must be interposed.

SPECIES 5. IMPETIGO *rodens*, CORRODING RUNNING SCALL.

Syn. Ecpyesis Exedens (*Good*).

This is a rare but intractable species of the disease, probably of a cancerous nature, in which the cellular membrane is affected, as well as the skin, and seems to shrink away as the ulceration and discharge go on. The disorder commences with a cluster of pustules, sometimes intermixed with vesicles, which soon break, and discharge for a long period of time an acrid humour, from open pores or from under scabs; and the skin and cellular texture are slowly, but deeply and extensively, corroded, with extreme irritation and pain, which are only to be alleviated by large doses of opium. The disease commonly begins on the side of the chest or trunk of the body, and gradually extends itself. I have not seen any instance of this disease, which is said to have always terminated fatally, and to have been benefited by no medicine, either external or internal, which had been employed.

Books which may be consulted on Impetigo.

PLUMBE on Diseases of the Skin, 2d edit. 1827.
RAYER, Traité des Mal. de la Peau, 8vo. 1826.
WILLAN, Practical Treatise on Impetigo, 4to. 1814.

Genus II. PORRIGO.

Syn. Ecpyesis porrigo (*Good*): Phlysis porrigo (*Young*): Tinea (*Auct. var.*): der Kleiengrind (*German*): Netek (*Hebrew*): Teigne (*F.*): *Moist Scall.*

Def. An eruption of straw-coloured pustules; concreting into yellow or brownish crusts or cellular scabs.

Porrigo * is a contagious disease, which may occur at any period of life, although it is more common under the age of puberty. It is principally characterized, as the definition states, by an eruption of the pustules, denominated *favi* and *achores* (Def. 5. *c, d*), unaccompanied by fever.

---

* This term is adopted, as a generic appellation, nearly in the same sense in which it was used by Celsus, who included the moist and ulcerating as well as the dry and furfuraceous eruptions of the scalp, under this denomination. (De Med. lib. vi. cap. 3.) The word *Tinea* is employed in the same generic sense by Sauvages; but being a term of no authority, and probably of Arabic origin †, it is properly superseded by the classical appellation. Numerous writers, ancient and modern, have designated the varieties of the disease by distinct names; such as crusta lactea, alopecia, pityriasis, favi, achores, scabies capitis, &c.: but the most intelligent observers have pointed out the identity of the nature and causes of these various eruptions. See Sennert. de Morb. Infant. p. ii. cap. 4.; and Pract. lib. v. p. iii. § ii. cap. 4. — Heister. Chirurg. p. i. lib. v. cap. x. — Tilingius, Lilium curiosum, cap. 17. — Vogel, de cognos. et cur. Hom. Morb. class. viii. § 713. — Stoll, Rat. Med. i. 49.

---

† Si eidem auctori (Avicenna) credamus, ab humore melancholico causam accipit, cutem corrumpit atque corrodit, hæcque est *alvathim* à quo nomine barbari, ut videtur, thim et thineum et *tineam* fecerunt. *Lorry de Morb. Cutaneis,* p. 463. T.

Q

The several appearances which the disorder assumes are reducible to six specific forms.*

  1. P. *larvalis*.   4. P. *scutulata*.
  2. P. *furfurans*.   5. P. *decalvans*.
  3. P. *lupinosa*.   6. P. *favosa*.

SPECIES 1. PORRIGO *larvalis*, MILK SCALL.

Syn. Ἀχὼρ (*Auct. Græc.*): Crusta lactea (*Auct. var. Lat.*): Tinea lactea (*Sauv.*): Scabies capitis simplex (*Plenck*): Tinea benigna (*Auctorum*): Ecpyesis Porrigo, α. Crustacea (*Good*): Teigne muqueuse. Tinea muciflua (*Alibert*): die Kopfraude, der Milchgrind (*German*): Croute de Lait (*F.*): Munday Cárápāng (*Tamool*).

This is the *Crusta lactea* of authors, (Plate XXXVII. of BATEMAN; Pl. 16. of THE ATLAS,) and is almost exclusively a disease of infancy. "It

---

* In a note, subjoined in this place, in the two preceding editions of this work, I remarked, that the non-contagious quality, and some other features of this disease, indicated an analogy to Impetigo. My subsequent experience has led me to question altogether the propriety with which Dr. Willan classed the crusta lactea under the genus *Porrigo*, and to believe that Impetigo *larvalis* would have been the more correct appellation. Even on the face and scalp, the character of the eruption is impetiginous; the pustules being psydracia, and not favi or achores; the crusts thin and laminated, not elevated and indented, like the honeycomb of Porrigo; and the subsequent oozing of ichor, from numerous points, and the repeated recession and renewal of the inflammation and incrustation, still more completely establish the identity of this disease with Impetigo, as well as its universal attacks over the whole body and extremities, fixing especially in the flexures of the large joints, and returning occasionally for several years, even till the age of puberty, in the spring and autumnal seasons; and from every successive irritation from both the processes of dentition, and other causes.—With these remarks, however, I leave the disease in its original place, in deference to my venerated preceptor, and in order to avoid the confusion of altered arrangement.

is generally supposed to be non-contagious; but Alibert mentions the case of an infant who was inoculated with the complaint, and took it. The same author remarks, that it most commonly appears in those who have golden-coloured hair." It commonly appears first on the forehead and cheeks, in an eruption of numerous minute and whitish pustules, which are crowded together, upon a red surface. These pustules soon break, and discharge a clear, viscid fluid, which concretes into thin yellowish or greenish scabs. As the pustular patches spread, the discharge is renewed, and continues also from beneath the scabs, increasing their thickness and extent, until the forehead, cheeks, and even the whole face, become enveloped, as by a mask (whence the epithet *larvalis*), the eyelids alone remaining exempt from the incrustation.* " The odour of the eruption is rank and peculiar." † The eruption is liable, however, to considerable variation in its course; the discharge being sometimes profuse, and the surface red and excoriated; a state to which young infants are very liable : at other times the discharge is scarcely perceptible, so that the surface remains covered with a dry and brown scab. When the scab ultimately falls off, and ceases to be renewed, a red, elevated, and tender cuticle, marked with deep lines, and exfoliating several times, is left behind;

* "Imo quandoque frontem occupant, et totam faciem, exceptis palpebris, *larvâ* tegunt." Plenck, p. 77.

† Celle du lait qui commence à s'aigrir ou à se putréfier." Alibert, liv. i. p. 11. T.

differing from that which succeeds to Impetigo, in-asmuch as it does not crack into deep fissures.

Smaller patches of the disease not unfrequently appear about the neck and breast, and sometimes on the extremities : and the ears and scalp are usually affected in the course of its progress. In general the health of the child is not materially affected, especially when the eruption does not appear in the early period of lactation ; but it is always ac-companied with considerable itching and irritation, which are most severe in young infants, and often greatly diminish the natural sleep, and disturb the digestion. " In children of full habits, as Mr. Plumbe justly remarks *, when the eruption occu-pies the fore part of the neck, ' extending from the chin and angles of the lower jaw to the clavi-cles,' the pain and irritation are most distressing to the little sufferers :" and much debility some-times ensues. The eyes and eyelids become in-flamed, and purulent discharges take place from them and from the ears; the parotid† and sub-sequently the mesenteric glands also inflame; and marasmus, with diarrhœa and hectic, cut off the patient.

Most commonly, however, the disease terminates favourably, though its duration is often long and uncertain. It sometimes suddenly puts on the ap-pearance of cessation, and afterwards returns with severity ; sometimes it disappears spontaneously

---

* Practical Treatise on Diseases of the Skin, 2d edit. 1827. p. 220.

† Plenck says, "Tumidæ simul sunt glandulæ jugulares raro parotides." Doct. de Morb. Cut. p. 77. T.

soon after weaning, or after the cutting of the first
teeth; and sometimes it will continue from two or
three months to a year and a half, or even longer.
"Dr. Underwood says, 'I never saw an infant much
loaded with it, but it has always been healthy, and
cut its teeth remarkably well.* In general, however, although it appears in the most healthy children, yet it is the consequence of repletion, and
the irritation of undigested food upon highly ex-
citable systems; and in these it probably prevents
the attack of more formidable diseases." It is remarkable, that, whatever excoriation may be produced, no permanent deformity ensues. Dr. Strack
has affirmed, that "when the disease is about to
terminate, the urine of the patient acquires the
odour of the urine of cats; and that, when the
usual odour remains unchanged, the disease will
generally be of long continuance."† "Dr. Strack's
opinion, however, on this part of the prognosis is
not to be depended upon, as he prescribed the
Viola *tricolor* as a specific in this disease; and it
is well known that that plant communicates to the
urine of those who take it the odour of the urine
of cats.

"The remote cause of this species of Porrigo
is improper diet, either as respects quantity or
quality, in strong and healthy children. I have
been able, frequently, to trace it to too free use of

* Underwood's Treatise on Diseases of Children, 8th edit. p. 170.

† See his Dis. de Crusta lactea infantum, et ejusdem specifico re-
medio : — also Lond. Med. Journal, vol. ii. p. 187.

acescent food, such as fruit tarts and puddings, sugar and the various articles of confectionary into which it largely enters, by children of full and gross habits of body. It frequently, also, appears to be the result of dentition, in children of full habits; and in this case is always beneficial." •

In the commencement of the Porrigo larvalis, while the discharge is copious and acrid, it is necessary to clear the surface two or three times a day by careful ablution with some tepid and mild fluid, as milk and water, thin gruel, or a decoction of bran * ; and to apply a mild ointment, such as the Unguentum Oxydi Zinci, or a combination of this with a Saturnine Cerate. " I have seen no ointment so quickly beneficial as the Unguentum Hydrargyri Nitratis diluted with seven parts of Spermaceti ointment. To aid in removing the crusts, a cataplasm of oatmeal water and butter, with the juice of the Nasturtium (Tropæolum *majus*), has been found very serviceable." The Saturnine Cerate will be useful to obviate excoriation, while the surface remains red and tender, after the discharge has ceased. " Plenck†, and several continental physicians, consider it dangerous to check suddenly

---

* The Hindoo physicians foment the parts with a decoction of the Sida *populifolia* (*toottie elley*); and touch excoriated parts, when the scabs are rubbed off, with " a little finely-prepared Castor oil." Ainslie's Mat. Indica, vol. ii. p. 530. T.

† Plenck, under the title *Crusta lactea infantum larvata*, says, — " Repressis autem papulis crustasis morbi glandularum, tussis, asthma, tabes sæpe oriuntur." He also says, — " Scabies capitis *retropulsa* exigit sinapismum, vel vesicatorium abraso capiti imponendum, ut revocetur scabies, vel denique novam infectionem ope applicatæ mitræ scabiosæ." Doct. de Morb. Cutaneis, p. 76.

the eruption by external applications; and imagine that it is likely to produce diseases of the
head and chest; as fever, ophthalmia, swelled
glands, cough, anasarca, hydrocephalus, and apo-
plexy. Dr. Granville thinks he has observed this
to be the case in the Dispensary for Children; but
in my own experience, which has been extensive
both in Dispensaries and in private practice, I have
seen no injury result from checking the eruption."

The removal of the disease is much accelerated
by the use of alterative doses of mercurial purgatives (especially where the biliary secretion is
defective, the abdomen tumid, or the mesenteric
glands enlarged), which should be continued for
three weeks or longer, according to circumstances.
Small doses of the Submuriate of Mercury may be
given twice a day, alone, or in combination with Soda
and a testaceous powder; or, if the bowels are very
irritable, the Hydrargyrus cum Cretâ, or the Cine-
reous Oxide, may be substituted. But if the general
health appear sound, the inflammatory condition
of the skin, and the profuse exudation, may be
alleviated by the internal use of Soda, with precipitated Sulphur, or with the Testacea.

When the state of irritation is removed, and the
crusts are dry and falling off, the Unguentum Hydrargyri Nitratis, much diluted, may be applied with
advantage. And now some gentle tonic, such as
Infusion of Calumba, the Decoction of Sarsaparilla,
the Decoction of the Water Dock, should be administered; or the Decoction of Cinchona, in com-

bination with Subcarbonate of Soda, or the Chalybeates (which are more readily taken by children),
especially the saturated solution of the Tartrate, or
the Vinum Ferri.

I cannot speak from experience respecting the
medicine recommended as a specific by Dr. Strack;
namely, a decoction of the leaves of the Viola tricolor of Linnæus, in milk.* In the course of the
first week, this medicine is said to increase the
eruption considerably; but at the same time the
urine acquires the smell above mentioned, and, at
the end of a fortnight, the crusts begin to fall off,
and the skin underneath appears clean. Professor Selle, however, has affirmed, that this plant
is either noxious, in this complaint, or wholly
inert.† " When the milk is thick, if the infant be
altogether nourished at the breast, the nurse must
be changed. If it be fed, much care must be taken
to repress a voracious appetite in the child, and to
make the food as light as possible."

SPECIES 2. PORRIGO *furfurans.*‡ FURFURACEOUS
SCALL.

---

* He prescribes a handful of the fresh, or half a drachm of the dried
leaves, to be boiled in half a pint of cow's milk, and the whole to be
taken night and morning.

† Medicina Clinica, i. 185.

‡ Sennert. de Curat. Infant. p. ii. cap. 4.— Sauvages, Nos. Method.
class. x. gen. xxix. spec. 6. Plenck, Doctr. de Morb. Cut. class. vii.
Alibert, plate 3., where it is well represented. — It may be observed that
the " T. amiantacée" of this writer (plate 4.) appears to be a variety of
P. furfurans.) It is, in fact, to a *furfuraceous* disease alone that the
translators of the Greek physicians, and many modern Latin writers,
apply the term Porrigo, deeming it synonymous with the Greek πιτυρίασις.
From the authority of Celsus, however, it is obvious that this is a mis-

Syn. Tinea furfuracea (*Sennert*) : Tinea porriginosa (*Astruc. Sauv.*) : Porrigo furfuracea (*Plenck*) : Ecpyesis porrigo, *ε.* furfuracea (*Good*) : Teigne furfuracée. Tinea furfuracea (*Alibert*) : Rache farineuse (*F.*).

In this form of the disease, (Plate XXXVIII. of BATEMAN ; Pl. 16. of THE ATLAS,) which commences with an eruption of small *achores*, the discharge from the pustules is moderate in quantity, and the excoriation slight ; the humour, therefore, soon concretes, and separates in innumerable thin laminated scabs, or scale-like exfoliations. At irregular periods, the pustules re-appear, and the discharge being renewed, the eruption becomes moist ; but it soon dries again and exfoliates. It is attended with a good deal of itching, and some soreness of the scalp, to which the disease is generally confined, " although I have seen it extend to the ears." The hair, which partially falls off, becomes thin, less strong in its texture, and sometimes lighter in its colour.* Occasionally the glands of the neck are swelled and painful.

---

application of the term ; and it is improper to comprehend the single dandriff, and the contagious scall, under the same generic appellation. See Pityriasis, above, page 45, *note.* Plenck, though applying the term to both, marks the distinction, calling the contagious disease, Porrigo furfuracea, seu *vera*, — and the other P. farinosa, seu *spuria*, which he considers as a mere accumulation of the secretion from the sebaceous glands.

* Alibert correctly remarks—" Toutes les fois que nous avons dépouillé le cuir chevelu des écailles qui le recouvroient, nous avons observé qu'il étoit dénué de son epiderme, qu'il avoit une couleur rosée, et offroit une surface lisse, polie, luisante, comme vernisée." Liv. 1. p. 7. — He also remarks that it is most common in those who have bright chesnut-coloured hair. T.

The P. furfurans occurs principally in adults[*], especially in females, in whom it is not always easily distinguished from the scaly diseases, Pityriasis, Psoriasis, or Lepra, affecting the capillitium. The circumstances just enumerated, however, will serve to establish the diagnosis: as in those diseases, no pustules appear in the beginning, — there is no moisture or ulceration, — and the hair is not detached, nor changed in texture and colour; — neither are they communicable by contact.

In the treatment of the P. furfurans, it is supposed to be absolutely necessary to keep the scalp closely shaven. " Many objections, however, are often made to shaving the head, which indeed is not absolutely requisite, if the hair be cut short, and the following lotion employed : —

> ℞ Potassæ Sulphureti (recentis prep.) ʒiij,
> Saponis Mollis ʒj,
> Aquæ Calcis f ℥viij,
> Spir. Rect. fʒij.   M. fiat lotio."

The branny scabs should be removed by gentle washing, with some mild soap and water, twice a day; and an oil-silk cap should be worn, partly for the purpose of keeping the surface moist as well as warm, and partly for the convenience of retaining an ointment in contact with it.

The nature of the ointments employed in this, as in the other species of Porrigo, must be varied, according to the period of the disease, and the irritability of the part affected. In the commencement

---

* Alibert nevertheless says, " Je n'ai jamais observé que la Teigne furfuracée attaquât les adultes." Liv. 1. p. 7. T.

of the eruption, when the surface is moist, tender, and somewhat inflamed, the Oxyd of Zinc ointment should be applied; or, what has been said to be more beneficial, an ointment prepared with the Cocculus Indicus, in the proportion of two drachms of the powdered berry to an ounce of lard. But when the scalp becomes dry and irritable, in the progress of the complaint, it may be washed with the common soft soap and water; or with a lather made by mixing equal portions of soft soap and Unguentum Sulphuris in warm water. More stimulant ointments will then be requisite, such as the Unguentum Hydrargyri Nitratis, Unguentum Hydrargyri Nitrico-oxydi, the Tar and Sulphur Ointments, or the Unguentum Acidi Nitrosi of the Edinburgh Pharmacopœia. These and other stimulant applications * succeed in different individuals in the inert state of the P. furfurans; but they must be intermitted, in case the inflammation and discharge return.

SPECIES 3. PORRIGO *lupinosa*, LUPINE-LIKE SCALL.

Syn. Scabies capitis lupina (*Plenck*): Tinea lupina (*Astruc. Sauv.*): Teigne faveuse †, Tinea

---

* A long catalogue of stimulants, of similar quality, may be collected from the writings of the Greeks, as remedies for the furfuraceous Porrigo: such as liniments of frankincense and vinegar, or the same gum with wine and oil; others prepared with oil of rue, litharge, and vinegar; or wish stavesacre and oil; lotions of the decoction of fœnugreek, the roots of beet, and of the cucumis silvestris, &c. See Oribas. Synops. lib. viii. cap. 25.—Aëtius, tetrab. ii. serm. ii. cap. 76.—Alex. Trall. lib. i. cap. 4.

† Alibert says, "La Teigne faveuse est celle qui s'est le plus fréquemment présentée à nos regards," p. 14. He also says, "J'ai observé

favosa (*Alibert*): Teigne annulaire; Teigne ru-
gueuse; Rache sèche (*F.*).

" This species of Porrigo (Pl. 15. of THE ATLAS,)
which is occasionally congenital, and sometimes
hereditary *," is characterised by the formation of
dry, circular scabs, of a yellowish white colour, set
deeply in the skin, with elevated edges and a
central indentation or cup-like depression, sometimes containing a white scaly powder, and resembling, on the whole, the seeds of lupines †, or
rather certain species of lichens. These scabs are
formed upon small separate clusters of *achores*,
by the concretion of the purulent fluid, which exudes when they break ‡; and they acquire, when
seated on the scalp, the size of a sixpence. Frequently there is also a thin white incrustation,
covering the intervening parts of the scalp, which
commonly exfoliates; but, if allowed to accumulate through inattention to cleanliness, it forms
an elevated crustaceous cap. The disease, however, is not exclusively confined to the head; but
sometimes appears on the chest, belly, shoulders,

---

cette affection sur des têtes dont les cheveux étoient noirs, blonds, et
même rouges." Liv. i. p. 15.   T.

  * Alibert mentions a case of it which appears to have been hereditary: " son père," says he, " en étoit atteint."   Liv. i. p. 13.   T.

  † From this resemblance, the same epithet was applied to the disease
by Haly Abbas, who has distinguished six species.   " Quinta est *lupinosa*, sicca, et colore alba, lupino similis, à qua quasi cortices et squamæ
fluunt albæ." (Theorice, lib. viii. cap. 18.)   See also Guid. Cauliac.
tract. vi. cap. 1. — Sennert. lib. v. p. i. cap. 32.

  ‡ Thenard and Vauquelin found that the purulent discharge in this
species affords much albumen.

loins, and the extremities, where the little white and indented scabs do not exceed two lines in diameter. "It is accompanied with great itching, and pediculi frequently infest the crevices of the crusts. The odour of the favi, Alibert compares to the urine of the cat; or chambers which have been infested with mice." This variety of Porrigo is liable to increase much if neglected; and is usually tedious, and of long duration. "When neglected, the acrid pus is absorbed, and swells the cervical glands. In old cases, in which the disease is abandoned to its progress, complete baldness or *alopecia* occurs."

The internal treatment in P. lupinosa does not differ from that necessary in P. larvalis. The first object in the local management of this form of the disease, is to remove the crusts and indented scabs, by a diligent application of soap and water, "or by a poultice of oatmeal, or of brown soap and oatmeal half boiled," or other emollient applications. If the scalp be the seat of the disease, the previous removal of the hair will be necessary. If the scabs are not penetrable by these ablutions or by ointments, or if any thick intervening incrustation is present, a lotion of the Liquor Potassæ *, or of the Muriatic Acid, or the Sulphuric Acid in a diluted state, may be employed. When the surface is cleared, "the rete mucosum is seen red and covered with

* An alkaline lotion may be made with the proportions of a drachm of the Aqua Kali Puri, two or three drachms of Oil, and an ounce of Water. — "Imprimis *salia lixivia*," says Prof. Selle, "ad crustam tam firmam atque alias insolubilem emolliendam sunt apta." Medic. Clin. 187

numerous small ulcers, which exude a viscid, fœtid, straw-coloured fluid.   At this time" the ointment of Cocculus Indicus may be applied to the red and shining cuticle ; and afterwards the more stimulant unguents, as in the case of P. furfurans, with regular daily ablution, will complete the cure.

SPECIES 4. PORRIGO *scutulata*, SCALLED HEAD, or RINGWORM OF THE SCALP.

Syn. Tinea ficosa (*Astruc. Sauv.*) : Achores, seu Scabies Capitis (*Plenck*) : Tinea granulata (*Alison*) : Ecpyesis Porrigo, 6. *Galeata* (*Good*) : Teigne granulée (*Alibert*) : Shirine (*Arab.*) : Kel (*Pers. Turk.*) : Grind ; Haarschuppen (*German*) : Tête Teigneuse (*F.*)

(Plate XXXIX. of BATEMAN ; Pl. 16. of THE ATLAS). This species of Porrigo appears in distinct and even distant patches, of an irregularly circular figure, upon the scalp, forehead, and neck. *

It commences with clusters of small light yellow pustules, which soon break and form thin scabs over each patch, which, if neglected, become thick and hard by accumulation. † If the scabs are removed, however, the surface of the patches is left red, and shining, but studded with slight elevated points, or papulæ, in some of which minute globules of pus again appear, in a few days. By these repetitions of the eruption of *achores*, the in-

---

* " Les enfans les plus sujets à la Teigne granulée, sont ceux dont la peau est brune ou basanée." Alibert, p. 15. T.

† Thenard and Vauquelin found the crusts in this species of Porrigo to be wholly gelatine.

crustations become thicker, and the areas of the patches extend, often becoming confluent, if the progress of the disease be unimpeded, so as to affect the whole head. As the patches extend, the hair covering them becomes lighter in its colour, and sometimes breaks off short ; and as the process of pustulation and scabbing is repeated, the roots of the hair are destroyed, and at length there remains uninjured only a narrow border of hair round the head. "Sometimes the achores are not perceptible in the commencement of the disease ; but the falling off of the hair is the first notice of its existence. The pustules are generally seated at the roots of the hairs, which are found penetrating the achores."

This very unmanageable form of Porrigo generally occurs in children of three or four years old and upwards, and often continues for several years. Whether the circles remain red, smooth, and shining, or become dry and scurfy, the prospect of a cure is still distant ; for the pustules will return, and the ulceration and scabbing will be repeated. It can only be considered as about to terminate, when the redness and exfoliation disappear together, and the hair begins to grow of its natural colour and texture.

The disease seems to originate spontaneously in children of feeble and flabby habits, or in a state approaching to marasmus, who are ill-fed, uncleanly, and not sufficiently exercised : but it is principally propagated "by contagion, both to the other parts of the head of the individual affected, by the conveyance of the matter from the diseased to the healthy parts," and to others, by the frequent contact of the heads of children, but more generally by the use of the same towels, combs, caps, and hats. Whence the multiplication of boarding-schools appears to have given rise to an increased prevalence of this disease, among the more cleanly classes of the community, at the present time. For such is the anxiety of parents to regain the lost years of education, that they too often send their children to these schools, when capable of communicating the infection, although supposed to be cured ; against which no vigilance on the part of the superintendants can afford a sufficient security.

The principles of local treatment already laid down, are particularly applicable in this species of Porrigo. While the patches are in an inflamed and irritable condition, it is necessary to limit the local applications to regular ablution, or sponging, with warm water or with lime-water, or some emollient fomentation. *　Even the operation of shaving

---

* This mode of treatment was recommended by some of the ancients. Oribasius observes, that "if there is much *heat* or *inflammation* connected with the achores, this must be first alleviated by a *moist sedative.*" (Synops. lib. viii. cap. 27.) Aëtius also observes, " Quod si incideris in achores *inflammatos* et *dolentes*, dolorem prius liquido medicamento concoctorio mollienteque ac leni mitigabis," &c. (tetrab. ii. serm. ii. cap. 68.) And among the moderns, Heister has made a similar discrimination respecting the treatment of Porrigo. He recommends, in all instances, in the commencement of the disease, the use of mild emollient applications; as cream with cerussa, oleum ovorum, " ung. de enula, de cerussa, diapompholygos, aliudve simile saturninum," while moderate alteratives, of calomel, antimony, &c. are given internally. He affirms

the head, which is necessary to be repeated at intervals of eight or ten days, produces a temporary increase of irritation. At this time, the patient should wear a light linen cap, which should be frequently changed; and all stimulant lotions and ointments, which tend only to aggravate the disease, should be proscribed.

In the progress of the disorder, various changes take place, which require corresponding variations of the method of treatment. By degrees the inflammatory state is diminished, and a dry exfoliation and scabbing ensue: but the pustular eruption returns, and the patches become again red and tender; or, in some cases, without much redness, there is an acrimonious exudation, with considerable irritability of the scalp. In other instances, the surface becomes inert, and in some degree torpid, while a dry scaly scab constantly appears, and active stimulants are requisite to effect any change in the disorder. It is very obvious, as Dr. Willan used to remark, that the adoption of any one mode of practice, or of any single pretended *specific*, under these varying circumstances of the disease, must be unavailing, and often extremely injurious.

that the application of mercurial and sulphur ointments, in the first instance, is exceedingly pernicious. Chirurg. part. i. lib. v. cap. 10. *Riedlinus* relates, that a gentlewoman whose son was afflicted with Porrigo had tried many applications in vain, and indeed had received no benefit until she was recommended to cover the whole head with a cataplasm composed of oatmeal, water, and butter, which soon succeeded in curing the disease, and restoring the healthy state of the scalp. Lin. Med. Ann. 6. Feb. 25. p. 215. seq.

R

In the more irritative states, the milder ointments, such as those prepared with Cocculus Indicus, "in the proportion of ʒij of the Pulvis Cocculi
to ℥j of Lard;" or with the Submuriate of Mercury, the Oxide of Zinc, the Superacetate of Lead,
or with Opium or Tobacco, should be employed;
or sedative lotions, such as decoctions or infusion
of Poppy-heads, or of Tobacco, may be substituted.
Where there is an acrimonious discharge, the Zinc
and saturnine with the milder mercurial ointments,
such as the Unguentum Hydrargyri præcipitati
albi, or the ointment of Calomel, or a lotion of
Lime-water with Calomel, "or a soap composed
of equal parts of soft Soap and of Sulphur ointment," are advantageous.

According to the different degrees of inertness
which ensue, various well-known stimulants must
be resorted to, and may be diluted, or strengthened,
and combined, according to the circumstances. The
Mercurial ointments, as the Unguentum Hydrargyri præcipitati, the U. Hydrargyri nitrico-oxydi,
and especially the U. Hydrargyri nitratis are often
effectual remedies: and those prepared with Sulphur, Tar, Hellebore, Turpentine, and Sabidilla,
the Unguentum Elemi, "or the Unguentum Sulphuris, with a small addition of the Calx Hydrargyri alba," &c. separately or in combination, occasionally succeed; as well as preparations of
Mustard *, Staves-acre, Black Pepper †, Capsicum,

---

* See Sennert. loc. cit. — Underwood on the Dis. of Children, vol. ii.

† There is an Unguentum Piperis nigri in the Dublin pharmacopœia,
of the efficacy of which Dr. Tuomy speaks highly. See his Essay on
the Diseases of Dublin.

Galls, Rue, and other acrid vegetable substances. *
Lotions containing the Sulphates of Zinc and of
Copper, or the Oxymuriate of Mercury, in solution,
are likewise occasionally beneficial. "Decoction of
Tobacco has been recommended; but it must be
applied with caution. Nitric Acid rubbed up with
Lard was tried by Alibert without permanent benefit.
Underwood, in cases of long standing, advises the
scalp to be shaved, then well washed with a strong
lather of soap; and, afterwards, the Unguentum
Picis made with Petroleum, instead of Pix liquida,
to be rubbed in for nearly an hour at a time, using
it hot, and covering the head with a bladder, both
to keep on the ointment and to promote the perspiration of the part. If the hairs loosen, they should
be pulled out by the roots. † Desault (*Journ. de
Chirurg.*) mentions a plaster composed of Ammo-
niacum and Vinegar, which being spread on linen,
is applied over the head, and left on it for two
months. Alibert mentions the good effects of a cataplasm of Hemlock : three cases out of four, he says,
were cured by this application in five months."

In the very dry and inert state of the patches,
the more caustic substances are often extremely

---

* The ancients were accustomed to employ a similar collection of
stimulants for the achores; among which were Sulphur Vivum, Atra-
mentum Sutorium (Sulphate of Iron), Tar, burnt Paper with Oil, Soap;
Oil of Rue and of Myrtle; Resin, Myrrh, and Frankincense, with Wine
and Vinegar, &c. Vinegar was deemed an efficacious remedy. "Acetum
vero acerrimum ad achoras omni tempore accommodatum est." See
Oribas. Synops. lib. viii. 27. Aët. tet. ii. serm. ii. cap. 68.

† Treatise on Diseases of Children, 8vo. 8th edit. p. 434.

successful. Thus I have seen a lotion, containing from three to six grains of the Nitrate of Silver in an ounce of distilled water, effectually remove the disease in this condition. Touching the patches with the muriated Tincture of Iron, or with any of the mineral acids, "particularly the Sulphuric," slightly diluted, in some cases removes the morbid cuticle, and the new one assumes a healthy action.* The application of a blister in like manner sometimes effectually accomplishes the same end. But, in many instances, the effect of these renovations of the cuticle is merely temporary, and the disease returns in a week or two, upon the new surface.

Professor Hamilton, of Edinburgh, who considers the ringworm of the scalp as "quite different from the scalled head," affirms, in a late publication, that he has seldom failed to cure the former by the use of the Unguentum ad Scabiem of Banyer. For delicate children, he dilutes this ointment with an equal portion of simple Cerate, and sometimes alternates the use of it with that of common Basilicon. †

---

* Mr. P. Fernandez mentioned to me an instance of speedy recovery which followed a single application of the strong Sulphuric Acid, which was instantaneously washed off. A new and healthy cuticle succeeded. The Acetic Acid, or Aromatic Vinegar, which acts as a more gentle, yet very effectual caustic, has proved an effectual remedy in a few instances.

† See his "Hints on the Management of Children." — The acrid ointment of Banyer consists of Ceruss. ℔ss, Litharg. Aur. ℥ij, Alum. Ust. ℥iss, Mercur. Sublim. ℥iss, Sevi Porcin. ℔ij, Terebinth. Ven. ℔ss. See his Pharmacopœia Pauperum. I have used this ointment, somewhat diluted, in a few cases of this disease, since the first edition of this Synopsis was published; and I have found it, like other applications, sometimes successful, but frequently inert and useless.

These various applications are enumerated, because not one of them is always successful, singly, even under circumstances apparently the same. They must be varied, and combined ; and the best criterion in the choice and combination* of them, is the degree of existing irritation in the morbid parts, or in the general habit. The rude and severe employment of depilatories, which some practitioners have recommended, is not always to be advised, as often inflicting great injury to the scalp, and retarding, rather than expediting, the progress to recovery. " They have been adopted on the supposition that the bulb of the hair is the seat of the disease. They are, nevertheless, recommended by some who do not refer the disease to the roots of the hair, but regard them only as sources of irritation in the diseased part. Mr. Plumbe * recommends, as a preliminary step to any method of local management, to discharge the contents of the pustules, to remove the hairs, and to wash the matter from the scalp. Having removed the hairs and discharged the pustules, he recommends the part to be rubbed with finely powdered Sulphate of Copper, which is afterwards to be washed off. This should be repeated as often as any new pustules make their appearance. Should the pustules recur when new hair grows on the spots, he recommends pressure by adhesive straps and cold lotions. A more easy method of getting rid of the hairs is that recommended by Mr. M. Mahon. The hair

* A Practical Treatise on Diseases of the Skin, p. 70.

is cut short, and the crusts and scurf removed by a cataplasm of Linseed meal applied every night for four or five days, and washing the scalp with soap and water. The affected parts are then to be anointed with a depilatory composed of weak (nearly carbonated) Quicklime, Silex, Alum, and Oxyd of Iron, a small quantity of Carbonate of Potass, some Charcoal, and a sufficient quantity of Lard. During the time of applying this, the hairs and scurf are to be removed by washing with soap and water. I have seen nearly the same advantages from using a lotion composed of one part of Liquor Potassæ, two parts of Alcohol, and two parts of Water. It is to be rubbed only on the diseased spot by means of a sponge."

I have said nothing respecting the administration of internal medicines in the Porrigo scutulata; because it is often merely local, being communicated by contagion to children in other respects healthy. But in those in whom it appears in combination with cachectic symptoms, chalybeate medicines, or the decoction of Cinchona and alteratives, must be prescribed, according to the particular indications; and the diet, clothing, and exercise of the patient must be carefully regulated. " The feet in particular should be kept warm and dry; and every means adopted to maintain a due equilibrium of the circulation and the insensible perspiration; at the same time all crude aliments, raw vegetable matter, and whatever is likely to irritate the stomach, should be carefully avoided. I have always found advantage from keeping the bowels open, by saline purgatives in stout children, and by those of a warm and tonic character in scrophulous subjects. The tepid bath, also, used in the morning, is beneficial.

SPECIES 5. PORRIGO *decalvans,* BALD or RING- WORM SCALL.

Syn. Area (*Celsus*): Alopecia areata (*Sauv.*): Trichosis Area (*Good*).

This singular variety of the disease (Plate XL. of BATEMAN; Pl. 16. of THE ATLAS,) presents no appearance whatever, except patches of simple baldness, of a more or less circular form, on which not a single hair remains, while that which surrounds the patches is as thick as usual. The surface of the scalp, within these areæ, is smooth, shining, and remarkably white. * It is probable, though not ascertained, that there may be an eruption of minute achores about the roots of the hair, in the first instance, which are not permanent, and do not discharge any fluid. † The disease, however, has been seen to occur, in one or two instances, in a large assemblage of children, among

* Celsus, and after him some other writers, have described this affec- tion under the appellation of " Area." Under this generic term, he comprises two varieties, called by the Greeks *Alopecia,* and *Ophiasis:* the former of which spreads in irregular patches; and the latter in a serpentine form, round both sides of the head, from the occiput. — De Medicina, lib. vi. cap. 4.

† It is not unfrequent in countries where the inhabitants live chiefly upon fish; as, for instance, formerly in the Shetland islands, where bald- ness from this cause was so common, that it was familiarly said, " that there was not a hair between them and Heaven." *Sir R. Sibbald's Description of Shetland,* fol. p. 25.

whom the other forms of the Porrigo prevailed.
But in other cases, and also in adults, it has appeared where no communication could be traced
or conjectured. The areæ gradually enlarge, and
sometimes become confluent, producing extensive
baldness, in which condition the scalp remains
many weeks, especially if no curative measures are
adopted. The hair which begins to grow is of a
softer texture, and lighter colour, than the rest;
and in persons beyond the middle age, it is grey.

If the scalp is cleared by constant shaving, and
at the same time some stimulant liniment be steadily applied to it, this obstinate affection may be at
length overcome, and the hair will regain its usual
strength and colour. In fact, until this change
takes place, the means of cure must not be intermitted. * Some of the more active ointments,
mentioned under the preceding head, may be employed with friction; but liniments, containing an
essential oil dissolved in spirit (for instance, two
drachms of the oil of Mace, in three or four ounces
of Alcohol), or prepared with Oil of Tar, Petroleum
Barbadense, Camphor, Turpentine, &c. are more
efficacious.

---

* All that can be prescribed respecting the treatment of this affection
has been expressed by Celsus with his usual terseness. " Quidam hæc
genera arearum scalpello exasperant: quidam illinunt adurentia ex oleo,
maximeque chartam combustum: quidam resinam terebinthinam cum
thapsia inducunt. Sed nihil melius est, quam novacula quotidie radere:
quia, cùm paulatim summa pellicula excisa est, adaperiuntur pilorum
radiculæ. Neque ante oportet desistere, quam frequentem pilum nasci
apparuerit. Id autem, quod subinde raditur, illini atramento sutorio
satis est." Loc. cit.

SPECIES 6. PORRIGO *favosa*, HONEYCOMB SCALL.'

Syn. Κηρίον (*G.*) : Favus (*Lat.*) : Tinea favosa (*Haly Abbas, Astruc. Sauv.*) : Tinea volatica, Ignis volaticus, Mentagra Infantum (*Auct. Var.*): Scabies, capitis favosa (*Plenck*) : Dartre crustacée flavescente ; Herpes crustaceus (*Alibert*) : Ecpyesis Porrigo, γ favosa (*Good*) : Teigne faveuse (*F.*): Pódóghoo (*Tam.*): Goorig (*Duk.*): Podooghoo Kūrāpānie (*Tel.*) : Badkhora (*Pers.*).

This species of the disorder (Plate XLI. of BATEMAN ; Pl. 16. of THE ATLAS,) consists of an eruption of the large, soft, straw-coloured pustules, denominated *favi*, without apparent previous inflammation. These are not in general globular, with a regularly circular margin ; but somewhat flattened, with an irregular edge, and surrounded by a slight inflammation. They occur on all parts of the body ; sometimes on the scalp alone, and sometimes on the face, or on the trunk and extremities only ; but most commonly they spread from the scalp, especially from behind the ears, to the face, or from the lips and chin to the scalp, and occasionally from the extremities to the trunk and head. * They are usually accompanied with considerable itching. Children from six months to four years of age are most liable to this eruption ; but adults are not unfrequently affected with it.

* When it thus spreads from one part to another, the names Tinea *volatica*, Ignis *volaticus*, &c., have been given by Sauvages and others.

" Cooks are very liable, according to Alibert [*] , to this species of Porrigo."

The pustules, especially on the scalp, appear at first distinct, though near together; but on the face and extremities they generally rise in irregular clusters, becoming confluent when broken, and discharging a viscid matter, which gradually concretes into greenish, or yellowish, semi-transparent scabs. The disease extends, by the successive formation of new blotches, which sometimes cover the chin, or surround the mouth, and spread to the cheeks and nose [†]; and, on the scalp, the ulceration ultimately extends, in a similar manner, over the whole head, with a constant discharge, by which the hair and moist scabs are matted together: " and a most disgusting odour is exhaled." Under the last-mentioned circumstances, pediculi are often generated in great numbers, and aggravate the itching and irritation of the disease. On the face, too, a similar aggravation of the symptoms is occasioned, in children, by an incessant picking and scratching about the edges of the scabs, which the itching demands, and by which the skin is kept sore, and the ulceration extended ; while the scabs are thickened into irregular masses, not unlike honeycomb, by the accumulating and concreting discharge. On the lower extremities considerable ulcerations sometimes form, especially about the

[*] Mal. de la Peau, p. 88.

[†] Rayer says, " Je l'ai vue occuper toute la partie postérieure jusqu'au sacrum." Traité des Mal. de la Peau, tome i. p. 497. T.

heels, and roots of the toes ; and the ends of the toes are sometimes ulcerated, the pustules arising at their sides, and even under the nails.

The ulcerating blotches seldom continue long, or extend far, before the lymphatic system exhibits marks of irritation, probably from the acrimony of the absorbed matter. When the scalp or face is the seat of the disease, the glands on the sides of the neck enlarge and harden, being at first perceived like a chain of little tumours, lying loose under the skin ; and the submaxillary and parotid glands are often affected in a similar manner.* At length some of them inflame, the skin becomes discoloured, and they suppurate slowly, and with much pain and irritation. The eruption, in these situations, is likewise often accompanied by a discharge from behind the ears, or from the ears themselves, with a tumid upper lip, and inflammation of the eyes, or obstinate ulcerations of the edges of the eyelids. When the eruption appears on the trunk, although the pustules there are smaller and less confluent, and the scabs thinner and less permanent, the axillary glands are liable to be affected in the same way.

The discharge from the ulcerated surfaces, espe-cially on the scalp, when the crusts and coverings are removed, exhales an offensive rancid vapour, not only affecting the organs of smell and taste, but the eyes, of those who examine the diseased

---

* Non criticè, non depuratoriè, sed mali communicatione." Lorry de Morb. Cutan. p. 466. T.

parts.* The acrimony of the discharge is also manifested by the appearance of inflammation, followed by pustules, ulceration, and scabbing, on any portion of the sound skin, which comes into frequent contact with the parts diseased: thus, in young children, the breast is inoculated by the chin, and the hands and arms by contact with the face. The disease is also contagious. The arm and breasts of the nurse are liable to receive the eruption; but it is not so readily communicated to adults as to children.

The duration of this form of Porrigo is very uncertain; but it is, on the whole, much more manageable than the P. scutulata and decalvans. Young infants often suffer severely from the pain and irritation of the eruption, and of the glandular affections which it induces; and those who are bred in large towns, and are ill fed and nursed, are thus sometimes reduced to a state of fatal marasmus.

The Porrigo favosa requires the exhibition of the same alteratives internally, which have been recommended for the cure of the P. larvalis, in doses proportioned to the age and strength of the patients. The diet and exercise should also be regulated with care: all crude vegetables and fruits on the one

* It has been supposed that the similarity of the odour of this discharge to that of garlic (*porrum*) gave rise to the appellation of Porrigo.

Rayer says that, after the application of poultices to detach the crust, this odour is " nauseabonde, et analogue à celle des os qu'on a fait bouillir avec leurs ligaments." — l. c. p. 499. T.

hand, all saccharine preparations and stimulating substances, whether solid or fluid, on the other, should be avoided; and milk, puddings, and a little plain animal food, should be alone recommended. If the patient be of a squalid habit, or if the glandular affections be severe, the Cinchona Bark and Chalybeates, or the solution of Muriate of Barytes united with the former, will contribute materially to the restoration of health. " Those cases that have come under my care have generally yielded to the administration of the Hydrargyrus cum Creta, in doses proportionate to the age of the patient, given every night; with the Carbonate or Subcarbonate of Soda, in full doses, given in the Infusion of Cinchona, or of Cascarilla Bark, three times a day."

There is commonly some degree of inflammation present, which contra-indicates the use of active stimulants externally. " Sulphur baths have been found sometimes injurious: but the simple warm bath and fomentations are serviceable." The Unguentum Zinci, or the Unguentum Hydrargyri præcipitati albi, mixed with the former, or with a saturnine ointment, will be preferred as external applications, especially where the discharge is copious: and the ointment of the Nitrate of Mercury, diluted with about equal parts of simple Cerate and of the Ceratum Plumbi Superacetatis, is generally beneficial; but the proportion of the Unguentum Ceræ must be varied according to the degree of inflammation. " The following is an old, but a useful ointment :

℞. Picis liquidæ ʒiv,
Ceræ flavæ ʒiv,
Solve lento igne,
et sperge ante frigescat
Sulphuris Vivi ʒj.
Tere ut fiat unguentum."

All stiff and rigid coverings, whether of oiled silk, or, according to a popular practice, of the leaves of Cabbage, Beet, &c. should be prohibited ; for they often excite a most severe irritation. I have witnessed, in several instances, an universal ulceration, with copious purulent discharge, and a highly inflammatory and painful state of the scalp, exciting even a considerable degree of symptomatic fever, produced by such applications. The substitution of a poultice, in these cases, removed this irritative condition in two or three days, and the disease was speedily subdued by the treatment above recommended.

It may be mentioned, in conclusion, that an eruption of *favi* is sometimes seen on the face (Plate XLII. of BATEMAN) ; on the ears, neck, and occiput, in adults * ; in whom it is preceded and accompanied by considerable derangement of the constitution, headach, pain of the stomach, loss of appetite, constipation, and some degree of fever. The pustules become confluent, discharge a viscid

* Of this form of Porrigo favosa on the cheek, the 16th plate of M. Alibert appears to be a representation. He calls it " Dartre crustacée flavescente."

humour, and scab, as in the eruption just described; but they are surrounded by more extensive inflammation, and become harder and more prominent, somewhat resembling, in this respect, the Ecthyma. Their course, however, is more rapid than that of the Ecthyma, or of the tubercular Sycosis, to which also the disease bears some affinity. A cathartic, followed by the Pilula Hydrargyri Submuriatis comp. of the last Pharmacopœia, or Dr. Plummer's Pill, and a vegetable tonic, especially the decoction of Sarsaparilla, will be found serviceable; and the mild external applications, above mentioned, must be employed according to the degree of inflammation present.

A sudden eruption of Porrigo *favosa*, accompanied by fever, occasionally takes place also in children. A considerable alarm was excited by such an occurrence, in a family which I was requested to see, in which the disease was deemed to be some new or anomalous contagion. The first patient, aged five, was seized with severe fever, in which the pulse was at one time 140, and continued at 110 for several days; at the same time, clusters of favous pustules appeared behind the ears, which were speedily followed by others on the scalp, and about the apertures of the nostrils, which they plugged up as the scabs were formed. A few days after the commencement of this attack, a younger child, aged two years, was seized in a similar manner; but in her, the pustules appeared also about the chest, the glands of the neck swelled, and the abdomen became tumid. The contagion was immediately, though but locally, received by the mother and the nurse; the former of whom was inoculated about the mouth, by kissing the children; the latter in the palm of the hand. These children were somewhat squalid, and apparently ill nursed, especially in respect to cleanliness and exercise.

" All the species of Porrigo are, sometimes, spontaneously cured, even after they have long resisted all remedies.

" Alibert mentions the case of a girl of sixteen who had a very obstinate attack of Porrigo favosa, which yielded to no remedies, but disappeared soon after she was attacked with fever and Erysipelas." [*]

Works which may be consulted on Porrigo.

ALIBERT, Maladies de la Peau, fol.
CAZENEVE et SCHEDEL, Abrégé Pratique des Maladies de la Peau, 8vo. 1828.
COOKE, W. on Tinea Capitis, 1810.
CRAMPTON, Transactions of the King and Queen's College of Physicians, Dublin, 1824.
DICT. des Sciences Méd. art. Teignes.
GALLOT, Recherches sur la Teigne, 8vo. 1805.
OLDENBOURG, de Porrigine, 1762.
PLUMBE on Diseases of the Skin, 2d edit. 1827.
RAYER, Traité des Maladies de la Peau, 8vo. 1826.
STRACK, de Crusta Lactea Infantum, &c. 1779.
TRANSACTIONS of King and Queen's College, Dublin, vol. iv.
WILKINSON on Cutaneous Diseases, 8vo, 1822.
WILLAN, A Practical Treatise on Porrigo, 4to. 1814.

[*] Malad. de le Peau, p. 93.

GENUS III. ECTHYMA.*

Syn. Εκθυμα (*G.*): Phlysis Ecthyma (*Young*): Ecpyesis Ecthyma (*Good*): Dartre crustacée, Faruncle atonique (*F.*) *Papulous Scall.*

Def. AN ERUPTION OF LARGE PHLYZACIOUS PUSTULES; EACH SEATED ON A HARD, ELEVATED RED BASE; AND TERMINATING IN A THICK, HARD, GREENISH OR DARK-COLOURED SCAB. THEY ARE DISTINCT, SPARINGLY SCATTERED, AND NOT CONTAGIOUS.

This eruption does not very frequently alone demand the assistance of medicine. It is commonly indicative of some state of distress, if that expression may be used, under which the constitution labours; and, although it is not attended by actual fever, yet a degree of general irritation, or erethism, is often present with it. " It attacks all

---

* The term εκθυμα seems to have been used by the Greeks in a general sense, and nearly synonymous with εξανθημα, or *eruption.* Perhaps the more elevated and inflammatory eruptions were particularly called *ecthymata;* since, as Galen has observed, in his Commentary on the third book of the Epidemics of Hippocrates, the term is derived from εκθυειν, " quod est εξορμαν (*impetu erumpere*) in iis quæ sponte extuberant in cute." (§ 51.) See also Erotian de voc. apud Hippoc.;—and Foës, Œconom. Hipp. ad voc. εκθυματα. This view of the subject has led many authors, Fernel, Paré, Vidus, Vidius, Sennert, Sebizius, &c. to believe, that the terms *ecthymata* and *exanthemata* were used specifically, as the denominations of smallpox and measles. " Variolas vocant εκθυματα, pustulas extumescentes, morbillos autem εξανθηματα nominant, maculas in cute apparentes," &c. See a learned Treatise of Melchior Sebizius, De Variol. et Morbil. Argent. 1642. These views sanction the appropriation of the term to the " pustulæ *extumescentes*" of this genus.

S

ages and constitutions; but young men are more liable to it than children of either sex." It shows itself under three or four different forms, and is usually attributed to long-continued exertion and fatigue, to much watching, to anxiety of mind, to imperfect nutriment, to the influence of a cold and moist atmosphere, to an abuse of spirituous liquors, to a state of pregnancy, or to the debilitating effects of previous malignant fevers, especially of smallpox, measles, and scarlatina. It occurs most frequently on the extremities, but sometimes over the whole body, face, and scalp. The diagnosis of this eruption from the contagious pustular diseases, as well as from some of the secondary appearances of syphilis, is of considerable importance in practice, which renders it necessary to notice this genus. " It may be mistaken for pustular scabies, from which, however, it is distinguished by the pustules appearing and running their course independent of one another, some being on the decline whilst others are just appearing; and by never being mixed with intervening vesicles. There is no itching, but a stinging pain in Ecthyma."

The genus comprehends four species :

  1. E. *vulgare.*   3. E. *luridum.*
  2. E. *infantile.*   4. E. *cachecticum.**

SPECIES 1. ECTHYMA *vulgare.*

* Rayer objects to this arrangement, and proposes to divide the genus into two species — *acute* and *chronic Ecthyma;* and although I retain the classification of Dr. Willan, here adopted by Dr. Bateman, yet I am decidedly of opinion that Rayer's is preferable. T.

Syn. Ecpyesis Ecthyma, *a.* vulgare (*Good*) :
L'Ecthyma aigu (*Rayer*) : *Common Papulous Scall.*

This (Plate XLIII. fig. 1. of BATEMAN; Pl. 17. of THE ATLAS,) is the slightest form of the disorder, and consists of a partial eruption of small hard pustules, on some part of the extremities, or on the neck and shoulders, which is completed in three or four days. In the course of a similar period, the pustules successively enlarge, and inflame highly at the base, while pus is formed in the apex; and in a day or two more they break, pour out their pus, and afterwards a thinner fluid, which speedily concretes into brown scabs. " The progress of the pustules is attended with sharp stinging pains." In a week more, the pains, soreness, and inflammation subside, and the scabs soon afterwards fall off, leaving no mark behind.

This eruption commonly supervenes on a state of languor, of some continuance, with loss of appetite, irregularity of the alvine evacuations, and pains in the stomach or limbs. Young persons are principally subject to it, and children are sometimes affected with it, especially in the spring or summer, after being over-heated, or fatigued, or from disturbing the digestive organs by improper food. The constitutional derangement is not immediately relieved on the appearance of the eruption, but ceases before its decline. The use of gentle purgatives, in the early stage, and of the decoction of Cinchona, or of the Sulphate of Quinia, in combination with the diluted Sulphuric Acid, after the maturation of the pustules, appears to comprehend all that is requisite in regard to medicine. " Mercurial preparations, if exhibited so as to affect the habit, invariably aggravate the disease."

Species 2. Ecthyma *infantile.*
Syn. Ecpyesis Ecthyma, 6. Infantile (*Good*): *Infantile Papulous Scall.*

This species occurs in weakly infants, during the period of lactation, when an insufficient nutriment is afforded them. It sometimes appears after the first teeth are cut. The pustules are, in appearance, the same as those of the preceding species, and go through similar stages of progress, in the same time. But the disorder does not terminate here: fresh eruptions of phlyzacia continue to rise in succession, and to a much greater extent than in the E. vulgare, appearing not only over the extremities and trunk, but on the scalp, and even on the face; in which situation the pustules do not occur except, sometimes, in the fourth species of Ecthyma. Hence also the duration of the eruption is much greater than in the preceding species, being occasionally protracted for several months. Yet the patients usually remain free from fever, and the pain and irritation seem to be inconsiderable, except when a few of the pustules become very large and hard, with a livid base, and ulcerate to some depth : in this case, also, a slight whitish depression is permanently left on the seat of the pustule.

The principal means of cure will be found in

changing the nurse: and the advantages of better aliment will be aided by proper clothing and exercise, as well as by moderate alteratives, and by the Cinchona, the Sulphate of Quinia, or chalybeates.

SPECIES 3. ECTHYMA *luridum.*

Syn. Melasma (*Plenck, Linn. Vogel*): Ecpyesis Ecthyma, γ. Luridum (*Good*): L'Ecthyma chronique (*Rayer*): *Lurid Papulous Scall.*

The most obvious peculiarity of this variety of the phlyzacious pustule (Plate XLIII. fig. 2. of BATEMAN; Pl. 17. of THE ATLAS,) is the dark red colour of its base, which is likewise hard and elevated. But the pustules of Ecthyma luridum differ also from the two preceding varieties, in being of a larger size; and from the first variety, in the slow but long succession in which they arise, and in the extent of surface over which they spread, the face alone being, generally but not always, exempt from their occurrence. This form of the disease is most frequently seen in persons of an advanced age, who have injured their constitutions by hard labour, intemperance in the use of ardent spirits, and night-watching; and it is most severe in the winter season.

Under these circumstances, the pustules, as might be expected, are slow in healing. They break in the course of eight or ten days, and discharge a curdly, sanious, or bloody matter: the ulcerated cavities, extending beyond the original boundary, soon become filled with hard, dark scabs, and re-

s 3

main surrounded by a deep-seated hardness in the flesh, and dark inflamed borders, until the scabs are about to separate, — a period generally of several weeks, and sometimes of many months. The scabs are commonly firmly seated ; but if removed by violence, they are not speedily reproduced ; on the contrary, tedious ulcers, with callous edges and a sanious discharge, are often thus occasioned.

The treatment of this Ecthyma must be chiefly directed to the amendment of the constitution, by means of good diet, by rest, the occasional use of the warm bath, and by the Cinchona Bark, the Sulphate of Quinia, and tonic vegetable decoctions, internally. " Sea-bathing has been found to produce highly beneficial effects, as an adjunct to tonics ; and, when it cannot be obtained, nearly the same benefit may be procured from sponging the trunk of the body with tepid salt and water before getting out of bed in the morning."

A *symptomatic* Ecthyma, which bears a considerable analogy to the E. luridum, sometimes occurs during the cachectic state which follows the measles, and occasionally after the scarlet fever and small-pox. It is accompanied with a hectic fever, laborious respiration, and swellings of the glands ; and is attended with extreme pain and soreness, sometimes with a tedious sloughing, in some of the larger pustules, which, in children particularly, are productive of considerable distress. The phlyzacia arise in various parts of the extremities and trunk, and are highly inflamed at their bases, even after the scabbing takes place. " Mr. Plumbe remarks, that when this symptomatic Ecthyma follows measles and other eruptive fevers, ' it is usually seen in its very earliest stage about the waist. It exhibits a few reddened and slightly-elevated spots, covered with a very thin lamina of cuticle, which readily separates. Some of these have a minute elevation in their centre resembling a vesicle : the latter, however, contains nothing like the serum of the herpetic vesicle, but a glutinous fluid, which dries upon the part, and forms with the morbid cuticle an elevated scab of a conical form, the basis of which, in a day or two, is surrounded by a small inflamed areola.' "* The whole duration of the disease is often from one to two months ; and the majority of patients struggle through it.

Opiates and the warm bath afford essential relief to the distressing irritation occasioned by this affection ; and a liberal use of the Cinchona Bark, where it can be administered, and of other vegetable tonics, both shortens and alleviates the disease.

SPECIES 4. ECTHYMA *cachecticum,* CACHECTIC PAPULOUS SCALL.

An extensive eruption of phlyzacious pustules (Plate XLIV. of BATEMAN ; Pl. 17. of THE ATLAS,) not unfrequently occurs, in connection with a state of cachexia, apparently indicative of the operation of a morbid poison in the habit : for the phænomena of the disease much resemble some of the

* Plumbe on Diseases of the Skin, 2d edit. p. 440.

s 4

secondary symptoms of syphilis, and it is often treated as syphilitic.*

The disorder usually commences with a febrile paroxysm, which is sometimes considerable. In the course of two or three days, numerous scattered pustules appear, with a hard inflamed base, sometimes first on the breast, but most commonly on the extremities : and these are multiplied day after day by a succession of similar pustules, which continue to rise and decline for the space of several weeks, until the skin is thickly studded with the eruption, under various phases. For, as the successive pustules go through their stages of inflammation, suppuration, scabbing, and desquamation, at similar periods after their rise, they are necessarily seen under all these conditions, at the same time; the rising pustules exhibiting a bright red hue at the base, which changes to a purple or chocolate tinge, as the inflammation declines, and the little laminated scabs are formed upon their tops: when these fall off, a dark stain is left upon the site of the pustules. In different cases the eruption varies in its distribution : it is sometimes confined to the extremities, where it is either generally diffused, or clustered in irregular patches; but it frequently

---

* A disease indicated by copper-coloured blotches, the size of a sixpence, on the nates and the soles of the feet, arising from a syphilitic taint in the parents, is not uncommon in London. It closely resembles this species of Ecthyma; but requires the aid of Mercury for its removal. I have generally removed it with small doses of Hydrargyrus cum Creta; and minute doses of the Oxymuriate of Mercury in Decoction of Elm Bark, or Emulsion of Bitter Almonds. T.

extends also over the trunk, face, and scalp. The pustules which occupy the breast and abdomen are generally less prominent than those on the face and arms, contain less matter, and terminate rather in scales than in scabs.

The febrile symptoms are diminished, but not removed, on the appearance of the eruption; for a constant erethism or hectic continues during the progress of the disease. It is accompanied by great languor, and by much depression both of the spirits and muscular strength. " Delirium occasionally attends the febrile state; and in habits with a predisposition to insanity, the depression of spirits is occasionally so great as to lead to suicide." The fever is throughout accompanied by headach and pains of the limbs, which are described as rheumatic; and by restlessness and impaired digestion, with irregularity of the bowels. There is commonly also some degree of ophthalmia, affecting both the conjunctiva and the tarsi; and the fauces are the seat of a slow inflammation, which is commonly accompanied by superficial ulcerations.

The duration of this disease seems to be from two to four months, in the course of which time, by the aid of the vegetable tonics, Cinchona, Sarsaparilla, Serpentaria, &c., with Antimonials, and the warm bath, the constitution gradually throws off the morbid condition which gives rise to it. The administration of Mercury is not necessary to its cure, nor does it appear to accelerate recovery.*

* The success attending the treatment pursued in the following case induces me to publish it. The patient, an unfortunate German gentle-

The diagnosis between this disease and the syphilitic Ecthyma, is to be collected rather from the
history of the disease, than from the prominent
symptoms: unless, indeed, we are ready to concede

---

man, having fallen ill of a fever, lost all his employment, and became so
depressed both in mind and body, that he sunk into a cachectic state of
habit, and was soon attacked with Ecthyma. He applied to me on the
27th of June 1828, two months after the disease had made its appearance. The eruption covered the whole of the body, with the exception
of the hands and the face. The stinging sensation was also accompanied
with itching, or rather a tingling, which induced an involuntary desire
to scratch, by which not only the heads of the pustules were rubbed off,
but large portions of skin, in some places two inches in length, and
nearly an inch in breadth, were torn off by the action of the nails during
sleep. Those pustules which had run their course had left dark stains
behind, so that the greater part of the entire skin was covered with these
and the crusted pustules. When the pustules were early rubbed, black
dots of effused blood remained. The thighs were covered with ulcers.
The body was greatly emaciated; there was a regular evening exacerba-
tion of fever; the tongue was clean, but red and glazed; the skin felt
dry and harsh; and the patient stated that the delirium attending the
fever and the depression of mind had driven him nearly to commit
suicide. The bowels were irregular. The following medicines were
ordered:

℞. Pulv. Jacobi veri gr. iij,
　　Extracti Stramonii gr. ½,
　　———— Hyosciami gr. iij: fiat pilulæ ij,
horâ somni omni nocte sumendæ.

℞. Magnesiæ Sulphatis ʒj,
　　Magnesiæ Carbonatis ℈j. M.
pulvis omni mane sumendus.

℞. Acidi Sulphurici diluti fʒxij,
　　Tincturæ Opii fʒiv. M.
Sumantur ℧ xx ex cyatho Decocti Corticis Cinchonæ Cordi-
　　foliæ ter quotidie.

When the irritation is severe, let the surface be sponged with hot
water. Let the diet be milk, fresh-boiled vegetables, and a moderate
share of mutton under-cooked.

July 5th. Few fresh pustules have appeared; and the dark colour of
the blotches is much less. The new pustules contain a mild pus. The
bowels are regulated by the aperient; and although the fever still re-

to a recent writer, that this and similar affections are never the result of the true syphilitic poison.*

---

turns every evening, yet the delirium which attended it has disappeared. He feels, occasionally, as if a cloud had settled upon him, and cut him off from all external impressions. The tingling and irritation are less, and return only in paroxysms, during which he still tears off large portions of the skin.

Cont. medicamenta.

> ℞. Plumbi Acetatis ℨss.
> Acidi Hydrocyanici f℥iij,
> Ung. Cetacei ℥iij. M.

Fiat unguentum partibus cutis nudatis applicandum.

18th July. He is much better in every respect, and the irritation is so much abated, that he can now sleep without excoriating his body. He is gaining both in flesh and strength.

Perstet in usu medicamentorum.

August 2d. The eruption is nearly gone, and the skin is regaining its natural aspect. He complains of watchfulness, and great depression; but the want of employment and distress of mind seem to be counteracting the full powers of the medicines.

Cont. medicamenta.

> ℞. Camphoræ gr. v,
> Pulveris Jacobi gr. iij.
> Extracti Hyosciami gr. iij.

Fiant pilulæ ij, h. s. sumendæ.

From this time the disease rapidly abated, and having discontinued his applications to me, he became fat, got into health, and is now in Germany.

The chief feature in the treatment of this case is the combination of the Tincture of Opium with the diluted acid, and the external application of the Hydrocyanic Acid, in the form of ointment. The Opium thus combined seemed to allay the irritation, and certainly augmented the tonic power of the Bark; whilst the ointment deadened the insupportable itching which had caused the tearing of the skin. T.

* See Part First of an "Essay on the Venereal Diseases, which have been confounded with Syphilis," by Richard Carmichael, President of the Royal College of Surgeons, Dublin, 1814. If I rightly comprehend this interesting but unfinished work, Mr. Carmichael maintains that the true syphilitic ulcer is followed exclusively by *one eruption*, the scaly copper blotch, or Lepra venerea, described by Dr. Willan. It will now scarcely be doubted, indeed, that the above-mentioned Ecthyma, and

Dr. Willan mentioned a *topical* variety of Ec-thyma, occurring on the hands and fingers of work-men employed among metallic powders, which I have never seen. As it commences in a vesicular form, and, though afterwards purulent, produces irregular patches of thin scabs, it should perhaps have been referred to Eczema.*

Books which may be consulted on Ecthyma.

CAZENEVE et SCHEDEL, Abrégé Pratique des Maladies de la Peau, 8vo.
HEWSON, North American Med. and Surg. Journal, 1826.
PLUMBE on Diseases of the Skin, 2d edit. 1827.
RAYER, Traité des Maladies de la Peau, 8vo. 1827.
WILLAN, on Ecthyma, 4to.

GENUS IV. VARIOLA.†

Syn. Euphlogia (*Rhazes*): Empyesis variola (*Good*): Kindspocken (*Germ.*): Petite verole, Picote (*F.*): Jedrie (*Arabic*): Perse ummay (*Tam.*): Bur-riseetle (*Duk.*): Pédumma (*Tel.*): Kruevan (*Bali*): Másoorikeh (*Sans.*): Kelumbuan-Chuchur (*Malay*): Gootry (*Bengalese*): *Smallpox.*

Def. AN ERUPTION OF PUSTULES APPEARING FROM THE THIRD TO THE FIFTH DAY OF A CONTAGIOUS FEVER, AND SUPPURATING FROM THE EIGHTH TO THE

---

some other eruptive diseases of an analogous character, are frequently, though erroneously, pronounced syphilitic; but we are not prepared by the present state of the evidence, to limit the syphilitic eruptions thus narrowly.

* A topical variety of Ecthyma is produced by Tartar Emetic oint-ment, and similar irritating applications. T.

† Variola, quasi parvi vari.

TENTH: THE FEVER IS FREQUENTLY ACCOMPANIED
WITH VOMITING AND PAIN WHEN PRESSURE IS MADE
ON THE EPIGASTRIUM.

" *Variola,* as the definition states, is a contagious
disease. The eruption attacks at once the skin and
mucous membrane of the lungs and of the primæ
viæ. The eruptive fever is not always evident: it
generally lasts about forty-eight hours: and towards
its close, in infants, vomiting and convulsions are
not unfrequent. The eruption appears first on the
face, thence it extends to the neck, the trunk of
the body and the arms, and lastly to the lower
extremities. It first shows itself in the form of
small, hard, red papulæ, which, about the fifth day,
become whey-coloured pustules, with a depression
in the centre, which is filled up on the eighth day.
The pustules are now spherical, turgid with pus,
and inflamed at the base. About the eleventh day
they spontaneously ooze out pus, which concretes
to a crust; this, after some time, falls off, and
leaves the skin of a reddish colour, which remains
for many days before the natural colour is restored.
The real variolous pustule is cellular, and tied
down in the centre*; the vesicle of Chickenpox,

---

* Dr. Macartney of Dublin thus describes the change of structure to
produce the smallpox pustule: " In the cellular tissue which surrounds
the villi of the cutis, a few blood-vessels are perceived determining to a
central point, and producing a pimple, which feels hard under the finger:
this acuminates; but by degrees the acumination disappears, and the
centre of the pimple is depressed, and a cellular, radiated arrangement
ensues. These cells, as well as the depression, are formed by the adhe-
sion of the central portion of the membrane to an inflamed part of the
villous surface of the true skin." T.

M. Velpeau, after many experiments on both the dead and living body,

Varicella, is a single cell; the pustule of modified·
smallpox is converted into a small horny button,
on the fifth day from the coagulation of the gelatinous lymph.

"Authors have spoken of two species of smallpox,
the *distinct,* and the *confluent ;* but these insensibly
run into one another, and are mere varieties of the
same disease, depending, in a great degree, on the
habit of body of the individual who is infected.
Another variety, of less frequent occurrence, is
marked by the pustules remaining solid throughout:
this has been termed the *Warty smallpox,* Variola
verrucosa.*

" The eruption, when the disease is produced by
infection, follows the general fever; when it is
communicated by inoculation, there is a local affection often extending beyond the points where the
virus was introduced previous to the formation of
the general fever.   It cannot be communicated by
the blood of an infected person, as was proved by
the experiments of Sutton the inoculator.

" VAR. 1. VARIOLA *discreta,* DISTINCT SMALLPOX
(ATLAS, Pl. XVIII.)   The fever, in this variety of
smallpox, is of the inflammatory type.   It is accompanied with pains of the back, limbs, and loins;

---

to discover the seat of the pustules, was led to conclude that they are
developed chiefly in the sebaceous follicles. — Bull. de Soc. Philomath.
Juin, 1825.   T.

* Dr. John Thomson has endeavoured to prove that variola and varicella are merely modifications of the same disease, and communicable
by the same virus.   As the question is still *sub judicè,* I refrain from
hazarding my opinion regarding it in this place.   T.

sometimes with pains, also, of the chest, dryness of the fauces, and coma. In the first day of the fever, the rigors are more or less prolonged, alternated with bursts of heat, general uneasiness, nausea, or a diminished appetite. On the second day, the nausea increases; arising sometimes to bilious vomiting: and, at the same time, a bilious diarrhœa supervenes. A little before the eruption appears, children are seized with an epileptic fit; sometimes there is only a convulsive twitching of the mouth and face: the face is flushed; the eyes are impatient of light; and there is an uneasy sense of oppression at the epigastrium, which is greatly increased by pressure.

Roseola sometimes accompanies or follows the first appearance of the eruption. The pustules at first are small, red, isolated, distinct points like fleabites; appearing on the face and hairy scalp, and extending over the whole body. This eruption is spread not only over the skin, but over the mucous membrane of the mouth, pharynx, and bowels, the prepuce and the vulva. On the second or third day of the eruption, the little tubercles are found to contain a fluid at the apex, which is, at first, nearly colourless and semitransparent, and depressed in the centre; but the eighth day they become spherical, and evidently contain pus. The face swells, and as it subsides, about the tenth or eleventh day, the hands and feet swell and continue swelled for some days; and if not in excess, these swellings are to be regarded indicative of a favourable termination of the disease. When the pustules are few, they become opaque, white, and ultimately yellow; and acquire the size of a small pea. After this, the shrinking and incrustation take place, as has been already described; the swelling of the face and other parts disappears; and a slight salivation and a hoarseness which accompany the swelling subside. The crusts generally drop about the fourteenth day of the disease, and leave brownish red blotches: convulsions seldom succeed to distinct smallpox.

The fever, in mild cases, seems to disappear after the eruption is fully formed; but it returns about the eleventh day; and when the pustules are numerous, is sometimes more severe than the eruptive fever.

VAR. 2. VARIOLA *confluens*, CONFLUENT SMALL-POX, (ATLAS, Pl. XVIII.) differs from the distinct, in the greater severity of all the symptoms. The head-ache is violent, often accompanied with delirium. The eruption appears earlier, and is less elevated above the surface of the skin than in the distinct Variola; the pustules are more numerous, sooner suppurate; and on the face they become flat and run together, or are confounded with one another, and have no inflamed base. The face continues longer swelled than in the other variety, and when the incrustation takes place, the whole visage seems as if covered with a single scab. The fever assumes the typhoid character, and a peculiar odour exhales from the surface of the body of the patient.

As the desquamation proceeds, the fever increases; and, sometimes, coma suddenly supervenes, and carries off the patient in forty-eight hours. In this form of the disease, when the crusts fall, they are replaced by scales which not unfrequently ulcerate and leave pits.

" The salivation is more distressing than in distinct Smallpox, the mouth and pharynx being covered with pustules: sometimes the cornea is the seat of a pustule, and becomes opaque, if it be not destroyed by the ulceration. Petechiæ appear in this form of the disease, when the strength fails. The matter in the pustules, instead of becoming yellow, remains white, or becomes brown, or almost black; and is, sometimes, mixed with extravasated blood. It is occasionally so acrid as to ulcerate deeply, and to destroy even the bones of the face. When the pustules are about to be confluent, the purging is often considerable; the stools are very fœtid, and, sometimes, mixed with blood.

" From these descriptions it will readily appear that the prognosis is not difficult in Smallpox. Danger is always to be dreaded in the confluent form of the disease; and a fatal termination is, too frequently, the consequence when the fever assumes, early, a typhoid character.

" Authors have pointed out several anomalous forms of Smallpox: but in a practical point of view these distinctions are of little value.

Measles and Smallpox, now and then, occur si-

T

multaneously*; but, in general, in such cases, the
progress of the Smallpox is arrested until the
Measles run their course, and then it goes on in
the usual way.

" Confluent Smallpox is apt to leave behind it
very distressing consequences when it does not prove
fatal : blindness ; a predisposition to inflammatory
affections ; obstructions of the glands ; and pulmonary consumption, are not unfrequently the
result of its attack. Dr. Tauchou has been led,
by the result of many dissections, to attribute the
fatal cases of Variola to inflammation of the arteries,
extending from those on the surface to the large
arterial trunks and the heart.

" The treatment of Variola is modified by the variety of the disease. The first object is to moderate
the eruptive fever, so as to diminish the number of
the pustules : but this is to be done with as little
expense of strength as possible. Free exposure to
cool air ; mild purging ; and, if the fever run high,
the cold effusion, are the most efficient means to
keep down, if not cut short the fever. In India,
the cold bath has been employed by the natives
during the eruptive fever, from time immemorial,
with the best effects. Whether the bath be used,
or the patient be merely exposed to cold air, it must

---

* M. Delagarde has lately recorded a case of this kind in the 13th
volume of the Medico-Chirurgical Transactions. Vogel mentions a case
in which Smallpox attacked the right side of the body and Measles the
left side, at the same time, the boundary of each disease being perpen-
dicular, drawn through the middle of the body.   T.

always be kept in mind that the patient should suffer no sensation of cold. His complaining of cold should be sufficient to terminate the use of that remedy; indeed, in every instance, caution is requisite. If the stomach is loaded, it ought to be relieved by an emetic; after which, saline draughts given in a state of effervescence, with Nitre, or the Tartarized Soda, will be found very serviceable. A moderate catharsis is necessary in the eruptive fever of Small-pox; but much purging is injurious. Sydenham recommended the free use of the lancet; but there are few cases that require or can warrant blood-letting in the eruptive fever of Variola : and if it be not admissible in the commencement of the disease, it is much less so in the termination. Local blood-letting, however, either by leeches or cupping, is useful, when the head is severely affected.

" Nothing is more useful in the eruptive fever than the use of the tepid bath, under 96.° It diminishes the febrile irritation; in general subdues the convulsions which precede the appearance of the eruption, particularly if the bowels have been previously cleared. The use of opiates is at least doubtful in the eruptive fever, unless there is reason to expect the confluent form of the disease : the pain is more effectually subdued, and the heat of surface diminished, by the use of the warm bath; and this is equally useful, after the maturation of the pustules, for removing the crusts, and lessening the risk of pitting.

" In the milder form of the disease, the patient

need not be confined to bed; but in the confluent
state, he should use no exertion, nor even be allowed to sit up longer than to have his bed made.
In this form of the disease also, cathartics are
recommended to be cautiously employed, and given
only to remove costiveness; but whatever may be
the form of the disease, cathartics are always beneficial in the eruptive fever. I have found six or
eight grains of Calomel, with twelve or fourteen
of the powder of Jalap, form the best purgative, if
the patient be not under six years of age : but this
should not be repeated, the saline purges being the
most useful after the intestines have been once
freely evacuated. If the strength does not admit
of purging, the bowels should be regulated by mild
cathartic clysters. The cold effusion is not admissible in the secondary fever; which, on the
contrary, in the confluent form of the disease,
requires the free exhibition of Wine, Bark, and
other tonics. The Sulphate of Quinia, in the solution of the Confection of Roses, acidulated with
the diluted Sulphuric Acid, is an excellent form of
tonic in confluent smallpox.

" It has long been a practice in eastern countries
to pierce the pustules with fine needles, in order to
lessen the violence of the secondary fever; for a
similar reason, M. Serres has lately observed that
Lunar Caustic applied to the pustules on the fourth
day, arrests their progress, cuts short the secondary
fever, and prevents pitting. The pustule is directed
to be opened, and the caustic introduced into it on
the end of a silver stilet. I have had no expe-

rience of the utility of this practice. I have seen much advantage derived from washing the surface during the state of incrustation of the pustules in Confluent Variola with a dilute solution of Chloruret of Soda of Labarraque. It lessens the acrimony of the pustular discharges, takes off the fœtor of the eruption, and, in every circumstance connected with the scabbing process, greatly mitigates the sufferings of the patient.

" When the fever has actually assumed the typhoid character, Cinchona Bark, or Sulphate of Quinia, Opium, and Wine are alone to be depended on. The empty vesicles are filled; the pus assumes a healthy appearance; and petechiæ disappear. When vomiting is a troublesome symptom, and the ordinary effervescing draughts fail to relieve it, Camphor, with the Tincture of Calumba in a glass of sound Sherry, may succeed. If a retrocession of the eruption occur, the best remedies are Wine and Opium; and the Semicupium should be employed, in conjunction with blisters, to the wrists and fore-arms.

" It may naturally be expected that I should here notice not only the effects of Vaccination as a preventive of Smallpox; but, also, that I should enter into the question of the nature of those cases which have occurred after vaccination, and have received the appellation ' modified Smallpox.' I shall notice the first under Vaccinia: and briefly state my opinion of the second under Varicella."

Genus V. SCABIES.*

Syn. Κνησμὸς; Ψωρα (*Gr.*): Pruritus (*Auct. var.*):
Psora (*Linn. Cull. Parr*): Ecpyesis Scabies (*Good*):
Phlysis scabies (*Young*): die Krätze (*Germ.*):
La Gale (*F.*): Nekeb (*Arab.*): Chéringoo (*Tam.*):
Chieri (*Malayalie*): Ghejæ (*Tel.*) Khārisht (*Duk.*):
Pāmā (*Sans.*): *The Itch.*

Def. A CONTAGIOUS ERUPTION OF MINUTE
PIMPLES, PUPULAR, VESICULAR, PUSTULAR, OR IN-
TERMIXED ACCORDING TO CIRCUMSTANCES; APPEAR-
ING CHIEFLY BETWEEN THE FINGERS, AND IN THE
FLEXURES OF THE JOINTS; TERMINATING IN SCABS,
AND ACCOMPANIED WITH INTOLERABLE ITCHING.

This troublesome disease, which, from its affinity
with three orders of eruptive appearances, Pustules, Vesicles, and Papulæ, almost bids defiance
to any attempt to reduce it to an artificial classifi-

---

* The Greek term *Psora* has been very generally, but incorrectly,
adopted for the designation of this disease, in consequence of the example of some of the early translators, who considered Scabies (quasi
scabrities) as synonymous with ψωρα, which, we have already seen,
(page 10. *note*) was universally employed by the Greeks as denoting a
scaly or scurfy disorder of the skin, more rough than Lichen, but less
scaly than Lepra. They did indeed occasionally use the term, in conjunction with the epithet ἑλκωδης, or *ulcerating*, as applicable to a pustular disease, apparently the Impetigo: but when used alone, it invariably implied the dry scaly or scurfy tetter, Psoriasis. (See above, ord. ii.
gen. 2.) Sir John Pringle, indeed, after noticing this inaccuracy,
concludes that the itch was probably unknown, or at least uncommon,
in ancient times. "The Psora of the Greeks has generally been supposed to be the Itch; but, as this does not appear by the description
they give of it, I should conclude," &c. (On Diseases of the Army,
part iii. chap. 5.)

cation, is not easily characterised in few words. An extreme latitude in the acceptation of the term has indeed been assumed by writers, from Celsus downwards; and no distinct or limited view of the disease has been given, until near our own times. Celsus has included other forms of pustular disease among the different species of Scabies; and some of the earlier writers, after the revival of learning, considered almost all the eruptions, to which the skin is liable, as modifications of this disease : even our countryman Willis, to whom the contagious nature of true Scabies, as well as its specific remedy, was well known, has not sufficiently separated it from some other pustular and pruriginous affections.*

The SCABIES, or *Itch*, appears occasionally on every part of the body, the face only excepted†; but most abundantly about the wrists and fingers, the axillæ, the fossa of the nates, and the flexures of the joints. ‡

Among the various forms which the disease

---

* See Celsus, lib. v. cap. 28.; Plater, de Superfic. Corp. Colorib. cap. 17.; Hafenreffer, Nosodoch. lib. i. cap. 15.; Willis Pharmac. Rational, part i. § iii. cap. 6.

† Some German authors, however, assert that they have seen Pustular Scabies affecting the ears and face. In one child who came under my care, it affected the side of the face, near the ear. T.

‡ " *Scabies* est pustularum *purulentarum*, vel *saniosarum*, vel *papularum siccarum*, ex duriore et rubicundiore cute, eruptio, — pruritum, sæpe quoque dolorem, creans, — interdum totum corpus, facie excepta, invadens, — sæpissimè tamen solos artus externos, digitorum imprimis interstitia, occupans." — Callisen, Syst. Chirurg. Hodiern. i. § 824.

assumes, four have been distinguished, with considerable accuracy, by the vulgar, who have, indeed, the most ample opportunities of becoming acquainted with its character: and to these they have given the epithets of *rank, watery, pocky*, and *scorbutic* Itch. Their subdivision was adopted by Dr. Willan, with the appropriate titles,

1. S. *papuliformis*.
2. S. *lymphatica*.
3. S. *purulenta*.
4. S. *cachectica*.

The characteristics of these species, and the diagnosis between them and the papular, vesicular, and pustular eruptions, which they resemble, I shall endeavour to point out; but must admit, at the same time, that the practical discrimination, in many of these cases, is more difficult than in any other Order of cutaneous disease.

SPECIES 1. SCABIES *papuliformis*, RANK ITCH.

Syn. Scabies sicca (*Plenck*): Ecpyesis scabies, *var. α.* papularis (*Good*).

This species consists of an extensive eruption of minute itching vesicles, which are slightly inflamed and acuminated, resembling papulæ when examined by the naked eye. They commonly arise first about the bend of the wrist and between the fingers, or in the epigastrium; on which parts, as well as about the axillæ and nates, and in the flexures of the upper and lower limbs, they are at all periods most numerous, and often intermixed with a few phlyza-

cious pustules, containing a thick yellow matter.
The itching is extremely troublesome in this form
of Scabies, more especially when the patient becomes warm after getting into bed.   The appearance of the disease is modified by the abrasion of
the tops of the vesicles and pustules, and even of
the rest of the skin, by the frequent scratching,
which cannot be withheld.   Hence long red lines
are here and there left, and the blood and humour
concrete upon the vesicles into little brown or
blackish scabs.

These mixed appearances, partly belonging to
the disease, and partly the result of abrasion by
the nails, being in some measure common to the
Lichen and Prurigo, where much scratching is
also often employed, render the diagnosis of the
Scabies papuliformis more difficult than it would
be from the mere similarity in the form of the
eruption.   But, as the most effectual remedy for
the Scabies is detrimental in the latter affections,
the distinction is of great practical importance.

With respect to the eruption itself, the unbroken
elevations in Scabies papuliformis, when carefully
examined, are found to be vesicular, and not papular; they are often intermixed, in particular situations, with pustules; and, when they break, are
succeeded by scabs: whereas in Lichen, the papulæ
terminate spontaneously in scurfy exfoliations.   In
Scabies, the eruption is unconnected with any constitutional or internal disorder, and the itching is
severe: but in Lichen there is commonly some

constitutional affection, and a tingling sensation, as well as itching. The highly contagious nature of Scabies will, in many cases, have already manifested itself, and removed all doubt; for the Lichen is not thus communicable.*

In Prurigo, the papulæ, where no friction has been applied, retain the usual colour of the skin, are commonly flatter, or less acuminated, and present no moisture or scab, except when their tops have been forcibly abraded; they are not particularly numerous in the parts above mentioned; and they remain long distinctly papular, without showing any contagious property. The eruption which I have called Lichen *urticatus*, and which often occurs in weakly children, and exhibits a troublesome series of papulæ, sometimes intermixed with minute vesicles, bears a close resemblance to Scabies, especially when it has been of some continuance. But the first appearance of these spots, in the shape of inflamed wheals, not unlike the inflammation produced by the bites of gnats, —their subsequent papular or vesicular appearance, with little or no surrounding inflammation,—the intermixture of these two states of the eruption, —the ultimate formation of a minute globular brown scab, which is set firm in the apex of each elevation, —and the absence of contagion, will serve as diagnostic marks.

---

* See the quotation from M. Lorry, *supra*, p. 12., *note.*

SPECIES 2. SCABIES *lymphatica*, WATERY ITCH.

This form of Scabies (Plate XLV. of BATEMAN; Pl. 18. of THE ATLAS,) is distinguished by an eruption of transparent vesicles, of a considerable size, and without any inflammation at their base. They arise in succession, with intense itching, chiefly round the wrists, between the fingers, on the back of the hands, and on the feet and toes: they often occur also about the axillæ, the hams, the bend of the elbows, and fossa of the nates, where they are intermixed with pustules: but they do not frequently appear, like the papuliform species, over the breast and epigastrium, nor on the thighs and upper parts of the arms.

In a day or two the vesicles break, and some of them heal, under the little scab that concretes upon them. But others inflame, and become pustules, which discharge at length a yellow matter, and extend into small ulcerated blotches, over which a dark scab is ultimately formed: so that, during the progress of the eruption, all these appearances are intermixed with one another; the vesicles, and pustules, the excoriated blotches discharging pus, the minute dry scabs, and the larger ones succeeding the ulceration, may be observed at the same time. This circumstance constitutes one of the points of diagnosis between this and other vesicular diseases. Of these, however, the Herpes and Eczema, especially the latter, are alone liable to be confounded with Scabies lymphatica:

whole family, it appeared on the side of the face in one of the children, a boy of six years of age." In several of these situations, where the pustules are largest and numerous, they coalesce, and form irregular blotches, which ulcerate to some extent, with hardness and elevation of the surface; but at length hard and dry scabs are formed, which adhere tenaciously for a considerable time.

The majority of the cases of Scabies purulenta, which I have seen, have occurred in children between the age of seven years and the period of puberty; and in them it not unfrequently assumes this form.

The Scabies purulenta cannot be easily mistaken for Impetigo, when it occurs in patches, in consequence of the large size, the greater prominence, and comparatively small number of its pustules; not to mention the absence of the intense itching, and of contagion, in the former. * From the Porrigo favosa affecting the extremities, it will be distinguished chiefly by its situation about the fingers, axillæ, fossa natum, and flexures of the joints, and by the total absence of the eruption from the face, ears, and scalp; by the nature of the discharge;

---

* Sauvages has described a variety of Scabies, which he terms *herpetica* (spec. 4.); Herpes, in his language, as in that of many other writers, signifying the same with Impetigo in the nomenclature of Dr. Willan. " Cognoscitur ex signis herpetis et scabiei simul concurrentibus, in amplos corymbos coeuntibus, papulis pruriginosis, rubris, quæ squamas albas, farinaceas deponunt." But this termination in branny scurf, and the commencement in papulæ, point out the eruption as a Lichen, probably the L. circumscriptus.

and by the thin, hard, and more permanent scab, which succeeds, instead of the soft, elevated, semi-transparent scab, formed by the viscous humour of the favi.

The only other disease, with which the Scabies purulentà has any affinity, is the Ecthyma: but the hard, elevated, vivid red or livid base, which surrounds the pustules of Ecthyma, — their slow progress both towards maturity and in the course of suppuration, — the deep ulceration, with a hard raised border, and the rounded, imbedded scab, which succeed, — as well as the distinct and separate distribution of them, — will afford the means of discrimination; to which the incessant itching, and the contagious property of Scabies, may be added.

SPECIES 4. SCABIES *cachectica.* This variety of Scabies exhibits, in different parts of the body, all the appearances which belong to the three foregoing species. It is occasionally also combined with patches resembling Lichen, Psoriasis, or Impetigo, especially in adults, or young persons approaching the term of puberty; whence it assumes an ambiguous character. In several instances, this form of Scabies has been obviously contagious in its double character; and after the scabious affection has disappeared, the impetiginous patches have remained for some time, in a drier form, and yielded very slowly to medicine. For although this form of Scabies does not so readily spread by contagion, it is much more obstinate under the use of remedies, than the preceding.

Another peculiarity of the S. cachectica is, that it often originates, independently of contagion, in weakly children, and also in adults, when the constitution is suffering under some chronic malady, or is debilitated by some previous acute disease*: and, however it is produced, it is liable to return at intervals, especially in the spring and autumnal seasons, after it has been to all appearance cured.†

A severe degree of this ambiguous and combined form of Scabies is often seen in this country, in persons who have come from India: I have chiefly had occasion to observe it in children brought from that country. The eruption is exceedingly rank and extensive, sometimes even spreading to the face, and giving a more dark and sordid hue to the skin than the ordinary Scabies: the intermixture of patches of an impetiginous character, where the pustules become confluent, is considerable. It is extremely contagious, and also obstinate in its resistance to the operation of remedies.‡

---

* Sir John Pringle observed, that, in military hospitals, the patients often became the subjects of itch after the crisis of fevers. Loc. cit. p. iii. cap. 8.

† " Quædam est etiam ejus species, quæ quanquam in ipso corpore non genita sit, sed aliunde advecta, quanquam et consuetis remediis primo sanata fueret, tamen non cessat redire semel vel bis quotannis." Heberden, Commentar. Perhaps the Scabies herpetica of Sauvages may include some of these cases of S. cachectica.

‡ Bontius, in his work De Medicina Indorum, lib. iii. cap. 17., has described this severe disease, under the appellation of " Herpes, seu

Another violent form of Scabies is excited by the contact of dogs, cats, hogs, and other animals, affected with *mange*. (Plate XLVI. fig. 2. of BATE-MAN.) This also extends over the whole body, the pustules being very rank and numerous, and more inflamed and hard at the base than in the ordinary eruption; the general surface of the skin is also rough, and of a browner hue; and the excoriations and abrasions more extensive, in consequence of the more violent and irresistible application of the nails.

The most ordinary cause of Scabies is contagion; the virus being communicated by the actual contact of those already affected with it, or of their clothes, bedding, &c. especially where there is much close intercourse. It seems to originate, however, in crowded, close, and uncleanly houses; and is, therefore, extremely prevalent in work-houses, jails, and hospitals, where the means of great cleanliness are not easily obtained, and is mostly seen among the families of the poor.* When the contagion has been introduced, however, into families, where every

---

Impetigo Indica," as frequent among the inhabitants of India, by whom it is denominated *Courap*, which is equivalent to our term *itch*. The cure of it, he says, is generally much neglected there, in consequence of a prevalent notion, that it renders a person secure from all violent diseases: yet the itching is severe and incessant, and so much abrasion is produced by scratching, that the linen often adheres to the excoriated parts, so as not to be removed without drawing blood. — This is the Scabies *Indica* of Sauvages, spec. 6.

* Plenck adds, "victu acri, salso, pingui nascitur. Hæc difficilius quam acquisitu curatur. *Doct. de Morb. Cut.* p. 42. T.

U

attention to cleanliness is enforced, it will frequently spread to all the individuals, children and adults, and continue, in spite of the utmost cleanliness, until the proper remedies are resorted to.

Some writers have ascribed the origin of the itch, in all cases, to the presence of a minute insect, breeding and burrowing in the skin; while others have doubted the existence of such an insect.* Both these opinions appear to be incorrect; and probably that of Sauvages is right, who considers the insect as generated only in some cases of Scabies, and therefore speaks of a Scabies *vermicularis,* as a separate species.†

The existence of such an insect, in some cases of Scabies, has been fully demonstrated; and, although never able to discover it in any patient myself, I have seen it, in one instance, when it had been taken from the diseased surface by another practitioner. In fact, it was first described by Abinzoar, or, as he is sometimes called, Avenzoar, a Hispano-Arabian physician of the twelfth century, and subsequently by Ingrassias of Naples, by Gabucinus, Laurence Joubert, and other writers of the fifteenth and sixteenth centuries, who are quoted by our countryman Moufet.‡ These writers describe the insects as *acari,* that is, very

* Dr. Heberden never saw any of these insects; and he was informed both by Baker and Canton, who excelled in the use of the microscope, that they had never been able to detect them. Loc. cit.

† Nosol. Method. loc. cit. spec. 11.

‡ See his " Theatrum Insectorum," printed in 1634, cap. 24. " de Syronibus, Acaris, Tineisque Animalium."

minute and almost invisible animalcula, burrowing under the cuticle, and exciting small pustules, filled with a thin fluid, and intense itching. Moufet states, that they do not reside *in* the vesicles or pustules, but *near* them; a remark which has been confirmed by Linnæus and Dr. Adams *, who ascertained that this acarus leaps; that they are not of the same genus with lice, which live exterior to the cuticle; — that they are similar to the acari, or *mites*, of cheese, wax, &c. but are called *wheal-worms* in man; — and that when they are pressed between the nails, a small sound is heard. Most of these points have been subsequently confirmed. The insects were accurately ascertained and figured (by the aid of the microscope) by Bonomo †, in 1683, whose account was afterwards published by Dr. Mead ‡. Schwiebe, Baker, and others: and Linnæus, De Geer §, Wichmann, &c. have since that period illustrated the subject of these Acari scabiei. ‖ The latest authors particularly confirm the observation of Moufet, that the insects are not to be found in the pustules, but in the reddish streaks or furrows near them, or in

* Observations, &c. p. 296.

† See his Letter to Redi —(Mr. Kirby remarks that his plates, as copied by Baker, are far from accurate) — also Miscel. Nat. Curios. ann. x. dec. 2.

‡ See Philosoph. Transact. vol. xxiii. for 1702.

§ De Geer's figure is the most correct; vide vol. viii. t. 5. f. 12. 14.

‖ See Linn. "Exanthemata Viva," 1757; — and Amœnit. Acad. vol. iii. p. 333., and vol. v. p. 95. — Wichmann, Aetiologie der Kraetze, Hanover, 1786; also in the Lond. Med. Journal, vol. ix. p. 28. — De Geer, Mémoires pour servir à l'Hist. des Insectes.

the recent minute vesicles : but I must acknowledge my own want of success to discover them in any of these situations.   I am disposed, therefore, to believe, that the breeding of these Acari in the scabious skin is a rare and casual circumstance, like the individual instance of the production of a minute Pulex in Prurigo, observed by Dr. Willan ; and that the contagious property of Scabies exists in the fluid secreted in the pustules, and not in the transference of insects.   " The opinions of Dr. Gales are in opposition to this idea, and strongly support the notion of a distinct animalcule.   His opportunities to ascertain this point at the Hospital of St. Louis were numerous, and he took every advantage of them.   He also produced the disease on himself by transferring the insect to his own skin.   Mr. Plumbe, also, states that he has seen great numbers of the insects extracted with the point of a needle. He supposes that the insect is unable to live in the fluid, which is the result of the irritation it induces; and therefore escapes from the vesicle."[*]

" Whatever may be the cause of the disease and the medium of its communication, it is very evident that the *same* virus will produce all the varieties of the disease ; and consequently these depend on the state of habit of the individual affected.   In one family which the editor attended, the four younger children had the purulent form of the disease ; and, in two of them, the pustules were mingled with

* Plumbe on Diseases of the Skin, 2d edit. p. 506.

disease and
ery evident
varieties of
end on the
d. In one
ur younger
ease; and,
ngled with

306.

There are few cases of Scabies which will not
yield to the steady employment of the Sulphur

* See Willis, Pharmaceut. Rational. part. ii. sect. iii. cap. 6.

† See Turner, de Morbis Cutaneis.

‡ Writers in general agree in asserting the greater facility of curing
the humid than the dry forms of Scabies. But under the term Scabies
sicca, it is obvious that they describe the Prurigo, and even some scaly
and furfuraceous eruptions, accompanied with itching, which are often
more difficult of removal than any variety of true Scabies. See Sauvages
and Sennert (loc. cit.), and Vogel, de curand. Hom. Morb.

u 3

ointment, continued a sufficient time, and rubbed
on the parts affected, nightly, with assiduity.   Five
or six applications are commonly sufficient for the
cure of the disease : but sometimes it is necessary
to persevere in the inunction for the space of a
fortnight, or even longer ; from which no detriment
ensues to the constitution.   " The quantity of the
Sulphur ointment to be used, and the mode of
using it, are of great consequence in the cure of
this disease.   I believe that if the whole body be
well rubbed over with it, and the patient be kept
in bed, in a flannel dress, for twenty-four hours, a
second application will seldom be necessary.   He
should immediately afterwards take a warm bath,
and cleanse the skin well with soap ; and be careful
not to put on his former clothes until they have
been several times fumigated with Sulphur."

The disgusting odour of the sulphur *, however,
has led practitioners to resort to various other stimulating applications ; some of which have been
recommended from ancient times, for the cure of
scabid and pruriginous eruptions.   Among these,
the root of the white Hellebore is possessed of con-

---

* Both the smell and sordid appearance of the Sulphur ointment may
be in a considerable degree obviated by the following combination :

℞ Potassæ Subcarbonatis ʒss,
   Aquæ Rosæ ʒj,
   Hydrargyri Sulphuretti Rubri ʒj,
   Olei Essentialis Bergamotæ ʒss,
   Sulphuris-sublimati
   Adipis Suillæ ā ā ʒix.   Misce secundum artem.

siderable efficacy, and may be applied in the form of the following ointment:

> R̥ Pulveris radicis Veratri albi Ʒjss.
> Hydrargyri præcipitati albi ʒj,
> Olei Citri Limonis fƷj,
> Adipis Ʒxiv.
>
> Tere ut fiat Unguentum, bis die utendum:

or in that of decoction. In the latter form I have generally found it advisable to employ a stronger decoction than that which is recommended in the Pharmacopœia of the College. Potass, in a state of deliquescence, was a favourite addition to these applications with Willis and his predecessors ; and Muriate of Ammonia, and some other saline stimulants, have been more recently used, and not without benefit.* , The strong Sulphuric acid, which was long ago recommended by Crollius, mixed with lard, in the proportion of fƷss. to Ʒj of lard, and applied by external friction, has also been employed † ; and it certainly possesses the recommendations of being inodorous and comparatively cleanly. But independently of its corrosive action on the patient's clothing, it has appeared to me to

---

* This salt, together with Hellebore, is said to constitute a part of a celebrated nostrum for Scabies, called the Edinburgh Ointment.

† See Hafenreffer de Cute, lib. i. cap. 14. The Sulphuric Acid was also recommended to be taken internally, as a remedy for Scabies, by Dr. Cothenius, who is said to have used it with success in the Prussian army, in 1756. See Edin. Med. Com. vol. i. p. 103. Dr. Albertus H. A. Helmich, of Berlin, also recommended it. The title of his treatise is, " Dissertatio Inauguralis Medica de usu interno Olei Vitrioli diluti in nonnullis Scabiei speciebus." But subsequent experience has not confirmed their reports.

be very uncertain in its effects. The Muriate of
Mercury, and the white precipitated oxide, are
very old remedies, and both possessed of considerable efficacy in the relief of Scabies. The testimonies in favour of the latter are very numerous. *
It seems particularly well adapted to the impetiginous form of the disease, which is liable to be
irritated by the more acrid applications. The Muriate has probably derived some of its remedial
character from its efficacy in the relief of Prurigo,
and other eruptions, accompanied by itching, with
little inflammation; but it is not altogether destitute of power in Scabies itself.

A committee of French physicians reported the
result of some experiments made with the root of
the Plumbago Europæa (pounded and mixed with
boiling oil) to the Medical Society of Paris; from
which they inferred, that it cured Scabies more
speedily than any other remedy. The third or
fourth inunction with this substance, they affirm, is
generally successful.† Several of the continental
writers recommend, in strong terms, the formula of
an " Unguentum ad Scabiem," prescribed by Jasser,
which directs equal parts of Sulphate of Zinc, Flowers
of Sulphur, and Laurel Berries, to be made into a

---

* See Willis, Vogel, Sauvages, Callisen, Heberden, &c. Prof. Selle
affirms, " Scabies è contagio externo maximè ex parte per solum merc.
præcip. albi usum tollitur." Med. Clin. 191. See also Fordyce, Frag-
menta Chirurgica. Turner, Treatise on Dis of the Skin, 4th edit. p. 58.
He combined it with Ol. Tart. per deliquium.

† See Mémoires de la Soc. Roy. de Médecine de Paris, tom. iii.; also
Lond. Med. Journal, vol. v.

liniment with Olive or Linseed Oil : " about the size of a bean is to be rubbed upon the palms of the hands every morning and night."*   From a few trials of this ointment, I am disposed to believe that it is possessed of considerable efficacy. " Dr. G. Pellegrini has extolled highly the external use of Conium, either the recent juice, or a solution of the extract, or a decoction of the dried plant. It is said to effect a cure in obstinate cases in five or six days. M. Derheims has found a solution of the Chloruret of Lime, in the proportion of ℥j to Oj of water, used twice or thrice a day, very beneficial. † The most cleanly method of treating Scabies is the Sulphur vapour baths."

Books which may be consulted on Scabies.

CAZENAVE et SCHEDEL, Abrégé pratique des Maladies de la Peau, 8vo. 1828.

ETMULLER, de Scabie programma, 1731.

HAFENREFFER, de Cute, 8vo.

HELMICH, de usu interno Olei Vitrioli diluti in nonnullis Scabiei speciebus, 4to. 1762.

KECK, de Scabie periodica, 1701.

LE ROUX, Traité sur la Gale, &c., 12mo. 1809.

PLENCK Doct. de Morbis Cutaneis, 8vo.

PLUMBE, on Diseases of the Skin, 2d edit. 1827.

RANQUE, Mém. et Obs. Cliniques sur un nouveau Procédé pour la Guérison de la Gale, 8vo. 1811.

RŒDERER, de Scabie, 1710.

TURNER, de Morbis Cutaneis, 4to.

ZIEGER, de Scabie artificiali, 1758.

* See Plenck, Doctr. de Morbis Cutaneis, p. 42.; Callisen, Syst. Chirurg. Hodiern.

† Journ. de Chim. Médicale, Decem. 1827.

Order VI.

VESICULÆ.

SYN. Die Wasserblattern (*German*): Vésiculeuses (*F.*): *Vesicles.*

Vesicles are small elevations of the cuticle, containing a transparent, serous fluid. After some time the fluid is often absorbed, and the cuticle separates in the form of white scales, occasionally in the form of thin, yellow, laminated crusts. The vesicles are sometimes seated upon an inflamed base, at others they exhibit only a very slight inflammatory areola. They appear on every part of the body. In general, vesicular diseases are not dangerous, and terminate by resolution: at other times, the fluid exudes and concretes into yellowish crusts. The Order comprehends seven genera:

1. VARICELLA.
2. VACCINIA.
3. HERPES.
4. RUPIA?
5. MILIARIA.
6. ECZEMA.
7. APHTHA?

GENUS I. VARICELLA.*

Syn. Crystalli, Variola spuria (*Auct. var.*): Variola lymphatica (*Auct.*): Variola pusilla (*Heber-*

* Since the introduction of vaccination, considerable differences of opinion have existed among medical practitioners, respecting the cha-

den): Exanthema varicella (*Parr*): Synochus varicella (*Young*): Cottamillie ummay (*Tam.*): Kāngé niāhn (*Duk.*): Cottāmillie (*Tel.*): Pittāmásoorikā (*Sans.*): Ravaglione (*Ital.*): die unächten Kindspocken (*German*): Vérole volante (*F.*): *Chicken-pox, Water jags.*

Def. ACCOMPANYING A SLIGHT ATTACK OF FEVER, AN ERUPTION OF SEMI-TRANSPARENT, GLABROUS VE-SICLES, SELDOM PASSING INTO SUPPURATION ; BUT, ON THE THIRD DAY, BURSTING AT THE TIP, AND CONCRETING INTO PUCKERED SCABS.

This disease is usually so slight as to require little medical assistance; but, in consequence of the resemblance of the eruption, under some of its varieties, to the Smallpox, it becomes important, as a point of diagnosis, to establish its character with accuracy.

Although its appearances were described by writers on the Smallpox three centuries ago, under the appellation of *Crystalli* *, and at a period not

---

racter of the eruption, which has occasionally appeared, after exposure to variolous infection, in persons previously vaccinated, some denominating it Chicken-pox and others Smallpox. The most careful observers must have admitted the difficulty of establishing a decisive distinction in many of these cases. A series of interesting observations which have lately been made at Edinburgh, have led the ingenious Prof. John Thomson to believe that the Chicken-pox itself is in fact a modified Smallpox. While the question is still *sub judice,* I leave Varicella in its nosological seat; but many facts crowd upon my own recollection, which incline me to believe that this suggestion will ultimately prove to be correct. See Edin. Med. and Surg. Journ. Oct. 1818.

* Vidus Vidius (De Crystallis) and Ingrassias (De Tumor. præt. Nat. lib. i. cap. 1.) describe these crystalli as white shining pustules, containing lymph, nearly as large as lupine seeds, and attended with little fever; " suntque hæ minus periculosæ (i. e. than smallpox), et sæpe citra notabilem febrem infantes prehendunt."

much later, it had even acquired popular names in Italy, France, and Germany, and subsequently in England * ; yet most of the systematic writers, down to the latter part of the eighteenth century, seem to have looked upon it as a variety of small-pox.   Dr. Heberden, in the year 1767, pointed out the distinction with his accustomed perspicuity.† Perhaps, however, as this learned physician, in his posthumous work, continues to designate the disease by the term Variola ‡, the employment of the same term by the systematic writers above alluded to, with the epithets *volatica*, *spuria* §, &c. cannot be deemed evidence, that they actually

* We have the testimony of many writers, in proof of the prior discrimination of the vulgar, in respect to this eruptive disease. Sennertus, who was a professor at Wittemberg, at the commencement of the seventeenth century, observes, in his treatise on smallpox and measles, that there are other varieties, " præter communes variolas et morbillos," which are popularly known, in Germany, by the terms *Schaffsblattern* (sheep-pox or vesicles), or *Windpocten* (wind-pox). See his Med. Pract. lib. iv. cap. 12. And Riverius, who was professor at Montpellier at the same period, speaks of the eruption as familiarly known by the common people, in France, by the appellation of *Verolette*. See his Prax. Med. cap. ii. In Italy it was called *Ravaglione*. Ibid.—See also Diemerbroeck, De Variolis et Morbis, cap. 2.—Fuller, in his " Exanthematologia," published in 1730, describes the eruption, and acknowledges himself indebted to the nurses for the appellation. " I have adventured to think," he says, " that this is that which *among our women* goeth by the name of chicken-pox," p. 161. And it is mentioned familiarly, at Edinburgh, in 1733, as " the bastard or chicken-pox." See Edin. Med. Essays, vol. ii. art. 2. At Newcastle, and in Cumberland, it is popularly known by the name of *Water-jags.* See Dr. Wood, in the Med. and Phys. Journal, vol. xiii. p. 58. *note.*

† See his paper in the Med. Transact. of the Coll. of Phys. vol. i. art. xvii.

‡ " *Variolæ pusillæ.*" See his Comment. de Morbis, cap. 96.

§ See Vogel, de cognoscend. et cur. Hom. Morb. § 128. (edit. 1772.) Burserius, Inst. Med. vol. ii. cap. 9. § 305. Sauvages, however, actually makes it a *species* of Variola, class. iii. gen. ii. spec. i. V. *lymphatica.*

considered the disease as generically the same with Smallpox. "This opinion, as Dr. Bateman has remarked in a note, p. 299, has been revived by Dr. John Thomson; and his opinion, founded on his own extensive observation, is supported by many practitioners. Dr. Thomson has remarked that the Variola, in its undoubted form, and Varicella, appear under the same exciting causes, whether the persons have been vaccinated or not: thence he concludes that they are merely varieties of the same disease. He also affirms that persons exposed to contagion of Varicella have had Variola, and that Varicella appears only in those whose constitutions have been modified by previous Variola or Vaccinia. But I believe vesicular Varicella has never been communicated by inoculation; that children have Chicken-pox, in the mildest form, who have not had Smallpox; but who afterwards take it. One might understand how Smallpox occurring a second time might be moderated into Chicken-pox: but, if the majority of children have Chicken-pox, in the mild form, under all circumstances, I cannot accord in the opinion of Dr. Thomson. Besides, Varicella has never been prevented by vaccination."

The three principal species of Chicken-pox were well known a century ago, and were distinguished in the north of England, and in some counties of Scotland, by the popular names of Chicken-pox, Swine-pox, and Hives. Dr. Willan proposed to distinguish them, according to the different forms of the vesicles, by the epithets,

1. V. *lentiformis.*
2. V. *coniformis.*
3. V. *globularis.**

SPECIES 1. VARICELLA *lentiformis*, LENTICULAR VARICELLA.

Syn. Varicella lymphatica (*Plenck*).

This species (Plate XLVII—VIII. of BATEMAN; Pl. 18. of THE ATLAS,) appears, on the first day of the eruption, " and is seldom preceded by any febrile symptoms," in the form of small red protuberances, not exactly circular, but tending to an oblong figure, having a nearly flat and shining surface, in the centre of which a minute transparent vesicle is speedily formed. " When the febrile symptoms which precede the eruption are obvious, they consist of rigor, lassitude, short cough, broken sleep, loss of appetite, and occasionally wandering pains. The best idea which can be given of the early appearance of the eruption is, that it resembles what might be conceived to be the effects of sprinkling boiling water over the skin from a loose brush." On the second day of the eruption, the vesicle is filled with a whitish lymph, and is about the tenth of an inch in diameter. On the third day it has undergone no change, except that the lymph is straw-coloured. On the fourth day, those vesicles which have not been broken begin to subside, and

* See his treatise " On Vaccine Inoculation," published in 1806, sect. vii.—Dr. Fuller, above quoted, described these three varieties under the appellations of Chicken-pox, Swine-pox, and Crystalli, p. 161—3.

are puckered at their edges. Few of them remain entire on the fifth day; but the orifices of several broken vesicles are closed, or adhere to the skin, so as to confine a little opaque lymph within the puckered margins. On the sixth day, small brown scabs appear universally in place of the vesicles. The scabs, on the seventh and eighth days, become yellowish, and gradually dry from the circumference towards the centre. On the ninth and tenth days they fall off, leaving for a time red marks on the skin, without depression. Sometimes, however, the duration of the disease is longer than the period just stated, as fresh vesicles arise during two or three successive days, and go through the same stages as the first. " The vesicles are seldom very numerous, and generally distinct; they appear first on the back, whereas the pustules of Smallpox appear first on the face, neck, and breast. The vesicles, even when they suppurate, rarely pit, or leave cicatrices."

SPECIES 2. VARICELLA *coniformis:* CONOIDAL VARICELLA: SWINE-POX.

Syn. Varicella verrucosa (*Plenck*)* : Pemphigus variolodes (*Frank.*): Variola lymphatica (*Sauv.*): Hydrachnis (*Cusson*): Vérolette (*F.*): Ravaglio (*Ital.*): *Swine-pox, Water-pox.*

In this form of the disease the vesicles rise suddenly, and have a somewhat hard and inflamed

* In Plenck's description of this species, he says, " supra cutem prominentes, in quibus nullus humor est," l. c. p. 52. T.

border: they are, on the first day of their appearance, acuminated, and contain a bright transparent lymph : " the eruption is sometimes preceded by a slight cough, restlessness, and fever." On the second day they appear somewhat more turgid, and are surrounded by more extensive inflammation : the lymph contained in many of them is of a light straw-colour. On the third day, the vesicles are shrivelled; those which have been broken exhibit, at the top, slight gummy scabs, formed by a concretion of the exuding lymph. Some of the shrivelled vesicles, which remain entire, but have much inflammation round them, evidently contain on this day whitish purulent fluid : every vesicle of this kind leaves, after scabbing, a durable cicatrix or pit. On the fourth day, thin dark-brown scabs appear intermixed with others, which are rounded, yellowish, and semi-transparent. These scabs gradually dry and separate, and fall off in four or five days. A fresh eruption of vesicles usually takes place on the second and third day; and, as each set has a similar course, the whole duration of the eruptive stage in this species of Varicella is six days. " In some cases minute red tubercles rise, but do not pass into vesicles, and disappear." The last formed scabs are not separated till the eleventh or twelfth day. " When the febrile symptoms are severe, and after the scabs fall off, in places subjected to pressure, inflammation and ulceration take place, sometimes; but there is no sloughing, as in Smallpox. These ulcers generally leave pits."

SPECIES 3. VARICELLA *globularis* : HIVES.

Syn. Varicellæ duræ ovales (*German*).

In this species the vesicles are large and *globular*, but their base is not exactly circular. There is an inflammation round them, and they contain a transparent lymph, which, on the second day of the eruption, resembles milk-whey. On the third day, the vesicles subside, and become puckered and shriveled, as in the two former species. They likewise appear yellowish, a small quantity of pus being mixed with the lymph. Some of them remain in the same state till the following morning; but, before the conclusion of the fourth day, the cuticle separates, and thin blackish scabs cover the bases of the vesicles. The scabs dry and fall off in four or five days.

Some degree of fever generally precedes the eruption of all the species of Varicella for a couple of days, which occasionally continues to the third day of the eruption. This is sometimes very slight, so that it is only recollected, as having been previously indicated by fretfulness, after the eruption appeared.* " The eruption usually commences on the breast and back, appearing next on the face and scalp, and lastly on the extremities. It is attended, especially in children, with an incessant tingling or itching, which leads them to scratch off

---

* Dr. Heberden observes, " These pocks come out in many without any illness or previous sign."—But Dr. Willan states, " I do not remember to have seen any case of Varicella without some disorder of the constitution." Loc. cit.

x

.the tops of the vesicles; so that the characteristics
of the disease are often destroyed at an early period.
Many of the vesicles thus broken and irritated, but
not removed, are presently surrounded by inflammation, and afterwards become pustules, containing thick yellow matter. These continue three or
four days, and finally leave pits in the skin."

The eruption is sometimes preceded, for a few
hours, by a general erythematous rash. It is usually fullest in the *conoidal* form of Varicella, in
which the vesicles are sometimes coherent, or seated
close together, but seldom confluent.* The incidental appearance of pustules, just mentioned,
among the vesicles, sometimes occasions a doubt
respecting the nature of the eruption. The following circumstances, however, if carefully attended
to, will afford sufficient grounds of diagnosis.

The " vesicle full of serum on the top of the
pock," as Dr. Heberden expresses it, on the first
day of the eruption; — the early abrasion of many
of these vesicles;—their irregular and oblong form;
—the shriveled or wrinkled state of those which
remain entire, on the third and fourth day, and the
radiating furrows of others, which have had their
ruptured apices closed by a slight incrustation; —
the general appearance of the small scabs on the
fifth day, at which time the Smallpox are not at the
height of their suppuration,—sufficiently distinguish
the eruption of Varicella, from the firm, durable,

* See Dr. Willan's treatise. A case of confluent chicken-pox, illustrated by a coloured engraving, was published by Mr. Ring, in the Med.
and Phys. Journal for 1805, vol. xiv. p. 141.

and slowly-maturating pustules of smallpox. Dr. Willan also points out a circumstance, which is very characteristic; *viz.* " that variolous pustules, on the first and second day of their eruption, are small, *hard*, globular, red, and painful: the sensation of them to the touch, on passing the finger over them, is similar to that which one might conceive would be excited by the pressure of small round seeds under the cuticle. In the Varicella almost every vesicle has, on the first day, a hard inflamed *margin ;* but the sensation communicated to the finger, in this case, is like that from a round seed, flattened by pressure."

Dr. Willan remarks likewise, that, as the vesicles of the Chicken-pox appear in succession during three or four days, different vesicles will be at once in different states of progress: and if the whole eruption, on the face, breast, and limbs, be examined on the fifth or sixth days, every gradation of the progress of the vesicles will appear at the same time. But this circumstance cannot take place in the slow and regulated progress of the Smallpox.

When the globular vesicles of the Hives appear (and they are occasionally intermixed both with the lenticular and conoidal vesicles), they afford a ready distinction from the Smallpox, to the pustules of which they bear little resemblance.

There is a variety of Smallpox, which is occasionally produced by variolous inoculation, and which has usually appeared where vaccination had only partially influenced the constitution: this commonly dries up on the sixth or seventh day, with out maturation. But the small, hard, tubercular form of this eruption is sufficiently distinct from every form of the vesicles of Chicken-pox.

It is unnecessary to say any thing respecting the treatment of Varicella; since nothing in general is requisite beyond an attention to the state of the bowels, and abstinence from animal diet for two or three days.

From some experiments made, in his own family, by an eminent surgeon, and from others performed at the Smallpox Hospital, it appears, that Varicella is communicable by inoculation with the lymph of the vesicles;—that it may be introduced while the constitution is under the influence of vaccination, without impeding the progress of the latter, or being itself interrupted; — that Smallpox, inoculated during the eruptive fever of Varicella, proceeds regularly in its course, without occasioning any deviation in that of the latter; — but that, when variolous and varicellous virus is inserted at the same time, the smallpox proceeds through its course, while that of the chicken-pox is in a great degree interrupted.* But the experiments have not been sufficiently numerous to warrant the accuracy of these general conclusions.

Books which may be consulted on Varicella.

CAZENAVE et SCHEDEL, Abrégé pratique des Maladies de la Peau, 8vo.
HEBERDEN, Med. Trans. of Col. of Phys., vol. 1. xvii.
RAYER, Traité des Maladies de la Peau, 8vo.
RING, Med. and Phys. Journ. vol. xiv.
THOMSON, Dr. J., on Varioloid Diseases, 8vo.
WILSON on Febrile Diseases.

* See Dr. Willan's Treatise on Vaccination, pp. 97—103.

GENUS II. VACCINIA. COW-POX.

Syn. Variola vaccina (*Jenner*): Vaccina (*Auct. var.*): Exanthema vaccina (*Parr*): Synocha vaccina (*Young*): Emphlysis vaccinia. γ. Inserta (*Good*): Pāssuvoo ummay (*Tamul*): Gȳke seetlā (*Dukanie*): Avoummā (*Tellingoo*): Ghoomāsoorikeh (*Sanscrit*): *Inoculated Cow-pox.*

Def. A CIRCULAR, SEMI-TRANSPARENT PEARL-COLOURED VESICLE, CONFINED TO THE PLACE OF PUNCTURE: DEPRESSED IN THE CENTRE; SURROUNDED WITH A RED AREOLA; CONCRETING INTO A HARD DARK-COLOURED SCAB AFTER THE TWELFTH DAY.

This disease appears naturally upon the teats of the cow, from which it is transferred to the human species; either by natural inoculation, when the milkers have chopped hands; or artificial, by inserting the virus, on the point of a lancet, under the skin. It appears on the day after that on which the inoculation took place, in the form of a small, hard tubercle, which about the fourth day has assumed the character of a small, semi-transparent pearl-coloured vesicle, with a circular or somewhat oval base; and with the upper surface, until the end of the eighth day, more elevated at the margin than in the centre, and with the margin itself turgid, shining, and rounded, so as to extend a little over the line of the base. This vesicle is filled with clear lymph, contained in numerous

x 3

little cells, that communicate with one another. After the eighth or ninth day, from the insertion of the virus, it is surrounded by a bright red, circumscribed areola, which varies in its diameter, in different cases, from a quarter of an inch to two inches, and is usually attended with a considerable tumour and hardness of the adjoining cellular membrane. This areola declines on the eleventh and twelfth day; the surface of the vesicle then becomes brown in the centre; and the fluid in the cells gradually concretes into a hard rounded scab, of a reddish-brown colour, which at length becomes black, contracted, and dry, but is not detached till after the twentieth day from the inoculation. "In the agglutinising process, the cells become gradually consolidated; and the fluid having become hard, a scab is formed, beneath which a small portion of the villi of the cutis is removed, and the loss of this causes the mark peculiar to the mild and regular vesicle." It leaves a permanent circular cicatrix, about five lines in diameter, and a little depressed, the surface being marked with very minute pits or indentations, denoting the number of cells of which the vesicle had been composed.*

A vesicle, possessing these characters, and passing through these regular gradations, whether accompanied by any obvious disorder of the constitution or not, was supposed effectually and per-

---

* See Dr. Willan's Treatise on Vaccination, p. 9.

manently to secure the individual from the danger, and almost universally from the contagion, of small-pox.* " This opinion, however, must be taken with great modification; and even Dr. Jenner himself, before his death, had reason to be satisfied that Smallpox may occur after the most perfect vaccination. Whether this depends on what has been termed the variolous diathesis, we shall not attempt to determine. In some instances it may depend on pre-occupation of the skin by some cutaneous eruption, overlooked by the vaccinator; for it is a well-known fact, that the presence of Herpetic or Psoriasitic eruptions will impede the constitutional influence of Vaccinia; and thence the propriety of early vaccination. It cannot, nevertheless, be denied that Smallpox has existed as an epidemic in many parts of Great Britain since Cow-pox was introduced; but it is satisfactory, in reviewing the history of these epidemics, to find, that of those persons who were attacked with Smallpox who had not been vaccinated, the proportion of deaths was as one in four; whilst of those who had undergone vaccination, the proportion was not one in four

* After so many years from the promulgation of the discovery, although this truth does not remain in full force, yet the very exceptions to it (and what result of human research is free from exceptions?) may be said, without a solecism, to corroborate it. For, in the very small number of cases (such as that of the son of Earl Grosvenor) where an *extensive* eruption of Smallpox has occurred subsequent to vaccination, the controlling influence of the Cow-pox has been invariably and strikingly manifested, by the sudden interruption of the Smallpox in the middle of its course, and the rapid convalescence of the patient.

hundred and fifty.   It is sufficient if Vaccinia
can modify smallpox so as to moderate its violence; the hope of eradicating it can scarcely be
entertained."

It is requisite that the vaccinator should attend
to the *irregular* appearances, which are produced
either by the insertion of matter, that is so far
corrupted or deteriorated, as to be incapable of
exciting the perfect disease, or by the inoculation
of proper lymph, under certain circumstances of
the habit, which interfere with its operation, and
which will be mentioned presently.

There is no uniform appearance which is characteristic of imperfect vaccination — on the contrary, three varieties of irregularity have been
noticed ; namely, pustules *, ulcerations, and vesicles of an irregular form.   The *pustule*, which is
sometimes produced instead of the proper vaccine
vesicle, is more like a common festering boil, occasioned by a thorn, or any other small extraneous
body, sticking in the skin, according to Dr. Jenner;
and it throws out a premature efflorescence, which
is seldom circumscribed.†   It is, as Dr. Willan
has stated, of a conoidal form, and raised upon a
hard inflamed base, with diffuse redness extending

---

* The pustules here mentioned occur on the inoculated part.   Those
pustules, which appeared over the body, in the first experiments with
the vaccine virus made, *in the Smallpox Hospital*, by Dr. Woodville, and
which puzzled the early vaccinators, were subsequently proved, and
admitted by Dr. Woodville himself, to have been genuine smallpox, the
result of the contagion of the place.

† See Med. and Physical Journ. vol. xii. for Aug. 1804, p. 98.

beyond it : it increases rapidly from the second to the sixth day, and is usually broken before the end of the latter, when an irregular, yellowish-brown scab succeeds.* *Ulceration,* occupying the place of a regular vesicle, must be obviously incorrect: it probably originates from the pustules just mentioned, which, on account of the itching that is excited, are sometimes scratched off at a very early period ; or, being prominent and tender, are readily injured and exasperated by the friction of the clothes, &c. †

With respect to the *irregular vesicles,* "which do not wholly secure the constitution from the Small-pox," Dr. Willan has described and figured three sorts. " The *first* is a single pearl-coloured vesicle, set on a hard dark red base, slightly elevated. It is larger and more globular than the pustule above represented, but much less than the genuine vesicle : its top is flattened, or sometimes a little depressed, but the margin is not rounded or prominent. The *second* appears to be cellular, like the genuine vesicle ; but it is somewhat smaller, and more sessile, and has a sharp angulated edge. In

---

* This premature advancement was pointed out by Dr. Jenner as a characteristic of the irregular pock, in his Paper of Instructions for Vaccine Inoculation, at an early period of the practice. He also justly remarked, in respect to the " soft, amber-coloured " scab, left by these pustules, that " *purulent* matter cannot form a scab so hard and compact as *limpid* matter," *loc. cit.* p. 99, *note.* In other words, that the scab succeeding a *pustule* is less hard and compact than the scab which forms on a *vesicle.*

† Dr. Willan, loc. cit.

the *first* the areola is usually diffuse, and of a dark
rose colour; in the *second*, it is sometimes of a
dilute scarlet colour, radiated, and very extensive,
as from the sting of a wasp.   The areola appears
(earlier) round these vesicles, on the seventh or
eighth day after inoculation, and continues more
or less vivid for three days, during which time the
scab is completely formed.   The scab is smaller
and less regular than that which succeeds the genuine vesicle; it also falls off much sooner, and,
when separated, leaves a smaller cicatrix, which is
sometimes angulated.   The *third* irregular appearance is a vesicle without an areola." *

There are two causes, as I have intimated above,
for these imperfect inoculations: the one is the
insertion of effete or corrupted virus, and the other
the presence of certain cutaneous eruptions, acute

* It appears to me that Mr. Bryce, in his able and valuable work on
the Inoculation of Cow-pox, has, without any sound reason, impugned
these observations upon the " irregular vesicles," and considered the
introduction of the terms as productive of " much injury to the true
interests of vaccination," and as serving " to screen ignorance or inattention in the operator:" and that his own reasoning, which amounts
to nothing more than a hypothetical explanation (and consequently an
admission) of the fact, is irrelevant.   He divides the vesicles " into constitutional and local ;" but at the same time admits, that he knows no
criterion by which they are to be distinguished, save the ultimate security against smallpox produced by the one, and not by the other.
(Appendix, No. x. p. 114. edit. 2d.) Now this is surely to screen ignorance
and inattention, by representing minute observation of appearances as
unnecessary.   However, he more than compensates for this error of
logic, by the ingenious test of a double inoculation, at the interval of
five or six days, which he has established, and which is sufficiently
mechanical to be employed without any unusual nicety of observation
or tact.

and chronic. "The period of life for vaccination is also of consequence. It is not easy to determine why the period of infancy between one and three months is the best, but experience has proved it to be so; and, probably, it is owing to the habit of the infant being more susceptible of that specific change which is requisite to secure it from small-pox than that of the adult. It cannot be owing to the degree of febrile action, for, in general, this is comparatively greatest in the adult."

The lymph of the vaccine vesicle becomes altered in its qualities soon after the appearance of the inflamed areola; so that, if it be taken for the purposes of inoculation after the twelfth day, or after the vesicle has suppurated, it frequently fails to produce any effect whatever; and in some cases it suddenly excites a pustule, or ulceration, in others an irregular vesicle, and in others Erysipelas. If taken when scabs are formed over the vesicles (as in the case of the pustules of Smallpox), the virus is occasionally so putrescent and acrid, that it excites the same violent and fatal disease, which arises from slight wounds received in dissecting putrid bodies.

Again, the lymph, although taken from a perfect vesicle on the sixth, seventh, or eighth day, may be so injured before its application, by heat, exposure to the air, moisture, rust, and other causes*, as to be rendered incapable of exciting the true disease.

* Dr. Willan, loc. cit.

"No lymph can be depended on which is taken after the eighth day. Many of the cases of Variola after Vaccinia may be attributed to the neglect of this rule. But although many practitioners are of opinion, that a vaccine vesicle produced by virus taken after the eighth day cannot be depended on for exciting that constitutional disease which is required for securing the habit from Smallpox; yet, Dr. George Gregory thinks this opinion fallacious, and that a vesicle produced by the scab, softened in water, is as good as one from recent six-day virus. The best period for taking the lymph is from the fifth to the ninth day. After this time it becomes opaque and purulent, and cannot be depended upon, either for producing a vesicle, or, if this occur, for securing the individual from Smallpox. The virus ought not to be kept in a heat exceeding 95° of Fahrenheit; for when this is the case, the most active vaccine virus loses its power of communicating the disease. When it is necessary to keep the virus, it should be preserved in little glass globules of the form or size of the marginal figure. The vesicle from which the virus is to be taken is punctured, and after warming the little ball, *a*, in the mouth to expel some of the air it contains, the open orifice *b*, should be applied to the exuded lymph, and the ball wetted: as the contained air cools, the lymph ascends into the tube and ball. The end of the tube *b*, must then be hermetrically sealed by melting it in the flame of a candle."

The most frequent causes of the imperfections in the progress of the vesicle, seem to be "dentition, inflammatory fever, or inflammation of any viscus, hooping-cough," the presence of chronic cutaneous eruptions, or the concurrence of eruptive fevers, or even of other febrile diseases. The chronic cutaneous diseases, which sometimes impede the formation of the genuine vaccine vesicle, have been described by Dr. Jenner under the ordinary indefinite term Herpes*, and Tinea capitis. In the more accurate phraseology of Dr. Willan, they are Herpes (including the *shingles* and *vesicular ring-worm*), Psoriasis, and Impetigo (the dry and humid *tetter*), the Lichen, and most frequently the varieties of Porrigo, comprising the contagious eruptions denominated by authors *crusta lactea, area, achores,* and *favi*. Dr. Willan thinks that the *Itch* and Prurigo likewise have the same influence.

Of the interference of the eruptive fevers, Measles, Scarlet fever, and Chicken-pox, with the progress of the vaccine vesicle, when they occur soon after vaccination, numerous instances have been recorded. The *suspension* of its progress, indeed, would be expected, under such circumstances, from the known facts respecting the reciprocal action of these contagious fevers on each other. But the action of the vaccine virus is not only suspended by these fevers, so that the vesicle is very slow in its pro-

---

* See his letter to Dr. Marcet, Med. and Phys. Journ. for May, 1803; also, the same Journal for Aug. 1804.

gress, and the areola not formed till after the fourteenth day or later, and sometimes not at all; but
it is occasionally rendered altogether inefficient.
Even Typhous fever, and the Influenza, have been
observed to produce a similar interruption in the
progress of vaccination.

Finally, the vesicle without an areola takes place
if the person inoculated have previously received
the infection of Smallpox, or if he be affected
with some other contagious disease during the progress of vaccination.*

Other irregularities may probably have occurred.
At all events, though the constitution is sometimes
fully secured from the infection of Smallpox, even
by the irregular vesicles; yet, as it is more commonly
but imperfectly guarded by such vesicles, the propriety of Dr. Jenner's caution is obvious; that,
" when a deviation arises, of whatever kind it may
be, common prudence points out the necessity of
re-inoculation."† " Dr. Jenner believed Smallpox
and Cow-pox to be varieties of the same disease;
an opinion which was said to have been confirmed
by some experiments lately made in Egypt, by
which it has been discovered, that by inoculating a
cow with Smallpox matter from the human body,
active vaccine virus is produced. Children were
successfully inoculated from this cow.‡ It is said,

---

* Dr. Willan, loc. cit.
† Paper of Instructions, before quoted.
‡ Letter from India. — London Medical Gazette, vol. i. p. 673.

however, that experiments of a similar nature made at the Veterinary College failed.

Books to be consulted regarding Cow-pox.

BRYCE's Practical Observ. on the Inoculation of Cow-pox, 8vo. 1809.
COXE's Pract. Obs. on Vaccination, 8vo. 1802.
JENNER, on the Variolæ Vaccinæ, 4to. 1800.
PRING, J., Treatise on Cow-pox, 2 vols. 8vo. 1805.
WILLAN, Treatise on Vaccine Inoculation, 8vo. 1806.

GENUS III. HERPES. *

Syn. Cytisma Herpes (*Young*): Lepidosis Herpes (*Good*): Neshr (*Arabic*): Zittermahl; die Flechte (*German*): Dartre (*F.*): *Tetter.*

Def. VESICLES IN DISTINCT, IRREGULAR CLUSTERS, UPON AN INFLAMED BASE, EXTENDING A LITTLE WAY BEYOND THE MARGIN OF EACH CLUSTER: ACCOMPANIED WITH TINGLING: CONCRETING INTO SCABS.

This appellation is here limited to a vesicular disease, which, in most of its forms, passes through a regular course of increase, maturation, and decline, and terminates in about ten, twelve, or fourteen days. The eruption is preceded, when it is

---

* Actuarius explains the origin of this term, as well as of the application of the word *fire*, to these hot and spreading eruptions. "*Herpes* dicitur eo quod videatur ἑρπειν (quod est *serpere* per summam cutem), modo hanc ejus partem, modo proximam occupans, quod semper, priore sanatâ, propinqua ejus vitium excipiat; non secus quam *ignis* qui proxima quæque depascitur, ubi ea quæ prius accensa erant, deficiente jam materiâ idoneâ, prius quoque extinguuntur." Meth. Med. lib. ii. cap. 12. — From this creeping progress, the disease was called *Formica* by the Arabians.

extensive, by considerable constitutional disorder, and is accompanied by a sensation of heat and tingling, sometimes by severe deep-seated pain, in the parts affected.* The lymph of the vesicles, which is at first clear and colourless, becomes gradually milky and opaque, and ultimately concretes into scabs : but, in some cases, a copious discharge of it takes place, and tedious ulcerations ensue. The disorder is not contagious in any of its forms.

The ancients, although they frequently mention Herpes, and give distinctive appellations to its varieties, have nowhere minutely described it : hence their followers have not agreed in their acceptation of the term. †   It has been principally

---

* This deep-seated pain has often been taken for Pleurisy, and, thence, we hear of cases of this disease cured by a critical eruption of Herpes.

† Although some of the ancients are more anxious to point out the nature of the morbid humour, to which the Herpes was to be imputed, than to describe its symptoms; yet, most of them speak of *small bullæ*, or *phlyctænæ*, as characteristic of the eruption.   See Galen de Tumoribus præt. Naturam ; — Aëtius, tetrab. iv. serm. ii. cap. 60. ; — Paulus, lib. iv. cap. 20. ; — Actuarius, lib. ii. cap. 12.)   Again, Scribonius Largus speaks of the most remarkable form of this vesicular disease (the Zoster, or shingles) as a species of Herpes. " Zona quam Græci ἑρπητα dicunt." See Scribon. de Compos. Medicam. cap. 13.   In describing the appearance of this disease, under the appellation of Ignis Sacer, Celsus has properly characterized it by the numerous and congregated eruption, the small and nearly equal size of the vesicles, and the situations which it most frequently occupies, &c. " Exasperatumque per pustulas continuas, quarum nulla alterâ major est, sed plurimæ perexiguæ : in his semper fere pus, et sæpe rubor cum calore est : serpitque id nonnunquam sanescente eo quod primum vitiatum est ; nonnunquam etiam exulcerato, ubi, ruptis pustulis, ulcus continuatur, humorque exit, qui esse inter saniem et pus videri potest. Fit maxime in pectore, aut lateribus, aut eminentibus partibus, præcipueque in plantis." Lib. v. cap. 28. § 4.

confounded with Erysipelas, on the one hand, and with Eczema, Impetigo *, and other slowly-spreading eruptions, on the other. But if the preceding character be well considered, the diagnosis between these affections and Herpes will be sufficiently obvious. From Erysipelas it may be distinguished by the numerous, small, clustering vesicles, by the natural condition of the surface in the interstices between the clusters, and by the absence of redness and tumefaction before the vesicles appear : and from the chronic eruptions just alluded to, by the purely vesicular form of the cuticular elevations in the commencement, by the regularity of their progress, maturation, and scabbing, and by the limitation of their duration, in general, to a certain number of days.

The ancient division of Herpes into three varieties, *miliary* (κεγχριας), *vesicular* (φλυκταινωδης), and *eroding* (εσθιομενος), may be properly discarded : for there appears to be no essential distinction between the first two, which differ only in respect to the size of the vesicles; and the last is incorrectly classed with Herpes, being perhaps referable rather to Pompholyx, or those larger bullæ, which arise in bad habits of body, and are followed by ill-conditioned ulcerations of the skin. † The va-

---

* See Dr. Cullen's definition of Herpes. Nosol. Method. gen. 147.

† Celsus, has, in fact, made this distinction between the Herpes esthiomenos, and the proper Herpes, ranking the latter under the head of Ignis sacer; a term which most of the translators of the Greek writings have incorrectly substituted for Erysipelas. Whereas he speaks of the H. esthiomenos as a deep-spreading ulcer, of a cancerous cha-

rious appearances of Herpes may be comprehended under the six following species : —

1. *H. phlyctœnodes,*	4. *H. labialis,*
2. *H. zoster,*	5. *H. prœputialis,*
3. *H. circinatus,*	6. *H. Iris.*

SPECIES 1. HERPES *phlyctœnodes,* MILIARY HERPES.

Syn. Herpes exedens, Serpigo (*Underwood*): Herpes miliaris (*Auct. var.*): Lepidosis Herpes. *a.* Miliaris (*Good*): die Flechte (*German*): Dartre phlycténoïde (*Alibert*).

This species of Herpes, (Plate XLIX. of Bateman; Pl. 20. of THE ATLAS,) including the miliary variety above mentioned, is commonly preceded by a slight febrile attack for two or three days. Small transparent vesicles then appear, in irregular clusters*, sometimes containing colourless, and sometimes a brownish lymph ; and, for

---

racter. "Fit ex his ulcus quod ἑρπηλα εσθιομενον Græci vocant, quia celeriter serpendo penetrandoque usque ossa, corpus vorat. Id ulcus inæquale est, cœno simile, inestque multus humor glutinosus, odor intolerabilis, majorque quam pro modo ulceris inflammatio. Utrumque, (*scil.* θηριωμα et ἑρπης) sicut omnis cancer, fit maxime in senibus, vel iis quorum corpora mali habitus sunt." Celsus de Medicina, lib. v. cap. 28. — See also Sennert. Pract. lib. v. part. i. cap. 17.

* Occasionally, however, the patches are of a *regular circular* form, and the areæ are completely covered with crowded vesicles: and in these cases the constitution is more violently disordered, and the heat and pain attending the eruption, amounting to a sensation of actual burning or scalding, are more severe, than in any other form of Herpes. To this variety of the eruption more particularly the popular appellation of *Nirles* has been given.

two or three days more, other clusters successively arise near the former. The eruption has no certain seat : sometimes it commences on the cheeks or forehead, and sometimes on one of the extremities; "sometimes about the fingers or toe-nails ;" and occasionally it begins on the neck and breast, and gradually extends over the trunk to the lower extremities, new clusters successively appearing for nearly the space of a week. It is chiefly the more minute or miliary variety which spreads thus extensively; for those which, at their maturity, attain a considerable size and an oval form *, seldom appear in more than two or three clusters together; and sometimes there is only a single cluster. The included lymph sometimes becomes milky or opake in the course of ten or twelve hours; and about the fourth day, the inflammation round the vesicles assumes a duller red hue, while the vesicles themselves break, and discharge their fluid, or begin to dry and flatten, and dark or yellowish scabs concrete upon them. These fall off about the eighth or tenth day, leaving a reddened and irritable surface, which slowly regains its healthy appearance. As the successive clusters go through a similar course, the termination of the whole is not complete before the thirteenth or fourteenth day.

* One of Alibert's best plates contains a representation of a vesicular disease of the face and neck, which might appear to be referable to this species of Herpes ; but, from his description of the disease, it is obviously a case of Pompholyx. He calls it " Dartre phlycténoïde confluente." See his plate 23.

The disorder of the constitution is not immediately relieved by the appearance of the eruption, but ceases as the latter proceeds. The heat, itching, and tingling in the skin which accompany the patches as they successively rise, are sometimes productive of much restlessness and uneasiness, being aggravated especially by external heat, and by the warmth of the bed.

The predisposing and exciting causes are equally obscure. The eruption occurs in its miliary form, and spreads most extensively, (sometimes over the greater portion of the surface of the body) in young and robust people, who generally refer its origin to cold. But it is apt to appear, in its more partial forms, in those persons who are subject to headachs, and other local pains, which are probably connected with derangements of the chylopoietic organs.

The same treatment is requisite for this as for the following species. "When this disease appears in children, Dr. Underwood recommends the expressed juice of Sium *nodiflorum* *, Creeping Water Parsnep." From one to four or five table-spoonfuls mixed with one or more spoonfuls of new milk may be given three times a day, according to the child's age and the state of its stomach, regulating the bowels. In obstinate cases, Hydrargyrus cum Creta will be found useful: and as a

---

* Dr. Underwood terms it *aquaticum*, which is the old name of Morison. It is common in rivulets, flowering in July and August. Underwood on the Diseases of Children, 8th edit. 8vo. p. 182.   T.

local application, the Unguentum Picis. Should the vesicles ulcerate, Solution of Sulphate of Zinc will be found useful; whilst the little ulcers may be touched with Butter of Antimony. Decoction of Sarsaparilla is a useful alterative.

SPECIES 2. HERPES *zoster* *, SHINGLES.

Syn. Zoster (*Pliny*): Zona ignea (*Hoffmann*): Dartre *phlycténoïde en Zone*, — Herpes *phlyctenoides Zonæformis* (*Alibert*): Le Zone Ceinture dartreuse (*F.*): die Fevergürtel (*German*): Zona (*Russell*): Erysipelas Zoster (*Sauv.*): Shingles.

This form of the eruption (Plate L. of Bateman; Pl. 20. of THE ATLAS,) which is sufficiently known to have obtained a popular appellation, the *Shingles* †, is very uniform in its appearance, follow-

* Ζωστηρ, Ζωνη, *a belt*. These terms have been applied to this form of Herpes, from the situation which it always occupies on the trunk of the body. It has been called simply *zoster* (see Plin. Nat. Hist. lib. xxvi. cap. 11.), and *zona*, or *zona ignea*, &c. by different writers; and its symptoms may be recognized, as I have stated above, in the first species of *sacer ignis*, described by Celsus. The disease has been described with different degrees of accuracy, by Tulpius (Obs. Med. lib. iii. cap. 44), Hoffmann (Med. Syst. Rat. tom. iv. part. i. cap. 13. § 6. & obs. 6.), De Haen (De Divis. Febrium, p. 112, &c.), Callisen (Syst. Chirurg. Hod. tom. i. p. 424.), Burserius Inst. Med. Pract. tom. ii. cap. 3.), and others. Sauvages has included it under two genera, with the appellations of Erysipelas *zoster* and Herpes *zoster*. (Nosol. Method. class. iii. gen. 7. & class. i. gen. 7.) Dr. Cullen has classed it with the former disease under the title of Erysipelas *phlyctænodes*; but at the same time expresses a doubt of the propriety of this classification. (Nosol. Meth. gen. xxxi. spec. 2.)

M. Alibert has given an indifferent representation of Herpes zoster, plate 24., under the title of "Dartre phlycténoïde en zone."

† Is this a corruption from the Latin *Cingulum*? Johnson held the

ing a course similar to that of Smallpox, and the other exanthematic fevers of the nosologists. It is usually preceded for two or three days by languor and loss of appetite, rigors, headach, sickness, and a frequent pulse, together with a scalding heat and tingling in the skin, and shooting pains through the chest and epigastrium. Sometimes, however, the precursory febrile symptoms are slight and scarcely noticed, and the attention of the patient is first attracted by a sense of heat, itching, and tingling, in some part of the trunk, where he finds several rèd patches of an irregular form, at a little distance from one another, upon each of which numerous small elevations appear, clustered together. These, if examined minutely, are found to be distinctly vesicular; and, in the course of twenty-four hours, they enlarge to the size of small pearls, and are perfectly transparent, being filled with a limpid fluid. The clusters are of various diameter, from one to two, or even three inches, and are surrounded by a narrow red margin, in consequence of the extension of the inflamed base a little beyond the congregated vesicles. During three or four days, other clusters continue to arise in succession, and with considerable regularity; that is, nearly in a line with the

---

affirmative: and it seems not less distinctly deducible from this word, than the vulgar terms *quinsey* and *megrim*, from their Greek roots *cynanche* and *hemicrania;* except that the latter had received a previous corruption by the French, in *esquinancie* and *migraine*, from which we doubtless took our words.

first, extending always towards the spine at one extremity, and towards the sternum, or linea alba of the abdomen, at the other, most commonly round the waist like half a sash, but sometimes like a sword-belt across the shoulder.* " Instead of the trunk, the clusters sometimes beginning on the loins or the nates, extend, in an oblique direction, down the thigh to the knee."

While the new clusters are appearing, the vesicles of the first begin to lose their transparency, and on the fourth day acquire a milky or yellowish hue†, which is soon followed by a bluish, or livid colour of the bases of the vesicles, and of the contained fluid.   They now become somewhat confluent, and flatten or subside, so that the outlines of many of them are nearly obliterated.   About this time they are often broken, and for three or four days discharge a small quantity of a serous fluid ; which at length concretes into thin dark

---

* " Hac tamen perpetua lege," says De Haen, " ut ab anteriore parte nunquam lineam albam, nunquam à postica spinam, transcenderent." (De Divis. Febrium, p. 112.) This observation, however, is not without exceptions ; although the rarity of the occurrence probably gave rise to the popular apprehension, which is as old as Pliny, that if the eruption completed the circle of the body, it would be fatal. " Zoster appellatur, et enecat, si cinxerit." (Plin. loc. cit.) I have seen the clusters extend across the linea alba in front ; and Turner asserts, that he has more than once observed it to surround the body. (On Dis. of the Skin, chap. v. p. 80.) Dr. Russell (De Tabe glandulari, hist. 33.) and Tulpius (Obs. Med. lib. iii. cap. 44.), also contradict the affirmation of Pliny.

Plenck says, " Sub umbilico et in regime ischiadica usque ad genua hunc morbum vidi. Doctrina de Morbis Cutaneis. Viennæ, 1783. p. 28. T.

† Can the fluid be now regarded sero-purulent?   T.

scabs, at first lying loosely over the contained matter, but soon becoming harder, and adhering more firmly, until they fall off about the twelfth or fourteenth day. The surface of the skin is left in a red and tender state; and where the ulceration and discharge have been considerable, numerous cicatrices or pits are left.

As all the clusters go through a similar series of changes, those which appeared latest, arrive at their termination several days later than the first; whence the disease is sometimes protracted to twenty or even twenty-four days, before the crusts exfoliate. In one or two instances I have seen the vesicles terminate in numerous small ulcers, or suppurating foramina, which continued to discharge for many days, and were not all healed before the end of the fourth week.

The febrile symptoms commonly subside when the eruption is completed; but sometimes they continue during the whole course of the disease, probably from the incessant irritation of the itching and smarting connected with it. In many instances, the most distressing part of the complaint is an intense darting pain, not superficial, but deep-seated in the chest, which continues to the latter stages of the disease, and is not easily allayed by anodynes* : sometimes this pain precedes the eruption.

* Hoffmann observes, " Inde quidem symptomata remiserunt, excepto exquisito ardente dolore, qui tantus erat, ut nec somnum capere, nec locum affectum contingere posset." Med. Syst. Rat. tom. iv. part. i. cap. 13. § 6. obs. vi.

Although the *Shingles* commonly follow the regular course of fever, eruption, maturation, and decline, within a limited period, like the eruptive fevers, or exanthemata of the nosologists * ; yet the disorder is not, like the latter, contagious, and may occur more than once in the same individual.† The disease, on the whole, is slight; it has never, in any instance that I have witnessed, exhibited any untoward symptom, or been followed by much debility : in the majority of cases, it did not confine the patients to the house. ‡

The causes of the *shingles* are not always obvious. Young persons from the age of twelve to twenty-five are most frequently the subjects of the disease, although the aged are not altogether exempt from its attacks, and suffer severely from the pains which accompany it. It is most frequent in the summer and autumn, and seems occasionally to arise from exposure to cold, after violent

* The regularity and brevity of its course have not been sufficiently attended to. Burserius has, however, observed, " *Zoster acutus* et *brevis* utplurimum morbus est ; nam, quanquam Lorryus et chronicum, et interdum epidemicum esse existimet, (quod de igne sacro latè sumpto fortasse ei concedendum est) hanc speciem tamen diutinam non vidi." Inst. Med. Pract. tom. ii. cap. 3. § 52.

† In the course of my attendance at the Public Dispensary, during twelve years, between thirty and forty cases of shingles have occurred, none of which were traced to a contagious origin, or occasioned the disease in other individuals.

‡ Some authors, as Platner and Hoffmann, have deemed the *Zoster* a malignant and dangerous disease ; and Langius (Epist. Med. p. 110.) has mentioned two fatal cases occurring in noblemen. But they have apparently mistaken the disease. Lorry, Burserius, Geoffroy, and others, (Hist. de la Soc. Roy. de Méd. ann. 1777-8) more correctly assert that it is free from danger.

exercise. Sometimes it has appeared critical, when supervening to bowel-complaints, or to the chronic pains of the chest remaining after acute pulmonary affections. Like Erysipelas, it has been ascribed by some authors to paroxysms of anger.[*]

It is scarcely necessary to speak of the treatment of a disorder, the course of which scarcely requires to be regulated, and cannot be shortened, by medicine. Gentle laxatives and diaphoretics, with occasional anodynes, when the severe deep-seated pains occur, and a light diet, seem to comprise every thing that is requisite in the cure. Experience altogether contradicts the cautionary precepts, which the majority of writers, even down to Burserius, have enjoined, in respect to the administration of purgatives, and which are founded entirely upon the prejudices of the humoral pathology.[†]

In general, no external application to the clustered vesicles is necessary: " the best plan is to prevent their breaking;" but when they are abraded by the friction of the clothes, a glutinous discharge takes place, which occasions the linen to adhere to the affected parts, producing some irritation. Under these circumstances, a little simple ointment, " or that of the Oxide of Zinc spread on lint," may be

---

[*] See Schwartz Diss. de Zonâ serpiginosâ, Halæ, 1745: he saw three instances, which followed violent fits of passion, p. 17; and Plenck affirms that he saw it occur twice after violent anger, and a copious potation of beer. (De Morb. cutan. p. 28.)

[†] De Meza relates an instance of a repelled Herpes being immediately followed by an intermittent. — Act. Soc. Med. Hafn. T. 1. N. 10. T.

interposed, to obviate that effect. With the view of clearing off the morbid humours, the older prac_titioners cut away the vesicles, and covered the surface with their unguents*, or even irritated it with the Nitrico-oxyd of Mercury, notwithstanding the extreme tenderness of the parts.† These pernicious interruptions of the healing process probably gave rise to ulceration, and prolonged the duration of the disease, and thus contributed to mislead practitioners in their views respecting its nature. ‡

SPECIES 3. HERPES *circinatus*, VESICULAR RINGWORM.

Syn. Formica ambulatoria (*Celsus*) : Herpes serpigo (*Sauv.*) : Annulus repens (*Darwin*) : Dartre encroûtée (*F.*).

This form of Herpes (Plate LI. fig. 1. of BATEMAN ; Pl. 20. of THE ATLAS,) is vulgarly termed a *Ringworm*, and is, in this country, a very slight affection, being unaccompanied with any disorder of the constitution. It appears in small circular patches, in which the vesicles arise only

---

* See Turner on Dis. of the Skin, chap. 5.

† "Illa autem ut inspicio," says Dr. Russell, " vesiculis depressis, et minimè tumentibus, at livescentibus inducta esse, (the natural decline of the eruption) atque acrem quendam ichorem substare cerno, proinde secantur vesiculæ, et præcipitato rubro, cum unguento aur. et cerato, ut medicamenta fixa atque immota emanerent, curantur." De Tabe glandulari, hist. 35.

‡ Plenck says, " Pinguia et humida, ut vidi, admodum nocent;" l. c. p. 28. T.

round the circumference: these are small, with moderately red bases, and contain a transparent fluid, which is discharged in three or four days, when little prominent dark scabs form over them. The central area, in each vesicular ring, is at first free from any eruption; but the surface becomes somewhat rough, and of a dull red colour, and throws off an exfoliation, as the vesicular eruption declines, which terminates in about a week with the falling off of the scabs, leaving the cuticle red for a short time.

The whole disease, however, does not conclude so soon: for there is commonly a succession of the vesicular circles, on the upper parts of the body, as the face and neck, and the arms and shoulders, which have occasionally extended to the lower extremities, protracting the duration of the whole to the end of the second or third week. No inconvenience, however, attends the eruption, except a disagreeable itching and tingling in the patches.

The *herpetic* ringworm is most commonly seen in children, and has been deemed contagious. It has sometimes, indeed, been observed in several children, in one school or family, at the same time: but this was most probably to be attributed to the season, or some other common cause; since none of the other species of Herpes are communicable by contact. It is scarcely necessary to point out here the difference between this *vesicular* ringworm, and the contagious *pustular* eruption of the scalp and forehead, which bears a similar popular appellation. *

The itching and tingling are considerably alleviated by the use of astringent and slightly-stimulant applications, and the vesicles are somewhat repressed by the same expedients. It is a popular practice to besmear them with ink : but solutions of the salts of iron, copper, or zinc, or of borax, alum, &c. in a less dirty form, answer the same end. Dr. Underwood remarks, "the use of a flesh-brush is a good prophylactic, in habits accustomed to the complaint." †

Another form of Herpes circinatus sometimes occurs, in which the whole area of the circles is covered with close-set vesicles, and the whole is surrounded by a circular inflamed border. The vesicles are of a considerable size, and filled with transparent lymph. The pain, heat, and irritation in the part are very distressing, and there is often a considerable constitutional disturbance accompanying the eruption. One cluster forms after another in rapid succession on the face, arms, and neck, and sometimes on the day following on the trunk and lower limbs. The pain, feverishness, and inquietude do not abate till the sixth day of the eruption, when the vesicles flatten, and the inflammation subsides. On the ninth and tenth days a scabby crust begins to form on some, while

* See Porrigo *scutulata*, above, p. 169.
† Treatise on the Diseases of Children, 8th edit. p. 459.

others dry, and exfoliate; the whole disease terminating about the fifteenth day.

All the forms of Herpes appear to be more severe in warm climates than in our northern lati-
tudes; and the inhabitants of the former are liable
to a variety of herpetic ringworm, which is almost
unknown here. This variety differs materially
from the preceding in its course, and is of much
greater duration, for it does not heal with the
disappearance of the first vesicles, but its area
continually dilates by the extension of the vesicular margin. The vesicles terminate in ulcerations,
which are often of a considerable depth; and
while these undergo the healing process, a new
circle of vesicles rises beyond them, which passes
through a similar course, and is succeeded by another circle exterior to itself: and thus the disease
proceeds, often to a great extent, the internal parts
of the ring healing, as the ulcerous and vesicular
circumference expands. *

SPECIES 4. HERPES *labialis*, HERPES OF THE LIPS.

A vesicular eruption upon the edge of the upper
and under lip, and at the angle of the mouth,
sometimes forming a semicircle, or even completing a circle round the mouth, by the successive
rising of the vesicles, is very common, and has

* Celsus appears to have described this form of Herpes as his second species of Ignis sacer. "Alterum autem est in summæ cutis
exulceratione, sed sine altitudine, latum, sublividum, inæqualiter tamen: mediumque sanescit, extremis procedentibus; ac sæpe id, quod
jam sanum videbatur, iterum exulceratur, &c. loc. cit. § 4.

been described by the oldest writers. At first the vesicles contain a transparent lymph, which in the course of twenty-four hours becomes turbid, and of a yellowish white colour, and ultimately assumes a puriform appearance. The lips become red, hard, and tumid, as well as sore, stiff, and painful, with a sensation of great heat and smarting, which continues troublesome for three or four days, until the fluid is discharged, and thick, dark scabs are formed over the excoriated parts. The swelling then subsides, and, in four or five days more, the crusts begin to fall off; the whole duration being, as in the other herpetic affections, about ten or twelve days.

The labial Herpes occasionally appears as an idiopathic affection, originating from cold, fatigue, &c., and is then preceded for about three days by the usual febrile symptoms, shiverings, head-ach, pains in the limbs and the stomach, with nausea, lassitude, and languor. Under these circumstances, a sort of *herpetic* sore-throat is sometimes connected with it; a similar eruption of inflamed vesicles taking place over the tonsils and uvula, and producing considerable pain and difficulty of deglutition. The internal vesicles, being kept in a state of moisture, form slight ulcerations when they break; but these heal about the eighth and ninth days, while the scabs are drying upon the external eruption.

The Herpes labialis, however, occurs most frequently in the course of diseases of the viscera, of

which it is symptomatic, and often critical; for
these diseases are frequently alleviated as soon as it
appears. Such an occurrence is most common in
bilious Fevers, in Cholera, and Dysentery, in Peritonitis, Peripneumony, and severe Catarrhs; but it is
not unfrequent in continued malignant Fevers, and
even in Intermittents. *

"This species of the disease has often proved obstinate, and resisted every form of management. I
have, however, found that it yields rapidly to moderate doses of the Hydrargyrum cum Creta and James'
Powder, in the proportion of sixteen grains of the
former and three grains of the latter, taken every
night at bed-time. During the day, it is necessary
to give the Liquor Potassæ in large doses, com-
mencing with fifteen minims, and gradually ascend-
ing to one hundred, in a large cupful of Decoction
of the Root of Rumex *acutus*. † This dose should
be repeated three times during the day: the food
should be light and free from acidity. Milk and a
light animal diet are to be preferred."

SPECIES 5. HERPES *præputialis*, HERPES OF THE
PREPUCE.

This local variety of Herpes (Plate LI. fig. 2. of
Bateman; Pl. 20. of THE ATLAS,) was not noticed
by Dr. Willan; but it is particularly worthy of

---

* See Huxham, De Aëre et Morb. Epid. vol. ii. p. 56. —Plenck, Doct.
de Morb. Cutan. p. 83.

† The decoction is made, by boiling one ounce of the root, *trans-
versely* sliced, in a quart of water, till it is reduced one third: then let
it be strained. T.

attention, because it occurs in a situation, where it is liable to occasion a practical mistake of serious consequence to the patient. The progress of the herpetic clusters, when seated on the prepuce, so closely resembles that of chancre, as described by some authors, that it may be doubted whether it has not been frequently confounded with the latter. *

The attention of the patient is attracted to the part by an extreme itching, with some sense of heat; and, on examining the prepuce, he finds one, or sometimes two, red patches, about the size of a silver penny, upon which are clustered five or six minute transparent vesicles, which, from their extreme tenuity, appear of the same red hue as the base on which they stand. In the course of twenty-four or thirty hours, the vesicles enlarge, and become of a milky hue, having lost their transparency; and on the third day, they are coherent, and assume an almost pustular appearance. If the eruption is seated within that part of the prepuce, which is in many individuals extended over the glans, so that the vesicles are kept constantly covered and moist (like those that occur in the throat), they commonly break about the fourth or fifth day, and form a small ulceration upon each patch. This discharges a little turbid serum, and

* As a similar description of this eruption will be found under the article Herpes, in Dr. Rees' New Cyclopædia, I might perhaps, in this as in some other instances, incur the charge of plagiarism, if I did not state that the articles " in *Medicine*," contained in that work, from letter C inclusive, were written by myself.

has a white base, with a slight elevation at the edges; and by an inaccurate or inexperienced observer it may be readily mistaken for chancre; more especially if any escharotic has been applied to it, which produces much irritation, as well as a deep-seated hardness beneath the sore, such as is felt in true chancre. If no irritant be applied, the slight ulceration continues till the ninth or tenth day nearly unchanged, and then begins to heal; which process is completed by the twelfth, and the scabs fall off on the thirteenth or fourteenth day. " An affection very similar in every respect sometimes occurs on the labia pudendi."

When the patches occur, however, on the exterior portion of the prepuce, or where that part does not cover the glans, the duration of the eruption is shortened, and ulceration does not actually take place. The contents of the vesicles begin to dry about the sixth day, and soon form a small, hard, acuminated scab, under which, if it be not rubbed off, the part is entirely healed by the ninth or tenth day, after which the little indented scab is loosened, and falls out.

This circumstance suggests the propriety of avoiding not only irritative, but even unctuous or moist applications, in the treatment of this variety of Hermes. And accordingly it will be found, that, where ulceration occurs within the prepuce, it will proceed with less irritation, and its course will be brought within the period above mentioned, if a little clean dry lint alone be interposed, twice a day, between the prepuce and the glans.

I have not been able to ascertain the causes of this eruption on the prepuce. Mr. Pearson is inclined to ascribe it to the previous use of mercury.* "I have seen it where no mercury had been taken, and no stricture of the urethra existed. Like the other species of Herpes, it evidently depends on some sympathy with the digestive organs, which are always in fault when this species of Herpes occurs." Whencesoever it may originate, it is liable to recur in the same individual, and often at intervals of six or eight weeks.

SPECIES 6. HERPES *Iris*, RAINBOW RINGWORM.
This rare and singular morbid appearance, (Plate LII. of BATEMAN; Pl. 20. of THE ATLAS,) which has not been noticed by medical writers, occurs in small circular patches, each of which is composed of concentric rings, of different colours. Its usual seat is on the back of the hands, or the palms and fingers, sometimes on the instep. Its first appearance is like an efflorescence †; but when it is fully

* Soon after the publication of the last edition, my friend, Mr. Copeland, surgeon, of Golden Square, informed me that he had observed this affection of the prepuce to be connected with an irritable state, or with actual stricture, of the urethra; and that by the removal of this condition, by means of the bougie, the recurrence of the Herpes had been prevented.

† Having at first seen it only in its incipient stage, Dr. Willan announced the Iris, on the cover of his second part, as a genus of the exanthematic order.

formed, not only the central umbo, but the surrounding rings become distinctly vesicular. The patches are at first small, and gradually attain their full size, which is nearly that of a sixpence, in the course of a week, or nine days, at the end of which time, the central part is prominent and distended, and the vesicular circles are also turgid with lymph; and, after remaining nearly stationary a couple of days, they gradually decline, and entirely disappear in about a week more. The central vesicle is of a yellowish white colour: the first ring surrounding it is of a dark or brownish red; the second is nearly of the same colour as the centre; and the third, which is narrower than the rest, is of a dark red colour; the fourth and outer ring, or areola, does not appear until the seventh, eighth, or ninth day, and is of a light red hue, which is gradually lost in the ordinary colour of the skin.

The Iris has been observed only in young people, and unconnected with any constitutional disorder, nor could it be traced to any assignable cause. In one or two cases, it followed a severe catarrhal affection, accompanied with hoarseness, and also with an eruption of Herpes labialis. In others, it had recurred several times in the persons affected, occupying always the same parts, and going through its course in the same periods of time.

No internal medicine is requisite in the treatment of the different species of Herpes, except when the constitution is disordered (and then the general antiphlogistic plan must be adopted); for, like the other eruptive diseases, which go through a regular and limited course, the eruptions cannot be interrupted, nor accelerated in their progress, by any medicinal expedient; but their termination may be retarded by improper treatment.

Works which may be consulted on Herpes.

BEDDOES, Considerations on Factitious Airs, &c. 8vo.
CAMPFEN's Dissertatio de Herpete, Duisbury, 1802.
GOLDBECK, Dissertatio de Herpete, 1797.
HENSLER, J. D. De Herpete, 8vo. 1802.
KIRSCHNER, De Zostere, 1816.
NYMMANN, Dissertatio de Herpete, 1594.
PLUMBE on Diseases of the Skin, 2d edit. 8vo. 1827.
RAYER, Traité des Maladies de la Peau, 8vo. 1827.
RUSSELL, " De Tectu Glandularum," 8vo.
WEDEL, Dissertatio de Herpete, 1703.

GENUS IV. RUPIA.

Def. AN ERUPTION OF FLAT, DISTINCT VESICLES, WITH THE BASE SLIGHTLY INFLAMED; CONTAINING A SANIOUS FLUID; SCABS ACCUMULATING, SOMETIMES IN A CONICAL FORM; EASILY RUBBED OFF, AND SOON REPRODUCED.

The eruptive disease, to which this appellation is appropriated *, was not noticed in the enumeration of the genera, formerly given by Dr. Willan. For practical purposes, it might have been included with the

* This term is arbitrarily formed from ρυπος, *sordes*, as indicative of the ill smell and sordid condition of the diseased parts.

Ecthymata, as it occurs under similar circumstances with the Ecthyma *luridum* and *cachecticum ;* but the different form of the eruption, for the sake of consistency of language, rendered the separation necessary.

The RUPIA is characterised by an appearance of broad and flattish vesicles, in different parts of the body, which do not become confluent : they are slightly inflamed at the base, slow in their progress, and succeeded by an ill-conditioned discharge, which concretes into thin and superficial scabs, that are easily rubbed off, and presently regenerated.* It comprehends the three following species :

  1. R. *simplex.*
  2. R. *prominens.*
  3. R. *escharotica.*

SPECIES 1. RUPIA *simplex,* SIMPLE RUPIA.

This species, which shows itself on many parts of the body, (Plate LIII. of BATEMAN ; Pl. 21. of THE ATLAS,) consists of little vesications, containing, on their first appearance, a clear lymph. In a short time, the fluid included in them begins to thicken, and becomes at length opaque and somewhat puriform : a slight ulceration of the skin takes place, with a sanious discharge, followed by scabbing ; and when this heals, it leaves the sur-

---

* This circumstance serves to mark the distinction between Rupia and Ecthyma, independently of the pustular form, and highly-inflamed hard base, of the latter : for the scab of Ecthyma is hard, deeply indented, and surrounded by a deep-seated hardness in the muscular flesh, especially in the larger forms of it.

face of a livid or blackish colour, as if from a thickening of the rete mucosum.

SPECIES 2. RUPIA *prominens*, CONICAL RUPIA.

This curious form of the disease (Plate LIV. of BATEMAN; Pl. 21. of THE ATLAS,) is distinguished by elevated, conical scabs, which are gradually formed upon the vesicated bases. A fluted scab is first generated, and with some rapidity (*e. g.* in the course of the night), as the fluid of the vesication concretes. This extends itself by the successive small advancement of the red border, upon which a new scab arises, raising the concretion above it, so as ultimately to form a conical crust, not unlike the shell of a small limpet. This scab is quite superficial, and if it be rubbed off, a new incrustation covers the excoriated spot in the space of six hours. The ulceration, however, is not phagedenic, but at length heals; although it often proves very tedious, especially in old and intemperate persons, in whom, and in young persons of delicate constitution, it most commonly occurs. "The persons most liable to this species of Rupia generally belong to the lower classes of society; and, if they be not intemperate in their habits, have, almost always, been in a half-starved state from extreme indigence; or have long laboured under some chronic disease, which has wasted down the body." *

* Mr. Plumbe says, "In the cases of this kind answering to the Rupia prominens, which have come under my notice in the St. Giles'

These varieties of Rupia are to be combated by the means recommended for the cure of Ecthyma; *i. e.* by supporting the system, by means of good, light, nutritious diet, " regulating the bowels," and by the use of alterative and tonic medicines; such as Plummer's pill, Cinchona, or rather Sulphate of Quinia, and Sarsaparilla. " Sometimes, however, they will not yield except to a mercurial course, continued until the mouth is slightly affected; after which the constitution should be supported, and the tone of the habit restored, by Sulphate of Quinia, or Decoction of Bark with diluted Sulphuric Acid. As the constitution improves, the local affection is advantageously treated by the application of the Nitrate of Silver to the ulcerated surface, from which the crust has been removed. It stimulates the relaxed surface, and disposes to cicatrization."

SPECIES 3. RUPIA *escharotica*, CACHECTIC RUPIA.

This species affects only infants and young children, when in a cachectic state, whether induced by previous diseases, especially the Smallpox, or by imperfect feeding and clothing, &c. ; whence, among the poor, where it is commonly seen, it often terminates fatally. — The vesicles generally occur on the loins, thighs, and lower extremities, and appear to contain a corrosive sanies : many of them terminate with gangrenous eschars, which

---

Infirmary, the patients have been not unfrequently the subjects of syphilis." PRACTICAL TREATISE, 2d edit. p. 445.   T.

leave deep pits. Nothing can ward off the fatal termination of this species of Rupia, except change of air; a good nutritious diet; sea-bathing; and the Cinchona Bark, or the Sulphate of Quinia, with the mineral acids.

Works which may be consulted on Rupia.

PLUMBE on Diseases of the Skin, 8vo. 2d edit. 1827.
RAYER des Maladies de la Peau, 8vo. 1827.

GENUS V. MILIARIA.

Syn. Miliaris, nova febris (*Syden.*): Purpura (*Hoff.*): Febris Miliaris (*Vogel, Webster*): Exanthema Miliara (*Parr*): Synochus Miliaria (*Young*): Emphlysis, Miliaria (*Good*): die Friselblattern der Friesel (*German*): Millet, fièvre miliare (*F.*): *Miliary Eruption.*

Def. AN ERUPTION OF MINUTE VESICULAR PIMPLES, FILLED WITH A COLOURLESS, ACRID FLUID; TERMINATING IN SCURF.

An eruption of miliary vesicles (Plate LV. fig. 1. of BATEMAN; Pl. 22. of THE ATLAS,) is perhaps invariably *symptomatic*, being connected with some feverish state of the body, previously induced; and it has occurred in every species of fever, continued, remittent, inflammatory, and contagious, as well as in other cases of disease, in which considerable heat of the skin and much sweating had been accidentally excited. The physicians and nosologists, who have described a miliary fever, as an idiopathic eruptive fever, like the Measles, Smallpox, and Scarlatina, have erred in different ways; some of them, in supposing it to originate from a specific virus, or acrimony, like the contagion of the diseases just mentioned*; and some by actually confounding the miliary eruption with the efflorescence of Scarlatina.†

The MILIARIA, of which we here speak, is characterised by a scattered eruption of minute round vesicles, about the size of millet seeds ‡, surrounded by a slight inflammation, or rash, and appearing at an uncertain period of febrile disorders. The eruption is immediately preceded by unusual languor and faintness, by profuse perspiration, which often

---

* Of the writers who have committed this error, a numerous host may be referred to. See Sir David Hamilton, De Febre Miliari, 1710; — Allionius, De Miliarium Orig. Progressu, Nat. et Cur. 1758; — Fordyce (Joan.) Hist. Febris Miliaris, 1758; — Collin, Epist. de Pust. Miliar. 1764; — Blackmore, on the Plague; — Macbride, Introduct. to Theor. and Pract. of Med. part ii. chap. 17; — Baraillon, in Mém. de la Soc. Roy. de Méd. de Paris, tom. i. p. 193; — An Essay on the Cure of the Miliary Fever, by a Subject of Mithridates, 1751; —Sauvages, Nosol. Meth. class. iii. gen. 5; — Burserius, Inst. Med. vol. ii. p. ii. cap. ii. &c. &c.

† In the history of the epidemic miliary fever, which occurred at Leipsic, about the year 1650, and which has been considered as the prototype of all miliary fevers, this mistake was obviously committed. See Godofr. Welsch, Hist. Med. novum istum puerperar. morbum continens, qui ipsis *der Friesel* dicitur; in Haller's Disput. Med. tom. v. § 174; — also Christ. Joan. Langius, Prax. Med. part. ii. cap. 14. § 9. De Purpura; — Etmuller de Febribus; —Schacher, de Febre acut. Exanthem. Lips. 1723, in Haller's Disp. v. § 175; — and Saltzmann, Hist. Purpuræ Miliaris albæ, *ibid.* § 176.

‡ Whence the denomination of the disease, from *milium*, the *millet*.

emits a sourish odour, and by a sense of great heat, with a prickling and tingling in the skin. It appears most abundantly upon the neck, breast, and back, sometimes in irregular patches, and sometimes more generally diffused, and remains on those parts during several days: on the face and extremities, it is less copious, and appears and disappears several times without any certain order. The vesicles, on their first rising, being extremely small and filled with a perfectly transparent lymph, exhibit the red colour of the inflamed surface beneath them; but, in the course of thirty hours, the lymph often acquires a milky opacity, and the vesicles assume necessarily a white or pearly appearance. This seems to have been partly the foundation of the epithets *rubra* and *alba,* which have been applied as specific appellations to miliary fevers.*
The tongue is furred, and of a dark red colour at the edges, and its papillæ are considerably elongated; and not unusually apthous vesicles and sloughs appear at the same time in the mouth and fauces.

The miliary eruption affords no crisis to the fever, in which it supervenes, nor any relief to the symp-

* I say *partly,* because it appears that, among those physicians, who confounded the efflorescence of Scarlatina with the miliary eruption, the terms of *red* and *white* miliary fever, or *red* and *white* Purpura, were used to denote the two eruptions respectively. And again, the miliary vesicles, like those of Varicella, were occasionally preceded by a diffuse efflorescence, which disappeared a few days after the rising of the vesicles; whence the *red* Miliaria has been said to be occasionally changed into the *white.*

toms; and its total duration, in consequence of a daily rising of fresh vesicles, is altogether uncertain; but frequently from seven to ten days, and sometimes much longer. Indeed, under the former treatment, when the sick lay "*drowning* in sweats," (as Sir Richard Blackmore says of one of his patients), it was not uncommon for these "crops" of vesicles to be repeated a second, third, or even fourth time, and the whole disease to be protracted to nearly fifty days.*

It is scarcely necessary now to enter into any detail of proofs, that the miliary eruption is the result of a highly heated and perspiring state of the skin; and that, in its severe and fatal degree, it is solely the effect of a stimulating regimen, in a confined atmosphere. The almost total annihilation of the disease, of late years, since the general adoption of a better practice, is of itself unequivocal evidence of its origin: while, on the other hand, the rarity of its occurrence, both before the abuse of hypothetical speculation had misled physicians from the path of observation, and in the practice of those who subsequently returned to that path, is an additional corroboration of the same truth. Hippocrates, whose mode of treatment in febrile diseases was not calculated to produce excitement, has once or twice but casually mentioned the miliary eruption.† And again, at the latter

* Blackmore, loc. cit. — Brocklesby, in the Med. Obs. and Inquir. vol. iv. p. 30.

† See especially the second book of Epidemics, sect. iii. where he

part of the seventeenth century, when, in the practice of the majority of physicians, the miliary fever was a frequent and fatal occurrence, Sydenham witnessed no such fever; but mentions the occasional appearance only of miliary vesicles, which he ascribes to their proper cause.* More than half a century elapsed, however, before the doctrine of Sydenham was established by De Haen, in Germany, and by Mr. White, of Manchester, Dr. Cullen, and others, in this country.†

As a symptomatic eruption, the Miliaria frequently appears during dentition, in blotches about the face and neck.

-states that, in a hot and dry summer, fevers were in some instances terminated by a critical sweat, and about the seventh, eighth, and ninth day, miliary elevations (τρηχισματα κεγχρωδεα) appeared on the skin, and continued till the crisis. See also the book of Prognostics, where he speaks of miliary sweats (ἱδρωτες κεγχροειδεες).

* Sir Richard Blackmore states, that miliary fever was " the most frequent in this country, of all the *malignant* kind;" and that, when the eruption was copious, it was " often fatal and always dangerous." (Loc. cit.) His contemporary, Sydenham, said of the miliary eruptions, "Licet suâ sponte nonnunquam ingruant, sæpius tamen *lecti calore* et *cardiacis* extorquentur." See his Sched. de Nov. Febris Ingressu.

† See De Haen, Theses sistent. Febrium Divis. § 4; and again in his Rat. Medend. vol. ii. p. 8; — White, on the Management of pregnant and lying-in Women, chap. ii.; — Cullen, First Lines, par. 723, and Nosol. Method. It appears, however, that, in the middle of the last century, the better educated members of the profession had already adopted the right opinions upon the subject. For a weak anonymous writer, of the Blackmore school, in 1751, in reprehending what he calls the " stupidity" and " unpardonable ignorance" of his brethren respecting the disease, ascribes it to " the *prevailing* opinion of some physicians that *this fever is a creature of our own making*," which, he believes, had " run through the whole College, and from thence the dangerous infection been conveyed to the apothecaries," &c. See the Essay by a Subject of Mithridates, *Pref.* p. iv.

Among the various circumstances under which the Miliaria was formerly excited, the *puerperal state* appears to have been most frequently the source of it; insomuch that it was first described as an epidemic among puerperal women. This is sufficiently accounted for by the treatment, which was unhappily pursued during the confinement after child-birth, and of which an impressive description is given by Mr. White. For not only was the mother immediately loaded with bed-clothes, from which she was not allowed to put out " even her nose," and supplied with heating liquors from the spout of a teapot; but to her room, heated by a crowd of visitors and a fire, all access of air was denied, even through a key-hole. From these causes fever was almost necessarily induced, with the most profuse sweats, oppression, anxiety, and fainting; and these again were aggravated by spicy caudles, spirits, opiates, and ammoniacal medicines. That numbers should perish, under such management, with every symptom of malignity, and that many who survived it should escape with broken constitutions, will surprise no person who is acquainted with the baneful influence of over excitement in febrile complaints.*

* The occurrence of this fatal Miliaria must be deemed one of the greatest *opprobria medicorum;* for it was the direct result of a mischievous practice, originating in a false hypothesis respecting the concoction and expulsion of morbid matter : and when we recollect that there was not a febrile disease in which this mischief was not more or less inflicted on the sick, we must blush for the character of our art. " Quid verò demum generi humano calamitosius," exclaims De Haen, " quam

With other fevers, in which a similar method of treatment was pursued, though in a less degree, and which confined the patient to bed, the miliary eruption, with its attendant languor and exhaustion, was frequently conjoined, especially with *catarrhal* and *rheumatic* fevers, and also with typhoid, remittent, and intermittent fevers. Whence the writers, who have described the miliary fever, speak of it as being disguised under, or counterfeiting the character of these fevers respectively. In the summer, indeed, where ventilation and coolness are not sufficiently attained or attended to, a slight miliary eruption is even now occasionally seen : and a Miliaria *clinica,* in fact, may be thus induced by any circumstance that confines a person to bed ; as an accident, or a surgical operation*, an attack of hysteria, a state of asthenia, &c. From the increase of cutaneous heat, connected with the exanthematous fevers of the nosologists, some degree of Miliaria is liable to occur in them all, but more especially in Scarlatina ; and a few larger pearl-coloured vesicles also occasionally appear.†

---

quòd, et plebe et medicis conspirantibus, tot melleni quotannis ægri, ab ipso principio acutorum, in sudores symptomaticos agitentur, ac veluti fundantur, ut coacta omnino crisis, in plerisque aut lethalis aut periculosa saltem, producatur; interea dum salutaria Naturæ molimina turbantur, confunduntur, ac penitus sufflaminantur. Faxit Deus, ut demum sapiant Phryges ! " — De Febrium Divis.

* Mr. White, loc. cit.

† See Fordyce (loc. cit.), " Nonnunquam bullæ insignes, apice digiti non minores, hic elevantur." — Also the Anon. Essay on the Cure of Mil. Fever ; — and Brocklesby, *loc. cit.*

It is unnecessary to dwell upon the method of treatment applicable to Miliaria; since, under the full employment of ventilation, and a cool regimen, the symptom will very rarely be produced. The room, in which a puerperal woman, or a patient under any febrile disease, is confined, ought to be as free from all unpleasant odour as any other apartment; and under the cordial influence of pure air, the support of spirituous and vinous liquors is so far from being requisite, that a small proportion of these stimulants will produce even a deleterious excitement.* Extreme cleanliness, a frequent change of linen, cool diluent drinks, light diet, and the other circumstances of what has been called the antiphlogistic regimen, will always be attended to with advantage, where the miliary eruption shows itself. The mineral acids, if no other symptom contraindicate the use of them, are advantageous.

* Mr. White observes, that a woman in child-bed is so much exhausted by the mode of treatment before described, " that the highest cordials have been necessary to support her; nay, I have been credibly informed," he adds, " that under these circumstances a patient has sometimes drunk a *gallon of wine* in a single day, *exclusive of brandy, and of the cordials from the apothecary's shop*, and all this too without intoxication." *loc. cit.* chap. viii.—Similar enormous potations of wine have been recommended by later practitioners in typhoid fevers, who have not been aware, that the very impunity, with which these doses have been administered, has arisen from the artificial exhaustion of the patient by external circumstances, and not from the necessary tendency of the disease. Many facts have occurred to my notice, in the course of my attendance at the Fever Institution, which have satisfied me of the correctness of this opinion, which I may probably illustrate at a future opportunity.

Books which may be consulted on Miliaria.

Balguy, de Febre Miliari.
Fordyce, J., M.D. Historia Febris Miliaris, &c. 8vo. 1750.
Hamilton, Sir David, A Treatise on Miliary Fever, 8vo. 1737.
Rayer, Traité des Maladies de la Peau, 8vo. 1827.

Genus VI. ECZEMA.*

Syn. Hidroa (*Sauv. Vog.*): Cytisma Eczema (*Young*): Ecphlysis Eczema (*Good*): Asef (*Arab.*): Schweis-blattern (*German*): Echauboulure, Dartre vive (*F.*): *Heat eruption.*

Def. An eruption of minute vesicles, not contagious, crowded together; and which, from the absorption of the fluid they contain, form into thin flakes or crusts.

This eruption is generally the effect of irritation, whether internally or externally applied, and is occasionally produced by a great variety of irritants, in persons whose skin is constitutionally very irritable. It differs from Miliaria, inasmuch as it is not the result of fever, and, unless it be very extensively diffused, is not accompanied with any

---

* Aëtius observes, that an eruption of hot and smarting phlyctænæ arises in all parts of the body, without proceeding to ulceration. " Eas εκζεματα ab *ebulliente fervore*, Græci vulgo appellant." Tetrab iv. serm. i. cap. 128. According to Paulus (lib. iv. cap. 10.), and Actuarius (lib. vi. cap. 8.), they were also called περιζεματα, and περιζεσματα, " quasi *vehementer ferventia.*" See Gorræus, Defin. Med.; and Sennert. Pract. Med. lib. v. part i. cap. 2.

derangement of the constitution: except in the most violent cases, the functions of the sensorium and of the stomach are seldom disturbed. "It may be confined to a small part of the surface of the body, or extended over the whole skin : it chiefly, however, affects the inside of the thighs, the axilla, and those places in which the mucous follicles are most abundant in men ; the under parts of the mammæ, the vulva, and the anus in women." When limited to the fingers, hand, and part of the fore-arm, it is not unfrequently mistaken for Scabies : but it may be distinguished by the appearance of its acuminated and pellucid vesicles; by the closeness and uniformity of their distribution ; by the absence of surrounding inflammation, and of subsequent ulceration ; and, in many cases, by the sensations of smarting and tingling, rather than of itching, which accompany them. According to the nature of the irritating cause, the extent and form of the disease are somewhat various ; and constitute three species of the genus :

1. E. *solare.*
2. E. *impetiginodes.*
3. E. *rubrum.*

SPECIES 1. ECZEMA *solare ;* SUN-HEAT.

This form of Eczema (Plate LVI. of BATEMAN ; Pl. 22. of THE ATLAS,) occurs in the summer season, and is the effect of irritation from the direct rays of the sun, or from the heated air. Hence it affects almost exclusively those parts of the surface which are exposed to their influence; as the face, the neck, and fore-arms, in women, but more particularly the back of the hands and fingers. The eruption is preceded and accompanied by a sense of heat and tingling, and these sensations are aggravated even to smarting, when the parts affected are exposed to the sunshine, or to the heat of a fire. The whole fingers are sometimes swelled *, and so thickly beset with the vesicles, as to leave no interstice of the natural appearance of the skin, nor any intervening redness. The vesicles themselves are small, and slightly elevated; they are filled with a thin, milky serum, which gives them a whitish colour, or sometimes with a brownish lymph; and they are without any surrounding inflammation. On the upper part of the arm, however, and, in women, on the breast, neck, and shoulders, the eczematous vesicles are sometimes surrounded by an inflammatory circle; when they are popularly termed *heat-spots*. It sometimes happens, indeed, in men of sanguine temperament, who use violent exercise in hot weather, that these vesicles are intermixed, in various places, with actual phlyzacious pustules, or with hard and painful tubercles, which appear in succession, and rise to the size of small

---

* As this eruption about the fingers, the ball of the thumbs, and the wrists, is often continued for several weeks, it is in this situation more particularly liable to be mistaken for the itch: but the circumstances just noticed, as well as those mentioned under the head of Scabies, will contribute to aid the diagnosis.

boils, and suppurate very slowly. This, however,
is a more frequent occurrence in the more local
forms of the disease, included under the second
head.

The eruption is successive, and has no regular
period of duration or decline: it commonly continues for two or three weeks, without any particular internal disorder. The included lymph
becomes more milky, and is gradually absorbed,
or dried into thin brownish scales, which exfoliate,
or into brownish yellow scabs, of the size of a small
pin's head, especially when the vesicles are broken.
But successive eruptions of the vesicles are apt to
appear, which terminate in a similar manner by
exfoliation or scabbing; and in those persons who,
by the peculiar irritability of their skin, are much
predisposed to the disorder, it is thus continued
many weeks, to the end of autumn, or even prolonged to the winter. When this happens, the
vesicles generally pour out an acrid serum, by
which the surface is inflamed, rendered tender,
and even slightly ulcerated, and the disease assumes the form of Impetigo.

The course of this disorder does not appear to be
materially shortened by the operation of medicine.
The mineral acids, with a decoction of Cinchona,
or other vegetable tonic, and a light but nutritious
diet, seem to be most effectual in diminishing the
eruption. When it has occurred after long-continued travelling, or any other severe fatigue, and
appears to be accompanied with some degree of

exhaustion of the powers of the constitution, a course of Serpentaria, or Sarsaparilla, is exceedingly beneficial. Active and repeated purgation is adverse to the complaint. Simple ablution with tepid water contributes to relieve the smarting and tingling of the parts affected, which do not bear unguents, or any stimulant application.

SPECIES 2. ECZEMA *impetiginodes*, IMPETIGINOUS ECZEMA.

A local Eczema (Plate LV. fig. 2. of BATEMAN; Pl. 22. of THE ATLAS,) is produced by the irritation of various substances, and, when these are habitually applied, it is constantly kept up in a chronic form, differing from the Impetigo only in the absence of pustules. Small separate vesicles, containing a transparent fluid, and, like the psydracious pustules, imbedded in the skin, or but slightly elevated, arise, and slowly increase: they are attended with pain, heat, smarting, often with intense itching, " and with swelling of the affected part." When they break, the acrid lymph, that is discharged, irritates and inflames the surrounding cuticle, which becomes thickened, rough, reddish, and cracked, as in the impetiginous state. The alliance, indeed, of this affection with Impetigo is further proved by the circumstance, that, in some cases, vesicles, and psydracious pustules are intermixed with each other; and, in different individuals, the same irritant will excite a pustular or a vesicular eruption respectively; the vesicular disease being always the most painful and obstinate. Of this we have an example in the affection of the hands and fingers, produced by the irritation of sugar, which is commonly called the *grocer's itch;* and which is in some persons vesicular, in others pustular. The acrid stimulus of lime occasions similar eruptions on the hands of *bricklayers :* and one of the most severe cases that I ever witnessed, occurred on the hands of a *file-maker,* being occasioned perhaps by the united irritation of the heat of the forge and the impalpable powder of steel, with which they were constantly covered during his work. In like manner, both vesicular and pustular affections are excited by the local irritation of blisters, stimulating plasters, and cataplasms of Mercury, the Ointment of Tartarized Antimony, the Oil of the Cashew nut, the Indian varnish, Arsenic, Valerian root, &c.* These often extend to a considerable distance beyond the part to which the irritants were immediately applied, and continue for some time, in a successive series, after the stimulus has been withdrawn, especially in irritable and cachectic habits. Thus, when a blister is applied to the pit of the stomach, an eruption of vesicles, intermixed often with ecthymatous pustules, and inflamed tubercles and boils, extends in some cases over nearly the whole abdomen, or to the top of the sternum ; or, if the blister be applied between the shoulders, the whole of the back and

---

* See Impetigo.

loins becomes covered with a similar eruption.
These tubercles and boils suppurate very slowly
and deeply in some habits, and are ultimately filled
with dry dark scabs, which do not soon fall off;
and when the sores are numerous, they produce
some degree of feverishness, and much pain on
motion. In other respects, the constitution suffers
no injury from this tedious eruption; although
from its duration, which is sometimes extended to
two or three weeks, it occasions more inconvenience
than the original applications.

" When this species of Eczema appears on the
wrists, the back of the hand, and between the fingers, it is often mistaken for itch. The stinging
sensation of Eczema, however, is sufficient to distinguish it from itch, were it not otherwise distin-
guishable: in itch the itching returns in paroxysms;
in Eczema the stinging sensation is continued.
It is, also, distinguished by its non-contagious
character."

The first step towards the cure of these varieties
of Eczema is to remove the irritating cause, where
that is obvious. The eruption, however, is not
easily removed: but the painful sensations connected with it are greatly alleviated by simple poultices, and by frequently washing the parts with
warm gruel, and milk or bran and water, " or with
the Emulsion of Bitter Almonds, containing, besides
the quantity natural to it, some Hydrocyanic acid,
to the extent of at least f$\mathfrak{z}$j to f$\mathfrak{z}$viij of the Emulsion. Cloths, also, moistened with a dilute solution of

acetate of Lead, should be applied over the parts, when the vesicles break, and ooze out their serum. A French author, M. Guillemineau, recommends strongly a solution of Nitrate of Silver.* The sulphur baths have been employed ; but are too irritating. Simple warm baths are more beneficial."

Where there is any other evidence of a cachectic condition of the patient, a tonic treatment must be prescribed for the improvement of the general health, as recommended in Ecthyma.† "Diluting, acidulated drinks must be prescribed. Nothing is more useful than diluted Sulphuric Acid, given in Infusion of Roses. — Calomel should be at first given, and afterwards a gentle purgative every morning."

SPECIES 3. ECZEMA *rubrum*.‡ INFLAMED ECZEMA.
SYN. Dartre squameuse humide (*Alibert*): Hydrargyria (*Alley*): Erythema Mercuriale (*Auct. Var.*): Lepra Mercuriale (*Moriarty*).

The most remarkable variety of the Eczema

---

* De l'Emploi du Nitrate d'Argent fonder dans le Traitement de quelques Maladies. 4to. Paris, 1826. T.

† The irritation produced by the attrition of the tight parts of our dress, as about the knees, neck, &c., which commonly produces a mere Intertrigo, occasions, in some persons, an eczematous eruption. Sauvages has hence made two species of Herpes, excited by the garter and the bandages of the neck, which he calls Herpes *periscelis* and H. *collaris*.

‡ There is, perhaps, a little incongruity in this species of Eczema, when the generic character is considered; but in every respect, except the surrounding redness, it accords with the genus, differing equally from the mere rash of the Erythemata, and from the symptomatic and febrile Miliaria.

rubrum is that which arises from the irritation of mercury.* (Plate LVIII. of BATEMAN; Pl. 22. of THE ATLAS.) But the disease is not exclusively occasioned by this mineral, either in its general or more partial attacks: it " is often associated with gastro-intestinal inflammation, without any mercurial preparation having been taken † ;" and it has been observed to follow exposure to cold, and to recur in the same individual, at irregular intervals, sometimes without any obvious or adequate cause.‡

The Eczema rubrum is preceded by a sense of stiffness, burning heat, and itching, in the part where it commences, which is most frequently the upper and inner surface of the thighs, and about the scrotum in men; but sometimes it appears first in the groins, axillæ, or in the bend of the arms, or about the wrists and hands, or in the neck. These sensations are soon followed by an appearance of redness, and the surface is somewhat rough

* Whence the disease has been called Eczema *mercuriale* (see Mr. Pearson's " Obs. on the Effects of var. Articles of the Mat. Med. in Lues Ven." chap. xiii. 2d edit.); — Erythema *mercuriale* (see Dr. Spens and Dr. M'Mullins in the Edin. Med. and Surg. Journ. vol. i. and ii.); — *Hydrargyria* (see Dr. Alley's " Obs. on the Hydrargyria, or that vesicular Disease arising from the Exhibition of Mercury," Lond. 1810.); — and *mercurial* Lepra (see a Tract of Dr. Moriarty of Dublin).

† See Medico-Chirurg. Trans. vol. ii. p. 73. T.

‡ See a description of two cases by Dr. Rutter (Edin. Med. and Surg. Journal, vol. v. p. 143.), and Dr. Marcet (Medico-Chirurg. Trans. vol. ii. art. ix.), under the appellation of Erythema, which recurred several times in both the patients to a severe degree. It is worthy of remark, however, that, in both these instances, the *first* attack of the disease occurred after a gonorrhœa; for which, in the one, some mercury had certainly, and in the other had probably, been administered.

to the touch. This, however, is not a simple Ery-thema; for on examining it minutely between the light and the eye, or with a convex glass, the roughness is found to be occasioned by innumerable, minute, and pellucid vesicles, which have been mistaken for papulæ. In two or three days, these vesicles, if they are not ruptured, attain the size of a pin's head; and the included serum then becoming somewhat opaque and milky, the character of the eruption is obvious. It soon extends itself over the body and limbs in successive large patches, and is accompanied by a considerable swelling of the integuments, such as is seen in smallpox and other eruptive fevers, and by great tenderness of the skin, and much itching. When the vesicles begin to lose their transparency, they generally burst, and discharge, from numerous points, a thin acrid fluid, which seems to irritate the surface over which it passes, and leaves it in a painful, inflamed, and excoriated condition. The quantity of this ichorous discharge is very considerable; and it gradually becomes thicker and more adhesive, stiffening the linen which absorbs it, and which thus becomes a new source of irritation : it emits, also, a very fœtid odour. This process takes place in the successive patches of the eruption, until the whole surface of the body, from head to foot, is sometimes in a state of painful excoriation, with deep fissures in the bends of the joints, and in the folds of the skin of the trunk; and with partial scaly incrustations, of a yellowish hue, produced by the drying of the humour, by which, also, the irritation is augmented. The extreme pain arising from the pressure of the weight of the body upon an extensive portion of such a raw surface is sufficient to give rise to an acceleration of the pulse, and white tongue; but the functions of the stomach and of the sensorium commune are not evidently disturbed by this disease.*

* The experience of the Editor obliges him to differ from this opinion of Dr. Bateman. In almost every case, which has come under his notice, there has been evident constitutional derangement, quick pulse, furred tongue, and impaired appetite, with considerable nervous irritability. Indeed, the latter state has been so frequently present, as to induce the Editor to regard an irritable state of the nervous system, such as produces hysteria in females, to be the predisposing cause of this disease when it occurs during a mercurial course. The following case will illustrate this opinion : —

A young woman was seduced from her parents and brought to London by one of those unprincipled men who sacrifice every moral and social feeling on the altar of self-gratification. Desire and the pleasure of possession having subsided, the wretched victim of unbridled passion was soon deserted, and fell into a course of life, which any deviation from the paths of virtue usually produces in the female sex thus situated. She went upon the town, as the term is, and in that wretched and precarious state of life contracted syphilis, for the cure of which she was placed under a course of mercury. Her father, whose paternal feelings were not destroyed by the stain which the misconduct of his child had affixed on the character of his family, had followed her to town; and in vain had endeavoured to discover her retreat. At length he met her in the street, when she was labouring not only under disease, but when her habit was charged with mercury for its relief; and when she was reduced to a state of extreme indigence. Her eye met that of her parent, and she fled as rapidly as she could from an interview which she dreaded; and although her father closely followed her, yet she secured her retreat to her lodgings for that night. On the following day she was too ill to move from home; her mouth was affected, and the salivation considerable; when late in the evening of that day she heard her father's voice at the door of the house in which she lodged. She instantly left her bed, and escaped into another room as he entered the one in which she

The duration of this excoriation and discharge is uncertain and irregular : when only a small part of the body is affected, it may terminate in ten days ; but when the disorder has been universal, the patient seldom completely recovers in less than six weeks, and is often afflicted to the end of eight or ten weeks. By so severe an inflammation the whole epidermis is destroyed in its organization ; and when the discharge ceases, it lies loose, assuming a pale brown colour, which changes almost to black before it falls off in large flakes. As in other superficial inflam-

---

had been lying, and ran into the street in a half-naked condition, during a heavy shower of rain. I was requested to see her on the following day. She was then covered in patches with an eruption, which, to the unassisted eye, much resembled that of scarlet fever. She complained of great heat, stiffness, and tingling upon the inner and upper surface of the thigh, and round the neck and waist. In these parts patches of extremely minute vesicles were apparent, gradually extending themselves over the whole body. The stinging and irritation increased to a degree almost insupportable. There was fever, which in a few days assumed an intermittent character ; and a very fœtid odour exhaled from the body. The viscid fluid which oozed from the patches dried and crusted, and the cuticle peeled off in large pieces. In this state the disease continued for ten days. The warm bath, anodyne fomentations, liniments of linseed oil and lime-water, were externally applied ; whilst saline purgatives, refrigerants, decoction of Cinchona bark, the mineral acids and opium were internally administered, without any beneficial result. In fifteen days from the commencement of the attack, the wretched girl died, in a state of suffering which no language can correctly describe.

In this case, the mental alarm had predisposed the body, under the influence of the mercury, to be excited by the sudden exposure to cold and damp in a peculiar manner ; for that it was not cold and damp alone is probable from the fact that the poor creature had been driven by strong necessity to walk the streets in all states of the weather, during the whole period in which she had been taking mercurials, without suffering, until the nervous system received the shock which has been described. T.

mations, however, the new red cuticle that is left is liable to desquamate again, even to the third or fourth time, but in smaller branny scales, of a white colour; and a roughness sometimes remains for a considerable period, like a slight degree of Psoriasis. In some instances, not only the cuticle, but the hair and nails are also observed to fall off; and the latter, when renewed, are incurvated, thickened, and furrowed, as in Lepra.

The Eczema rubrum, however, even from the irritation of Mercury, is often limited to a small space; and then the discharge is slight, and its whole duration short. Similar local attacks of it occur in irritable constitutions, especially in hot weather, affecting the hands and wrists, the neck and external ear, and other parts, but without any constitutional disorder. Successive crops of the vesicles arise, in irregular patches, with a red blush around them, which produce partial incrustations, as the ichor, that issues, is dried: and by these vesications and desiccations of the matter the affection is kept up for some weeks.

The treatment of this species of Eczema may be comprised in few words; for it is principally palliative. But although medicine may not possess the power of shortening the period of its duration, yet, the omission of the palliative measures will allow an extreme aggravation of the sufferings of the patient to take place, and probably prolong it beyond its natural course, as well as contribute to wear out the vigour of his constitution.

" The first step is to omit the further use of the Mercury, and to remove the patient from the atmosphere in which the disease was generated, and to soothe every anxiety of the mind as far as possible."

The misery and exhaustion, resulting from the excessively tender and irritated state of the skin, may be greatly alleviated by frequent ablution or fomentation with warm gruel, or strained bran and water; or by the frequent use of the warm bath, which has the advantage of cleansing the surface, without occasioning any abrasion by friction. A constant application of poultices has produced considerable ease to the patient, when the affection was confined to the extremities. Where the cuticle has exfoliated, Mr. Pearson recommends the application of a mild cerate, consisting of litharge plaster, wax, and oil, spread thickly on linen rollers, and renewed twice a day. With the same view of diminishing the irritation of the surface, the bed and body linen of the patient, which becomes hard and stiff as the discharge dries upon it, should be frequently changed.

Every additional irritation from stimulating food and drink should be avoided; the bowels should be kept open by the administration of occasional laxatives; and some saline diaphoretic, or an antimonial, should be given regularly, to which an opiate may be added, for the purpose of soothing the sensations of the patient. The Sulphuric Acid is grateful and refreshing; and, in the decline of the swelling and discharge, it may be combined advantageously with the liberal exhibition of Cinchona, or the Sulphate of Quinia, and Sarsaparilla.

Books to be consulted on Eczema.

ALLEY, Observations on the Hydrargyria, 8vo. 1810.
BUTTER's Treatise on the Venereal Rose, 1799.
EDINBURGH Med. and Surg. Journ. vol. ii.
MORIARTY, A Description of Mercurial Lepra, 8vo. 1804.
MATHIAS, (And.) on the Mercurial Disease, 8vo. 1811.

———————

GENUS VII. APHTHA.

Syn. 'Αφθας, (*Gr.*): Febris Aphthosa (*Vogel*): Typhus Aphthoidéus (*Young*): Emphlysis Aphtha (*Good*): Pustulæ oris (*Haly Abbas*): Achirum, Parititooroo (*Tam.*): Achir (*Duk.*): Achérum (*Tel.*): Mookāpākum (*Sans.*): Ninanwan (*Hind.*): Aphthes (*F.*): die Mundschwämchen (*German*): Thrush.

Def. AN ERUPTION OF GRANULAR, PEARL-CO-LOURED VESICLES *, ON THE INSIDE OF THE CHEEKS,

---

* The vesicular character of the aphthous eruption has been pointed out by several accurate observers; especially by Van Swieten, in commenting upon the word *ulcuscula* used by Boerhaave, aph. 978.; by Sauvages, who considers their character as *phlyctænous;* and by Prof. Arnemann, who describes them as small elevations, of a greyish-white colour, " *seroso* quodam *liquore* referti." (Comment. de Aphthis, § ii.) See also Welti, Diss. de Exanthem. Fonte Abdominali, § vi.; Callisen, Syst. Chir. Hod. § 834.; and Plenck, Doctr. de Morb. Cutan. class. x., who still more distinctly describes them. " *Incipiunt* aphthæ *sub forma*

AND OF THE LIPS, EXTENDING OVER THE WHOLE OF THE MOUTH, THE FAUCES, AND INTO THE INTESTINAL CANAL, TERMINATING IN SLOUGHS, OR WHITISH CRUSTS.

This affection of the mouth, which has been described by medical writers from Hippocrates downwards, has been almost universally noticed as a frequent occurrence during the period of infancy *, and generally ascribed to disorder of the first passages, or considered as the result of gastric and eruptive fevers. In truth, it occurs in connection with various states of disease, both acute and chronic, and at all ages, where great debility is induced. It consists of the following species:—

1. A. *lactantium.*
2. A. *adultorum.*
3. A. *anginosa.*

SPECIES 1. APHTHA *lactantium* †, INFANTILE THRUSH.

Syn. Aphtha infantiles (*Plenck*): Aphtha infan-

---

vesicularum miliarium albarum, quæ in apice foraminulum gerunt, dein collabuntur et aliquantum latescunt." — Some English writers have called them " little white *specks*," (see Underwood, vol. i. p. 62.) little white " specks or sloughs," (Armstrong on the Man. of Children, p. 18.) or merely " a white fur," (Syer, on Man. of Infants, p. ii. chap. 3.) having attended only to the ultimate state of the eruption.

* Hippoc. aph. 24. sect. iii. &c. — Celsus, lib. ii. cap. 9. and lib. viii. cap. 42. — Aëtius, tetr. ii. serm. iv. cap. 39. — Julius Pollux, Onomast. lib. iv. cap. 24.

† The appellation of *lactumina*, or *lactucimina*, was given to the infantile Aphthæ by Amatus Lucitanus (Curat. Medic. cent. v.), upon the supposition that they originated from a vitiated condition of the milk.

tum (*Cullen*): Aphtha lactucimen (*Sauv.*): Emphlysis Aphtha; *a. infantum* (*Good*) : *White Thrush.*

Aphthous eruptions are most frequently seen in
infants, in whom they sometimes appear without
any considerable indisposition; but they are often
accompanied by restlessness and slight febrile
symptoms, especially when the stomach and bowels
are much deranged. The nurse is led to suspect
their occurrence by the difficulty and apparent pain
with which the infant sucks, and by the heat of its
mouth, as perceived by the nipple, which at length
becomes inflamed, and even excoriated. The Aphthæ appear first on the edges of the tongue, or at
the angles and inside of the lips, and often extend
over the whole surface of the tongue, palate, inside
of the cheeks, and into the fauces : the surface on
which they arise is of a red or purplish hue; the
tongue is sometimes slightly tumid, and its papillæ,
especially near the extremity, are elongated and
inflamed, protruding their red tips above the rest
of the surface, nearly as in scarlet fever. The
aphthous vesicles are of a white colour, and semi-
opake, and speedily put on the appearance of
minute fragments of curd, adhering to the surfaces
just mentioned. At various periods, from twelve
hours to several days, these specks become loose
and fall off, leaving the surface smooth and red.
Others, however, commonly spring up, and go
through a similar course, while at the same time
new ones appear on other parts ; so that at length
the whole surface of the tongue and mouth is often

covered with a sort of whitish granulated crust, formed of the coherent Aphthæ. Sometimes these crops are renewed several successive times; and not unfrequently the removal and repullulation are only partial, and the general crust remains for several weeks. The Aphthæ appear to extend down the œsophagus, and are supposed to affect the internal surface of the stomach, and of the whole intestinal canal, when tenesmus ensues, with a redness and partial excoriation about the anus: these latter symptoms, however, may be occasioned by the irritation of the morbid excretions from the bowels, which are usually discharged under the occurrence of severe aphthous eruptions. The trachea is occasionally affected with the Aphthæ; but they very rarely extend to the cavity of the nose.[*]

The Aphthæ of infants are most commonly the result of disorder in the stomach and bowels, combined with debility. Hence they occur in sucking infants, where the supply of milk afforded by the nurse is inadequate, or imperfect in its qualities; " a consequence not unfrequently of an over-anxious and irritable temper in a nursing mother," but still more frequently and severely, where a child is brought up, without being suckled, upon unnatural or improper food. In either case, the tendency to Aphthæ is increased by whatever contributes to impair the general health; as want of cleanliness, confined air, neglect of giving exercise, allowing the child to sleep too much under the bedclothes,

[*] Callisen, loc. cit.

&c. Indigestion and its consequences, especially acidity, are occasioned by giving the food too thick, too hot, or too sweet, or in any other way widely different from that which the provision of nature suggests.

The Aphthæ of infants, when accompanied with slight general indisposition, or only with acidity at the stomach, and especially when they are few and scattered, are not indicative of danger, nor productive of much inconvenience. But when they are very copious, coalescing into an extensive coating over the tongue, mouth, and throat, or are accompanied with a red, shining appearance of the tongue, with an obstinate and irritating diarrhœa, fever, and restlessness, — or when they supervene on the state of debility and emaciation which is left by measles, Erysipelas, and other acute diseases, or on a chronic marasmus, — they not only betoken a dangerous state of constitutional distress, but contribute, by the inability of taking nourishment which they occasion, to augment that state. They are also unfavourable when they assume a dark hue.

In the milder degrees of Aphtha lactantium, just mentioned, slight remedies are sufficient to alleviate or remove the disease. The acidity in the first passages is often readily corrected by some testaceous powder, which, if the bowels be not irritable, may be joined with a little Rhubarb or Magnesia; or by the Pulvis Contrayervæ compositus, if they are in the opposite state, and the child weakly. "In the latter case, I have derived more benefit from a mixture of Carbonate of Soda and Calumba in powder, and in doses proportionate to the age of the infant, than from any other remedy. It is requisite to clear the bowels with a dose of Castor Oil every morning, which prevents diarrhœa. When the alvine discharges are so acrid as to cause heat and soreness round the anus, much comfort is derived from glysters composed of equal quantities of mutton broth and starch." At the same time, the nutriment of the patient should be regulated, by attending to the diet and general health of the nurse, " who should abstain from the use of wine and porter or ale." If the child be not suckled, a wet-nurse should be procured, where that is practicable, which often speedily cures the complaint. " If the infant be suckled by the mother, it is of importance to enquire into the state both of the health of the body and that of the mind of the mother; and, in all cases when the disease does not yield to the usual remedies, and the strength of the infant fails, the nurse, whether mother or a hireling, should be changed; ·for in many instances little more is required than a sufficient supply of healthy nutriment for the effectual removal of the disease."

Various local applications have been employed for the removal of Aphthæ from the earliest times, of a gently astringent nature; and when they are not made too stimulant, especially in the commencement of the eruption, they not only serve the good purpose of coagulating and removing the mucous and clammy discharge, but also diminish the tendency to resprout in the aphthous surfaces. The most effectual detergent of this kind is Borax, recommended by Mr. Gooch, of Norwich*, and now in the hands of every nurse. It is conveniently combined with water, mucilage, syrup, or honey, in the proportion of one-twelfth, or even one-eighth part of the salt. It is unnecessary to describe the compositions of honey of Roses, syrup of Mulberries, &c. with small proportions of Muriatic or Sulphuric Acid, or of the Sulphate of Zinc, or of some absorbent powder, which different practitioners have preferred. Where the surface is exceedingly tender and excoriated, some mild and lubricating application, such as the compound of cream, with the yolk of eggs and Syrup of Poppies, recommended by Van Swieten †, should be first employed, and the restringents gradually introduced, as the irritability is diminished.

At a later period of infancy, the Aphthæ partake more of the nature of those which appear in adults: they seldom occur, except as symptomatic of some more serious derangement of the organs of nutrition, or as the sequelæ of febrile disease; and are consequently indicative of great danger, and more difficult of cure. If the child have been long at the breast, it is probable that the milk has become deteriorated in quality, or insufficient in quantity; and weaning, or a change of nurse, may be neces-

* See his Surg. Observations.   † Comment. ad Aph. 990.

sary.   If a state of marasmus, with emaciation, tumid abdomen, and morbid excretions from the bowels, have supervened, the usual course of absorbents and alteratives, the Hydrargyrus cum Creta, or the grey Oxide with Soda and testaceous powder, must be carefully administered, and followed by mild tonics.   Where the Aphthæ assume a brown hue, or appear in the state of debility consequent on acute diseases, the general strength must be supported by light tonics and cordials, with proper diet ; such as a weak decoction of Cinchona or Cascarilla, or the solution of the Tartrate of Iron, with Rhubarb, light animal broths, and preparations of milk with the starches. *

SPECIES 2. APHTHA *adultorum :* THRUSH OF ADULTS.

Syn. Aphtha maligna (*Sauv.*) : Emphlysis Aphtha, ε. *maligna* (*Good*) : *Black Thrush.*

In children grown up, and in adult persons, Aphthæ occur under a great variety of circumstances, being symptomatic of numerous diseases, both acute and chronic.   They not only occur after Smallpox, Measles, Erysipelas, and Scarlet Fever ; but seldom fail to appear, whenever the constitution has been weakened by old age, by long confinement from wounds and accidents, from dropsical, gouty, and dyspeptic complaints, from diarrhœa, chlorosis, consumption, and hectic fever

* Such as Arrow-root, Tapioca, Sago.

of every kind *; in the latter diseases, indeed, the
Aphthæ are usually indications of the approach of
dissolution. The particular tendency of autumnal
fevers, in cold and damp seasons, to produce Aphthæ, especially when combined with affections of
the bowels, or occurring in puerperal women, has
been noticed by many writers; as well as the connection between the aphthous and miliary eruptions, under a heating regimen.† The Aphthæ,
like the Miliaria, when they supervene in these
fevers, never produce any amendment of the symptoms, as the continental writers have stated, but
rather seem to aggravate them, and to prolong
their duration. They always, indeed, imply a dangerous state of the system, when they accompany
other diseases; and especially when they appear
first in the pharynx, and ascend from the stomach;
when there is much anxiety, pain, and heat of the
præcordia, with sickness and hiccup; and when
they are among the sequelæ of fevers, the pulse at
the same time remaining small and frequent, and
the appetite failing to return.

The principal objects of medicine, in these cases,

* See Callisen, loc. cit. — " Neque infrequenter (aphthæ) in adultis
metastasi imperfectæ, infidæ, in febribus continuis, exanthematicis, pu-
tridis, inflammatoriis, lentis, à suppuratione internâ seu pure resorpto,
vel alvifluxu, vires pessundanti inductæ, debentur." — See also Willan,
Reports on Dis. of London, p. 114., and Arnemann, loc. cit. § iii. de
Aphthis adultorum.

† See Arnemann and Willan, *ibid.* — Van Swieten ad Aph. 983.—
Sydenham, sect. iv. cap. iii.—Stoll, Rat. Med. tom. ii. p. 167.—Huxham,
de Aëre et Morb. Epidem. lib. ii. p. 29. — Frank, de curand. Hom. Morbis, lib. iii. § 366.

are to restore the energy of the constitution, and
relieve the local complaint. The former indication
is to be fulfilled by means of Cinchona and the mineral acids, where the bowels will admit of them,
by light but nutritious diet, and by the exercise of
gestation, when it can be obtained. For the latter,
frequent ablution of the mouth and throat with
cold water, and the use of the various linctuses and
lotions, before enumerated, must be resorted to.

SPECIES 3. APHTHA *anginosa*, APHTHA OF THE
THROAT.

This appellation may be given to a species of
sore throat, which is not unfrequently observed
during damp and cold autumnal seasons, especially
in women and children. It is preceded by slight
febrile symptoms, which seldom continue many
days: on the second or third day, a roughness and
soreness are perceived in the throat, which, on
inspection, is found to be tumid, especially the
tonsils, uvula, and lower part of the velum pendulum, and considerably inflamed, but of a purplish
red colour. The same colour extends along the
sides of the tongue, which is covered in the middle
with a thin white crust, through which the elongated and inflamed papillæ protrude their red points.
Small whitish specks form on these parts, which
usually remain distinct, and heal in a few days,
but occasionally coalesce, and produce patches of
superficial ulceration. The complaint is sometimes
continued three weeks or a month, by successive

appearances of the Aphthæ, but without any constitutional disturbance.

This disease appears to arise from the influence of cold and moisture, unwholesome diet, and acrid effluvia taken into the lungs. In the latter mode, it is produced in persons who attend on patients affected with confluent smallpox, Scarlatina anginosa, or other malignant fevers. Although there is no clear evidence of its propagation by contagion, it is frequently seen to attack several children in the same family about the same time, or in very quick succession.

There appears to be no danger in this affection, and medicine does not materially abbreviate its duration. A light diet, with diluent drinks, and gentle laxatives, where there is a disposition to inactivity in the bowels, constitute the only treatment required for its cure. Leeches and blisters seem to be rather detrimental than advantageous; and Cinchona, with mineral acids, to be useless, until the decline of the disorder, when they contribute to restore the strength.*

Books which may be consulted on Aphtha.

BAILLIE, Series of Engravings, &c. Fasc. iii.
DIEZ, Dissertatio de Aphthis, 8vo. 1771.
HARRIS, de Morbis Acutis Infantum.
HEBERDEN, Commentarii de Morborum, &c. 8vo.
UNDERWOOD, Treatise on the Diseases of Children, 8vo. 1828.
WILSON, A Treatise on Febrile Diseases, 8vo. 1804.

* See Dr. Willan's Reports on Dis. in London, p. 111.; — and my Reports of the Public Dispensary, Edin. Med. and Surg. Journal for Jan. 1813.

Order VII.

TUBERCULA.

TUBERCLES.

SYN. Des Knotes (*German*) : Bouton, Inflammation Tuberculeuses (*F.*).

Def. SMALL, HARD, SUPERFICIAL TUMOURS, CIRCUMSCRIBED AND PERMANENT, OR SUPPURATING PARTIALLY.

The Order of Tubercles comprehends nine genera : but as some of them require only surgical treatment, some are of rare occurrence, and some are unknown in this country, they will not require a very ample discussion in this place. The following are the Genera of Tubercles :

1. PHYMA.
2. VERRUCA.
3. MOLLUSCUM.
4. VITILIGO.
5. ACNE.
6. SYCOSIS.
7. LUPUS.
8. ELEPHANTIASIS.
9. FRAMBOESIA.

GENUS I. PHYMA.

Syn. Die Erbsenblattern; Eiter-blasem (*Germ.*): Charbon (*F.*).

Def. IMPERFECTLY SUPPURATING CUTANEOUS OR SUBCUTANEOUS TUMOURS : FORMING AN ABSCESS THICKENED AND INDURATED AT THE EDGE, OFTEN WITH A CORE IN THE CENTRE.

Under the genus PHYMA*, Dr. Willan intended to comprise the Terminthus, the Epinyctis, the lesser species of boil (Furunculus), and the carbuncle of authors. These tubercular affections are commonly treated of in chirurgical works, and I have nothing to add to the general information on the subject.

———

GENUS II. VERRUCA.

Syn. Phymosis verrucosa (*Young*): Porri (*Auct.*): die Warze (*Germ.*): Verrue (*F.*): Shullul (*Arab.*): *Warts.*

Def. A FIRM, HARD, ARID EXTUBERANCE OF THE SKIN, CHIEFLY ON THE HANDS.

The same considerations induce me to omit details relative to the varieties of VERRUCA, which is here understood in its ordinary sense, denoting the cuticular excrescences called *warts.*

The most common variety of wart is that which is hard, has a broad base, and is covered with the cuticle. They in general disappear before the age

---

* According to Paulus, the term φυμα was employed to signify in general a suppurating tumour, but in particular a suppurating tumour in a glandular part. (De Re Med. lib. iv. cap. 22. See also Oribas. de Morb. Cur. lib. iii. c. 34.; and Actuar. Meth. Med. lib. ii. cap. 12.) Hippocrates uses the term in the general sense (aph. 20. § iii. and aph. 82. § iv.), and speaks also of scrofulous phymata, φυματα χοιρωδεα, in Prædict. lib. ii. § ii. 77. Foës. See also Celsus, lib. v. cap. 18.

of puberty. The best application is to touch the
wart, daily, with the strong Acetic Acid, taking care
not to touch the sound skin. The destroyed surface should always be rubbed off before the re-
application of the acid.

Genus III. MOLLUSCUM.

Syn. Encystis (*Vog. Parr*): Lupia (*Sauv*).:
Steatoma (*Sharp*): Emphyma encystis (*Good*):
Atheroma (*Auct.*): *Wen.*

Def. A MOVABLE TUMOUR; LITTLE SENSIBLE;
OFTEN ELASTIC TO THE TOUCH.

This form of tubercular disease is noticed rather
as a singularity, which occasionally occurs, and of
which a few instances are recorded, than as an object of medical treatment. It is characterised by
the appearance of numerous tubercles, of slow
growth and little sensibility, and of various sizes,
from that of a vetch to that of a pigeon's egg.
(Plate LX. Fig. 1. of BATEMAN; Pl. 21. of THE
ATLAS). These contain an atheromatous matter,
and are of various forms, some being sessile, globular, or flattish, and some attached by a neck, and
pendulous. The growth of the tubercles is apparently unconnected with any constitutional disorder;
they show no tendency to inflammation or ulceration; but continue through life, having apparently
no natural termination. A very extraordinary in-

stance of this cutaneous deformity, which occurred in a poor man, who was living in good health, at Muhlberg, in 1793, and whose body, face, and extremities were thickly studded with these atheromatous tubercles, has been described by Prof. Tilesius, who has given portraits of the naked patient in three positions, in a pamphlet, edited at Leipsic, in that year, by Prof. Ludwig.

Since the second edition was printed, a patient was sent to me by a distinguished physician, affected with a singular species of molluscum, which appears to be communicable by contact. (Plate LXI. of BATEMAN; Pl. 21. of the ATLAS). The face and neck of this young woman were thickly studded with round prominent tubercles, of various sizes, from that of a large pin's head to that of a small bean, which were hard, smooth, and shining on their surface, with a slight degree of transparency, and nearly of the colour of the skin. The tubercles were all sessile, upon a contracted base, without any peduncle. From the larger ones a small quantity of milk-like fluid issued, on pressure, from a minute aperture, such as might be made by a needle's point, and which only became visible on the exit of the fluid. The progress of their growth was very slow: for the first tubercle had appeared on the chin a twelvemonth ago, and only a few of them had attained a large size. Some of the latter had recently become inflamed, and were proceeding to a slow and curdly suppuration; and the cervical glands, lying under those on the neck, were also swollen, and discoloured, as if proceeding to suppurate. The eruption was still increasing much, and not only disfigured her greatly, but had recently impaired her general health, and occasioned a considerable loss of flesh, by the irritation which it produced.

She ascribed the origin of this disease to contact with the face of a child, whom she nursed, on which a large tubercle of the same sort existed; and on a subsequent visit she informed me, that two other children of the same family were disfigured by similar tubercles; and besides, that the parents believed that the first child had received the eruption from a servant, on whose face it was observed. Since my attention was drawn to this species of tubercle, I have seen it in another instance, in an infant brought to me with Porrigo larvalis; and, on investigation, it was found that she had apparently received it from an older child, who was in the habit of nursing it. In this case the milky fluid issued from the tubercles, and may be presumed to be the medium of the contagion.

Of the best mode of managing this singular Molluscum I have not had sufficient experience to speak. Nothing remedial was administered to the children; but, in the adult patient, I had the satisfaction to find, that, after the liquor arsenicalis had been taken in small doses for a month, the tubercles were universally diminished both in number and magnitude, most of them having gradually subsided: a few, especially on the neck, had suppurated.

Genus IV. VITILIGO.

Syn. Epichrosis *leucasmus* (*Good*).

Def. White, shining, smooth tubercles arising in the skin, about the ears, neck, and face;
terminating without suppuration.

Dr. Willan adopted this generic term from Celsus, but proposed to appropriate it to a disease
somewhat different from those to which that classical writer applied it, and which is not of frequent
occurrence. There is, indeed, a substantial reason
for not adopting the term in the acceptation in
which it is used by Celsus; namely, that he has
comprehended under it three forms of disease, two
of which are generically distinct from the third.
The two former, *alphos* and *melas*, are superficial,
scaly diseases, *i. e.* only slighter varieties of Lepra
and Psoriasis; whereas the last, *Leuce*, deeply
affects the skin and subjacent structure, occasioning a loss of sensibility, and ultimately of vitality, in
those parts.*

The disease which is here intended to be designated by the term Vitiligo, (Plate LX. Fig. 2. of
Bateman; Pl. 21. of The Atlas,) is, as I have
already stated, somewhat rare, and perhaps but little

---

* See Lepra *alphoides*, above, p. 30. After having described the characteristics of the three forms of Vitiligo, Celsus thus points out the
circumstances which mark the greater severity of the last: " *Alphos* et
Melas in quibusdam variis temporibus et oriuntur et desinunt: *Leuce*
quem occupavit, non facile dimittit. Priora curationem non difficilli-
mam recipiunt; ultimum vix unquam sanescit; ac siquid ei vitio demp-
tum est, tamen non ex toto sanus color redditur." De Medicinâ, lib. v.
cap. 28.

known. It is characterised by the appearance of smooth, white, shining tubercles, which rise on the skin, sometimes in particular parts, as about the ears, neck, and face; and sometimes over nearly the whole body, intermixed with shining papulæ. They vary much in their course and progress: in some cases they reach their full size in the space of a week (attaining the magnitude of a large wart), and then begin to subside, becoming flattened to the level of the cuticle in about ten days : in other instances, they advance less rapidly, and the elevation which they acquire is less considerable ; in fact, they are less distinctly tubercular. But in these cases they are more permanent; and as they gradually subside to the level of the surface, they creep along in one direction, as, for example, across the face or along the limbs, chequering the whole superficies with a veal-skin appearance.* All the hairs drop out, where the disease passes, and never sprout again, a smooth shining surface, as if polished, being left, and the morbid whiteness remaining through life. The eruption never goes on to ulceration.

There is no considerable constitutional disorder combined with this affection ; but it has proved exceedingly unmanageable under the use of both internal and external medicines. The mineral acids internally, and the application of diluted caustic

---

* This white and glistening appearance, bearing some resemblance to the flesh of calves (vituli), seems to have given rise to the generic term.

and spirituous substances externally, have been chiefly employed, but with little obvious effect.

Book which may be consulted on Vitiligo.

BLANCKAERTT, (E. L.) de Vitiligine, 4to. 1764.

V. ACNE.*

Syn. Vari Ionthi (*Auct.*): Psydracia Acne (*Sauv.*) Boutons (*F.*): die Finnen (*German*).

Def. TUBERCULAR TUMOURS; SLOWLY SUPPUR-ATING; CHIEFLY COMMON TO THE FACE.

This genus, as the definition describes, is characterised by an eruption of distinct, hard, inflamed tubercles, which are sometimes permanent for a considerable length of time, and sometimes suppurate very slowly and partially. They usually appear on the face, especially on the forehead, temples, and chin, and sometimes also on the neck, shoulders, and upper part of the breast; but never descend to the lower parts of the trunk, or to the extremities. As the progress of each tubercle is slow, and they appear in succession, they are generally seen at the same time in the various stages of growth and decline; and, in the more violent cases,

---

* This term is borrowed from Aëtius, who mentions it as a synonyme of ιονθος, by which most of the Greek writers designate the disease. Aët. tetrab. ii. serm. iv. cap. 13. The Latins denominated the tubercles *vari.* See Celsus, lib. vi. cap. 5.—Plin. Hist. Nat. lib. xxiii.—Sennert having spoken of the affinity of *vari* with the pustules about the head, called *psydracia* by some writers, Sauvages made the eruption a species of the latter, Psydracia *acne.* Nosol. Meth. class i. ord. ii. gen. 9. See Jul. Pollux, Onomasticon, lib. iv. cap. 25.

are intermixed likewise with the marks or vestiges
of those which have subsided. The eruption occurs
almost exclusively in persons of the sanguine tem-
.perament, and in the early part of life, from the age
of puberty* to thirty or thirty-five ; but in those of
more exquisite temperament, even later. It is common to both sexes ; but the most severe forms of it
are seen in young men.

There are four species of this eruption : —

    1. A. *simplex.*   3. A. *indurata.*

    2. A. *punctata.*   4. A. *rosacea.*†

SPECIES 1. ACNE *simplex,* SIMPLE PIMPLE.

Syn. Dartre pustuleuse miliaire ; Herpes pustulosus miliaris (*Alibert*).

This is an eruption of small vari, which appear
singly, and are not very numerous, nor accompanied
by much inflammation, nor by any intermediate
affection of the skin. (Plate LXII. of BATEMAN ;
Pl. 23. of THE ATLAS.) When it has continued some
time, indeed, a little roughness of the face is produced, where the larger tubercles have disappeared,
in consequence of a slight cracking or disposition

* From this circumstance, both the Greek appellations appear to have
originated ; ιονθος, from its occurring during the growth of the *lanugo,*
or first beard, which the word also signifies ; — and ακνη, quasi ακμη,
from its appearance at the *acme,* or full growth and evolution of the
system. " Ionthi, flores cum papulis circa faciem, *vigoris signum,*" is
the definition given by Julius Pollux (loc. cit.). And Cassius, in his
33d problem, explains, " Cur in facie vari prodeunt ferè in ipso ætatis
flore vigoreque (quapropter et ακμος, id est, *vigores,* idiotarum vulgus eos
nuncupat)? "

† Alibert has not figured any specimen of Acne, unless an ill-defined
plate (22d), representing what he calls " Dartre pustuleuse miliaire," on
the forehead, be intended for Acne simplex.

to exfoliate in the new cuticle; but these marks are not permanent.

Many of the tubercles do not proceed to suppuration; but gradually rise, become moderately inflamed, and again slowly subside, in the course of eight or ten days, leaving a transient purplish red mark behind. But others go on to a partial suppuration, the whole process of which occupies from a fortnight to three weeks. The tubercles are first felt in the skin, like a small hard seed, about the size of a pin's head, and enlarge for three or four days, when they begin to inflame: about the sixth or seventh day they attain their greatest magnitude, and are then prominent, red, smooth, and shining, and hard and painful to the touch. After two or three days more, a small speck of yellow matter appears on the apices of some of the tubercles; and when these afterwards break, a thinner humour is secreted, which soon dries into a yellowish scab. The inflammation now gradually declines, the size and hardness of the tubercles diminish, and the small scab becomes loosened at the edges, and at length falls off about the third week. The individual tubercles, which rise and suppurate in succession, pass through a similar course.

This eruption recurs frequently, at short intervals, in some individuals, who have it partially; but in others, who are more strongly predisposed to it, it is more extensive, and never wholly disappears, but is, at uncertain periods, more or less troublesome. Such persons often enjoy good health, and cannot refer the cutaneous complaint to any obvious exciting cause; whence Dr. Darwin* has constituted it a distinct species, with the epithet, " hereditary ;" which, in fact, is to ascribe it solely to the temperament of the patient, or to consider the predisposition, arising from the great vascularity of the skin in sanguine habits, as adequate to give rise to the eruption, under ordinary stimulation.   There appears, however, to be no clear distinction between the *stomachic* and *hereditary* cases of Acne, as Dr. Darwin supposes; for it is only where there is a strong constitutional predisposition, that substances which disorder the stomach excite the eruption of Acne; and in those who are so predisposed, the vari occasionally appear after eating heartily, or drinking an unusual portion of wine, or from any slight cause of indigestion; as well as after any inordinate excitement of the cutaneous circulation from violent exercise in hot weather, or in heated rooms, especially when followed by a copious draught of cold liquor. In some cases, a sort of critical eruption of vari has suddenly occurred, after severe indigestion, or continued pains in the stomach, which have been imme-

---

* Dr. Darwin names the genus Gutta Rosea, of which he says, there are three species:— 1. The Gutta Rosea *hepatica*, connected with diseased liver in drunkards : 2. G. R. *stomatica*, which is occasioned by taking cold drink, eating cold raw turnips, &c. when the body is much heated by exercise: and 3. The G. R. *hereditaria*, or Puncta rosea (the Acne simplex), which consists of smaller pimples, that are less liable to suppurate, and which seems to be hereditary, " or at least has no apparent cause, like the others." See Zoonomia, class ii. 1. 4. 6. — and class iv. 1, 2. 13. and 14.

diately relieved; and in such instances, there is occasionally also an eruption of lichenous papulæ on the body and limbs.

Being generally, however, a local disease, the Acne simplex is to be treated chiefly by external applications. Except in females, indeed, this variety of the eruption seldom calls for the attention of medical men. Celsus observes, that, in his time, the Roman ladies were so solicitous of maintaining their beauty, that he deemed it necessary to mention the remedies for this affection, which otherwise he considered as too trifling for the notice of the physician.* The ancients agree in recommending a number of stimulant applications, with the view of discussing the "thick humours" which were supposed to constitute the vari. Lotions and liniments containing vinegar and honey, sometimes combined with an emulsion of Bitter Almonds, and sometimes with Turpentine, Resin, Myrrh, and other gums, or with Alum, Soap, and Cimolian earth, or the bruised roots of the Lily, Cyclamen, Narcissus, &c. were the substances which they principally employed.† They were, doubtless, correct as to the principle; as a gentle stimulus to the skin is

* " Pene ineptiæ sunt, curare varos, et lenticulas, et ephelidas: sed eripi tamen fœminis cura cultus sui non potest." De Med. lib. vi. cap. v.

† See Celsus, loc. cit. — Oribas. Synops. lib. viii. cap. 34.; and De Loc. Affect. lib. iv. cap. 51. — Aëtius, tetrab. ii. serm. iv. cap. 13. — Paulus, lib. iii. cap. 25. — Actuarius, lib. iv. cap. 12. By the older modern writers, who were chiefly their copyists, the same applications were prescribed. See Hafenreffer, Nosodochium, lib. ii. cap. 14.

the most safe and effectual remedy. The apprehensions, which have been strongly expressed by the humoral pathologists, of producing internal disorder by the sudden repulsion, as it has been called, of these cutaneous eruptions, are not altogether hypothetical. Headache, and affections of the stomach and bowels, have sometimes been thus produced, which have ceased on the re-appearance of the eruption: but, on the whole, as far as my observation goes, this alternation of disease is less frequent and obvious in this form of Acne, than in the pustular and crustose eruptions of the face and head.

The stimulant applications, which are most easily proportioned to the irritability of the tubercles, are lotions containing Alcohol, which may be reduced or strengthened, according to circumstances, by the addition of any distilled water. It is not easy to describe the appearances of the eruption, which indicate any certain degree of strength in the lotion; but a little observation will teach this discrimination. If the tubercles are considerably inflamed, and a great number of them pustular, a dilute mixture will be requisite; containing, for example, equal parts of spiritus tenuior, and of Rose or Elder-flower water. The effect of a very acrid lotion, under such circumstances, is to multiply the pustules, to render many of them confluent, and to produce the formation of a crust of some extent, as well as to excite an inflammatory redness in the adjoining skin.* A slight increase of the inflammation, indeed, is sometimes occasioned by the first applications of a weak stimulus; but this is of short duration, and the skin soon bears an augmentation of the stimulant; until at length the pure spirit is borne with advantage, as the inflammatory disposition subsides. Under the latter circumstances, even a considerable additional stimulus is often useful; such as from half a grain to a grain or more of the Muriate of Mercury, in each ounce of the spirit; or a drachm or more of the Liquor Potassæ, or of the Muriatic Acid, in six ounces: "perhaps the best vehicle for either the Chloride of Mercury or the Liquor Potassæ is the Emulsion of Bitter Almonds, containing ten minims of Hydrocyanic acid to each fluid ounce of the Emulsion." Acetous acid, as recommended by the ancients, and the Liquor Ammoniæ Acetatis, afford also an agreeable stimulant, in proper proportions. Sulphur yields a small portion of its substance to boiling water, poured upon it, and allowed to infuse for twelve or fourteen hours, a quart of water being added to about an ounce of broken Sulphur. A lotion of this nature has been found advantageous

---

* It must be admitted, however, that the eruption is sometimes materially diminished, after the violent action of an irritating application has subsided. I lately saw a lady, who considered herself much benefited after a severe inflammation, and even excoriation, of the face, which had been produced by a poultice of bruised *parsley*. Dr. Darwin affirms that blistering the whole face, in small portions, successively, is the most effectual remedy for this Acne (loc. cit.). But the "cura cultus sui" generally renders patients of this class unwilling to employ harsh remedies.

in slight cases of Acne simplex, and especially in removing the roughness and duskiness of the face connected with it. *

SPECIES 2.   ACNE *punctata*, MAGGOT PIMPLE.

Syn. Punctæ mucosæ (*Darwin*): Ionthus varus punctatus (*Good*): Crimones (*Underwood*): *Grubs.*

The eruption, in this variety of the disorder, (Plate LXII. of BATEMAN ; Pl. 23. of THE ATLAS,) consists of a number of black points, surrounded by a very slight raised border of cuticle.   These are vulgarly considered as the extremities of small worms or grubs, because, when they are pressed out, a sort of wormlike appendage is found attached to them : but they are, in fact, only concreted mucus or sebaceous matter, moulded in the ducts of the sebaceous glands into this vermicular form, the extremity of which is blackened by contact with the air.   In consequence of the distention of the ducts, the glands themselves sometimes inflame, and form small tubercles, with little black points on their surface, which partially suppurate, as in the foregoing species ; but many of them remain stationary for a long period, without ever passing into the inflammatory state.   Not unfrequently they are intermixed with a few tubercles, in which the puncta have not appeared.

These concretions may be extracted, by pressing on both sides of the specks with the nails, until the

* This lotion has been recommended by Dr. Clarke of Dublin, as containing a sufficient impregnation of sulphur for the cure of Scabies in children. See Med. Facts and Observ. vol. viii. p. 275.

hardened mucus is sufficiently elevated to be taken hold of. A blunt curved forceps may be employed with advantage for this purpose.* When the puncta are removed, the disease becomes Acne simplex, and requires the same treatment with the preceding species.

Dr. Underwood has recommended the use of a solution of Carbonate of Potass internally, in these cases †; and Dr. Willan was in the habit of occasionally prescribing the Oxymuriatic Acid. One or two tea-spoonsful of this liquid, taken in a glass of water three times a day for a considerable period, has sometimes appeared to benefit the health, and improve the colour and smoothness of the skin; but, on the whole, it is not easy to discover any sensible operation of this medicine, and its only effect is, perhaps, that of a tonic to the stomach. Medicines of this nature are more adapted to the subsequent species of the complaint, especially to the A. rosacea.‡

* Such a forceps has been contrived by a surgeon's instrument-maker, of the name of Hattersley, in South-Molton-Street.

† See some observations relative to " *crinones*, or grubs," which, he says, he had often found troublesome, especially in females, about the time of puberty. Treatise on the Dis. of Children, vol. ii. p. 167. 5th edit.

‡ The Editor cannot concur in this opinion of Dr. Bateman: he has seen the skin completely cleared by the use of the following Alkaline Tonic for six weeks; at the same time regulating the bowels:—

 ℞ Sulphatis Zinci gr. xxiv,
  Liquoris Potassæ f℥xij. Solve.
 Sumantur guttæ xxx ex cyatho aquæ bis quotidie.

The skin should be well cleaned with soap and hot water, or a solution of pure Potass, or Ox-gall; and well rubbed with a rough towel, night and morning.

SPECIES 3. ACNE *indurata*, STONE-POCK.

In this form of Acne (Plate LXIII. of BATE-
MAN; Pl. 22. of THE ATLAS,) the tubercles are
larger, as well as more indurated and permanent,
than in A. simplex. They rise often in considerable numbers, of a conical, or oblong conoidal
form, and are occasionally somewhat acuminated,
as if tending to immediate suppuration, being at
the same time of a bright roseate hue: yet many
of them continue in a hard and elevated state for a
great length of time, without any disposition to
suppurate. Others, however, pass on very slowly
to suppuration, the matter not being completely
formed in them for several weeks, and then only a
small part of the tubercles are removed by that
process. Sometimes two or three coalesce, forming a large irregular tubercle, which occasionally
suppurates at the separate apices, and sometimes
only at the largest. In whatever mode they proceed, the vivid hue of the tubercles gradually
becomes more purple or even livid, especially in
those which show no tendency to suppurate. Slight
crusts form upon the suppurating tubercles, which
after some time fall off, leaving small scars, surrounded by hard tumours of the same dark red colour; and these sometimes suppurate again at
uncertain periods, and sometimes slowly subside
and disappear, leaving a purple or livid discoloration, and occasionally a slight depression, which is
long in wearing off.

The tubercles, even when they do not suppurate, but especially while they continue highly red, are always sore and tender to the touch; so that washing, shaving, the friction of the clothes, &c. are somewhat painful. In its most severe form, this eruption nearly covers the face, breast, shoulders, and top of the back, but does not descend lower than an ordinary tippet in dress: yet this limitation of the disorder is independent of the exposure of those parts; for it occurs equally in men and women. In a few instances in young men, I have seen an extensive eruption of Acne indurata affecting these covered parts, while the face remained nearly free from it. By the successive rise and progress of the tumours, the whole surface, within the limits just mentioned, was spotted with the red and livid tubercles, intermixed with the purple discolorations and depressions left by those which had subsided, and variegated with yellow suppurating points and small crusts, so that very little of the natural skin appeared. Sometimes the black puncta of the sebaceous ducts were likewise mixed with the vari and their sequelæ.

The general health does not commonly suffer, even under this aggravated form of the eruption.* If a fever or other severe disease should take place,

* Forestus, and several other physicians of the sixteenth century, assert that *vari* are the precursors of Elephantiasis, and indicate its approach. Sennertus asserts the same of *vari*, that are accompanied with puffy swelling (inflatio) of the face, and hoarseness. But these assertions

indeed, the tubercles often subside and disappear;
so that their recurrence, under such circumstances,
is to be deemed a sign of returning health. I
have seen the erethism of a mercurial course, administered for other purposes, occasion the disappearance of this Acne, which returned with the
restoration of flesh and strength, after the omission
of the medicine. Many persons, however, who are
affected with the eruption, are liable to disorders of
the bowels and stomach, to Hæmorrhoids, and some
to Phthisis pulmonalis. Its first appearance, too, is
commonly ascribed to some irregularity of diet, or
to some cold substance swallowed when the person
had been overheated, and was in a free perspiration.
Hence the first eruption is not unfrequently sudden.

The Acne indurata is often much alleviated " in
the first or inflammatory stage of the eruption by
poultices, made with the decoction of Poppy Cap-
sules, boiled until they are quite soft, and then
strained by pressure through a cloth. After the
tubercles have suppurated and discharged their
contents, or have been opened," the disease is
sometimes entirely removed by the steady use of
external stimulants, combined with a proper regulation of the diet and exercise. The eruption will

---

are obviously either the result of mere hypothesis, founded on the resemblance of the larger vari to the incipient tubercles of Elephantiasis;
or of practical error, in applying the appellation of vari to the early
symptoms of the latter disease. See Forest. Obs. Chirurg. lib. v. obs. 7.
Sennert. Med. Pract. lib. v. part ii. cap. 23.

bear a more acrid stimulus, even from the beginning, than the inflamed Acne simplex. A spiritous lotion, at first a little diluted, and containing the Oxymuriate of Mercury, in the proportion of a grain or somewhat less to the ounce of the vehicle, is often extremely beneficial. Gowland's lotion, an empirical preparation, which is said to contain this mercurial salt in an emulsion of Bitter Almonds *, is popularly used ; and where its strength happens to accord with the degree of irritability in the eruption, and it is not applied to the other varieties of it, it is doubtless beneficial. Many other stimulants, some of which have been already named, may be substituted, of course, with similar effect ; but it is unnecessary to specify them. It will be proper to remark, that, in general, it is requisite to augment the activity of all these applications in the progress of the treatment, partly in consequence of the diminished effect of an accustomed stimulus, and partly on account of the increasing inertness of the tubercles, as the inflammatory state subsides, which must be determined by the appearances.

Frequent purgatives, which are often resorted to in these cases, especially by unprofessional persons, among whom the dregs of the humoral pa-

---

* The Bitter Almond was a favourite application with all the ancient physicians in inflammatory cutaneous eruptions. Its emulsion is prescribed, as a vehicle of more active substances, in every tract which they have left on these subjects. Yet it is probably a mere agreeable mucilage.

This note was written before the fact that the Bitter Almond contains a large portion of Hydrocyanic acid was known. T.

thology still remain, are of no advantage; but, on
the contrary, often augment the disease in feeble
habits. "On the contrary, even where the tongue
is furred, and indicates the use of an alterative, a
tonic taken in conjunction with five or six grains
of Plummer's pill at bed-time, for ten or twelve
successive nights, proves often highly beneficial.
As far as my experience has enabled me to decide,
the Carbonate of Soda, in doses of a drachm in
twelve fluid drachms of Infusion of Cascarilla Bark,
taken at noon and about four o'clock in the after-
noon, daily, is the best tonic in this affection. The
irritability of the stomach is allayed at the same time
its tonic power is augmented." The copious use
of *raw* vegetables in diet, which the misapplication
of the term "scurvy" has introduced, is to be de-
precated, as well as the free use of vegetable acids,
especially in constitutions that are predisposed to
indigestion. These substances not only afford little
nutriment, under such circumstances, but tend to
increase the indigestion : and it is a fact, which it
may not be easy to explain, that under many modifications of cutaneous inflammation, especially
about the head and face, that inflammation is immediately increased in sympathy with the offended
stomach, when these substances are eaten.* It
were totally superfluous to remind professional
men of the very opposite nature of inflammatory
and suppurating affections of the skin, to that of
petechiæ and ecchymoses, the mere effusions of

extravasated blood under the cuticle, which belong to the proper, or, as it has been called, the *putrid* scurvy. And this negative inference at least must be deduced from the fact, that it is almost impossible, that these two opposite states of disease should be benefited by the same remedies. The diet, in these cases of Acne, should be good, *i. e.* light and nutritious, but not stimulating ; consisting of animal food, with well-dressed vegetables, and the farinaceæ ; wine and fermented liquors being omitted, or taken with great moderation.

Internally, medicines effect little ; but I have had an opportunity, in several severe cases of Acne *tuberata*, of witnessing the increased amendment of the disorder, under the external treatment already mentioned, when small doses of Soda, Sulphur, and Antimony were at the same time administered ; by which plan the skin has been totally cleared.

SPECIES 4. ACNE *rosacea* *, ROSY DROP.

Syn. Bacchia (*Linn.*): Gutta Rosea (*Sauv. Darwin*): Gutta Rosacea Œnopotarum (*Plenck*): Ionthus Corymbefer (*Good*): Roth-gesicht, Roth-nase Kupferbandel (*German*): Couperose Rougeurs, Goutte Rose (*F.*): *Carbuncled face.*

This form of Acne (Plate LXIV. of BATEMAN; Pl. 23. of THE ATLAS,) differs in several respects

---

* This is the *Gutta rosea*, or *rosacea* of authors; some of whom, however, (as Dr. Darwin, to whom I have already referred,) comprehend all the varieties of *vari* under that appellation.

from the preceding species. In addition to an
eruption of small suppurating tubercles, there is
also a shining redness, and an irregular granulated
appearance of the skin of that part of the face
which is affected. The redness commonly appears
first at the end of the nose, and afterwards spreads
from both sides of the nose to the cheeks, the whole
of which, however, it very seldom covers. In the
commencement it is not uniformly vivid; but is
paler in the morning, and readily increased to an
intense red after dinner, or at any time if a glass
of wine or spirits be taken, or the patient be heated
by exercise, or by sitting near a fire. After some
continuance in this state, the texture of the cuticle
becomes gradually thickened, and its surface uneven or granulated, and variegated by reticulations
of enlarged cutaneous veins, with smaller red
lines stretching across the cheeks, and sometimes
by the intermixture of small suppurating *vari*,
which successively arise on different parts of the
face.

This species of Acne seldom occurs in early life,
except where there is a great hereditary predisposition to it: in general it does not appear before
the age of forty; but it may be produced in any
person by the constant immoderate use of wine
and spirituous liquors. The greater part of the
face, even the forehead and chin, are often affected
in these cases; but the nose especially becomes
tumid, and of a fiery red colour; and, in advanced
life, it sometimes enlarges to an enormous size, the

nostrils being distended and patulous, or the alæ fissured, as it were, and divided into several separate lobes.* At that period of life, too, the colour of the Acne rosacea becomes darker and more livid ; and if suppuration take place in any of the tubercles, they ulcerate unfavourably, and do not readily assume a healing disposition.

In young persons, however, who are hereditarily predisposed to this complaint, irregular red patches not unfrequently appear in the face, which are often smooth, and free from tubercles, and sometimes throw off slight exfoliations at intervals. These patches may be gradually extended, if great temperance both in food and drink be not observed, until the whole face assume a preternatural redness.

As this eruption is chiefly sympathetic of some derangement of the chylopoietic viscera, or of a peculiar irritability of the stomach, little advantage can be expected from local applications: and, in fact, the stimulants, which are beneficial, under proper regulations, in most of the other forms of Acne, are generally prejudicial in this, and aggravate the complaint. The misapplication of the

---

* Sennert mentions a case, in which the enlarging nose made such an approximation in magnitude to Strasburg steeple, as to impede the exercise of vision, and to require lopping. " Sumunt tubercula ista interdum incrementum, ut facies inæqualis et horrida evadat, et nasus valde augeatur. Vixit superiori adhuc anno, non procul a Dresdâ, vir, cui hoc malo affecto, nasus ita incrementum sumsit, ut eum in legendo impediret; quod malum ipsum eo adegit, ut anno 1629 particulas quasdam de naso sibi amputari curaret." Pract. Med. lib. v. part. i. cap. 31.

nostrum, before mentioned, to this variety of the eruption, is one among the numerous practical errors which originate from the indiscriminate recommendations of empiricism. On the other hand, all strong sedatives or restringents, if they succeed in repressing the eruption, are liable to aggravate the internal disorder.

The perfect cure of Acne rosacea is, in fact, seldom accomplished; for, whether it originate in a strong hereditary predisposition, or from habitual intemperance, the difficulties in the way of correcting the habit of body, are almost insurmountable. The regulation of the diet, in both cases, is important; " the bowels should be regulated by gentle aperients; for instance, the Hydrargyrum cum Creta, in doses of from ten to twelve grains, may be given every night at bed-time :" and when the stomach or liver is disordered, the symptoms may be sometimes palliated by the Liquor Potassæ, or other antacids, which seem also to have some influence in lessening inflammatory action in the skin. " The Editor is of opinion that much of the difficulty attending the treatment of Acne rosacea has arisen from giving the Liquor Potassæ in too small doses : he has seldom seen it fail to relieve the disease when the dose has been gradually carried to sixty or eighty drops three times a day. The best vehicle for giving the Liquor Potassæ in is the Bitter Almond Emulsion." The gentlest restringents should be used externally to the patches of reticulated veins; such as very dilute spirituous or acetous lotions, with or without a small proportion of the Acetate of Lead; or simple ointments combined with Alum, Acetate of Lead, &c. in small quantities. The more purely local and primary the eruption appears to be, the more active may be the astringency of the substances applied to it.

Genus VI. SYCOSIS.

Def. AN ERUPTION OF INFLAMED, FLESHY, DARK-ISH-RED TUBERCLES ON THE BEARDED PORTION OF THE FACE, AND ON THE SCALP; GREGARIOUS; OFTEN COALESCING: DISCHARGE PARTIAL AND SANIOUS.

Although this eruption was not mentioned in the enumeration of Tubercles, on the cover of Dr. Willan's publication, I believe he intended, after the example of the old writers, to introduce it in this place, in consequence of its affinity to Acne.

Celsus has correctly stated, that some difference takes place in the appearance and progress of the eruption, when it is seated in the chin, and in the scalp; whence it may be divided into two species*:

1. S. *menti.*
2. S. *capillitii.*

---

* "Sub eo vero duæ sunt species. Altera ulcus durum et rotundum est; altera humidum et inæquale. Ex duro exiguum quiddam et glutinosum exit: ex humido pus, et mali odoris. Fit utrumque in iis partibus quæ pilis conteguntur: sed id quod callosum et rotundum est maxime in barba; id vero, quod humidum, præcipue in capillo." loc. cit.

Species I. Sycosis * *menti*, Sycosis of the Beard.

Syn. Sycosis Barbæ (*Celsus*): Mentagra (*Plenck*): Dartre pustuleuse mentagre; Herpes pustulosus mentagra (*Alibert*): Boutons bilieux (*M. Retz.*): Phyma Sycosis Barbæ (*Good*): der Kieferaustatz (*German*).

In this species (Plate LXV. of Bateman; Pl. 24. of The Atlas,) the tubercles arise first on the under lip, or on the prominent part of the chin, in an irregularly-circular cluster; but this is speedily followed by other clusters, and by distinct tubercles, which appear in succession, along the lower part of the cheeks up to the ears, and under the jaw towards the neck, as far as the beard grows.† The tubercles are red and smooth, and of a conoidal form, and nearly equal to a pea in magnitude. Many of them continue in this condition for three or four weeks, or even longer, having attained their

---

* This denomination has been given to the disease, from the granulated and prominent surface of the ulceration which ensues, and which somewhat resembles the soft inside pulp of *a fig* (συκον). " Est etiam ulcus, quod a *fici* similitudine συκωσις à Græcis nominatur, quia caro in eo excrescit." Celsus, lib. vi. cap. 3. The later Greeks, however, apply the terms συκα and ογκοι συκωδεις (*fici*, and *ficose tumours*,) to excrescences of the eyelids, as well as to the proper *Sycosis* of Celsus. See Aëtius, tetrab. i. serm. ii. cap. 80 & 190; — also tetr. ii. serm. iii. cap. 43; Paul. Ægin. lib. iii. cap. 22; — and Actuarius, lib. ii. cap. 7. Paul, however, describes the Sycosis of the face as an eruption of " round, red, somewhat hard, painful, and ulcerating tubercles." (lib. iii. cap. 3.) And Aëtius, in another place, mentions the eruption as " one of the affections of the chin, which," he says, " differs from Acne, in the nature of the humour which it discharges, and in its greater tendency to ulceration." (tetrab. ii. serm. iv. cap. 14.)

† An indifferent representation of this disease is given by Alibert, plate 20, under the appellation of " Dartre pustuleuse mentagra."

full size in seven or eight days; but others suppurate very slowly and partially, discharging a small quantity of thick matter, by which the hairs of the beard are matted together, so that shaving becomes impracticable, from the tender and irregular surface of the skin. This condition of the face, rendered rugged by tubercles from both ears round to the point of the chin, together with the partial ulceration and scabbing, and the matting together of the unshaven beard, occasions a considerable degree of deformity; and it is accompanied also with a very troublesome itching.

This form of the Sycosis occurs, of course, chiefly in men; but women are not altogether exempt from it, though it is commonly slight, when it appears in them. Its duration is very uncertain: it is commonly removed in about a fortnight; but sometimes the slow suppuration goes on for many weeks; and sometimes the suppurating tubercles heal, and again begin to discharge. Occasionally the disease disappears for a season, and breaks out again.

SPECIES II. SYCOSIS *capillitii* *, SYCOSIS OF THE SCALP.

Syn. Sycosis capilli (*Celsus*): Phyma sycosis capilli (*Good*): Pian ruboide (*Alibert*).

This species (Plate LXVI. of BATEMAN: Pl. 23.

---

* M. Alibert has figured a disease of the scalp, under the appellation of "Pian ruboide," in plate 35, which resembles the Sycosis of the scalp, if it be not a case of neglected or mismanaged Porrigo favosa.

of THE ATLAS,) is seated chiefly about the margin of
the hairy scalp, in the occiput, or round the forehead
and temples, and near the external ear, which is also
liable to be included in the eruption.   The tubercles
rise in clusters, which affect the circular form ; they
are softer and more acuminated than those on the
chin ; and they all pass into suppuration in the course
of eight or ten days, becoming confluent, and producing an elevated, unequal, ulcerated surface,
which often appears granulated, so as to afford some
resemblance to the internal pulp of a fig.   The ulceration, as Celsus states, is generally humid ; for
there is a considerable discharge of a thin ichorous
fluid, which emits an unpleasant rancid odour.

The Sycosis, under its first-mentioned form, may
be distinguished from Acne indurata by its seat
being exclusively on the bearded part of the face,
— by the softer, more numerous, and clustered
tubercles, — and by the ulceration which they tend
to produce.   And, under its second form, in which
it is somewhat assimilated to the eruption of favous
pustules, or Porrigo favosa, affecting the face and
the borders of the capillitium, it may be discrimi-
nated by the tuberculated and elevated base of the
suppurating tumours ; not to mention the adult
age of the patient, and the absence of contagion.

The cure of Sycosis is generally much more
easily accomplished than that of Porrigo favosa ;
but the method of treatment required for it is not
very different.   When the tubercles are numerous,
inflamed, and confluent, and especially when the

suppuration is either beginning or considerably advanced, the most speedy benefit is derived from the application of poultices at night, of linseed powder, bread and milk, or other simple ingredients.* In the less severe forms, warm ablutions or fomentations may be substituted. " The tubercles should be punctured, and the hairs extracted." When the inflammatory symptoms are reduced, and in cases where they are from the first moderate, the healing process is much promoted, and the discharge moderated and restrained, by the application of the Unguentum Hydrargyri Nitratis, diluted with three or four parts of simple ointment, or by the Ung. Hydrargyri præcipitati united with an equal portion of the Zinc ointment, or the cerate of Acetate of Lead. At the same time it is useful to prescribe Antimonials, with alterative doses of Mercury, followed by Cinchona, or Serpentaria, and the fixed alkalies, especially where there appears to be any affection of the digestive organs, which, not unfrequently, concurs with this eruption.

Books which may be consulted on Sycosis.

BIETT, Dictionnaire de Médecine, *art.* Mentagra.
PLUMBE (SAM.) A Practical Treatise of the Diseases of the Skin, 8vo. 1827.
RAYER, Traité des Maladies de la Peau, 8vo. 1826.

---

* Super utrumque oportet imponere elaterium, aut lini semen contritum et aqua coactum, aut ficum in aqua decoctam.—*Celsus.* T.

Genus VII. LUPUS.

Syn. Cancer Lupus (*Sauv.*) : Ulcus Tuberculosus (*Good*): Formica corrosiva ; Ignis sacer ; Noli me tangere (*Auct. Var.*): Dartre rongeante idiopathique, Herpes exedens idiopathicus (*Alibert*): Dartre rongeante (*F.*).

Of this disease I shall not treat at any length ; for I can mention no medicine which has been of any essential service in the cure of it, and it requires the constant assistance of the surgeon, in consequence of the spreading ulcerations, in which the original tubercles terminate.* (Plate LXVII. of Bateman.)

The term was intended by Dr. Willan to comprise, together with the "*noli me tangere*" affecting the nose and lips, other slow tubercular affections, especially about the face, commonly ending in ragged ulcerations of the cheeks, forehead, eyelids, and lips, and sometimes occurring in other parts of the body, where they gradually destroy the skin and muscular parts to a considerable depth. Sometimes the disease appears in the cheek circularly, or in the form of a sort of ringworm, destroying the substance, and leaving a deep and deformed

---

* Alibert has two admirable portraits of Lupus in the face, in plates 19 *bis,* and 21 ; the former of Noli me tangere, which he calls " Dartre rongeante scrophuleuse;" and the latter of a less malignant variety, which he terms " Dartre pustuleuse couperose." His 19th plate is apparently an incipient Lupus of the ala nasi, under the appellation of " Dartre rongeante idiopathique."

cicatrix: and I have seen a similar circular patch of the disease, dilating itself at length to the extent of a hand-breadth or more upon the pectoral muscle. " Alibert mentions having seen instances in which it attacked the loins; and in one case the thigh was the site, and the disease proved fatal."

By surgical means, *i. e.* by the knife or the caustic, a separation has sometimes been made of the morbid from the sound parts, and the progress of the disease arrested. " I have employed the Nitrate of Silver with much advantage in some cases, extending the application beyond the limits of the ulceration. Mr. Plumbe states that in two cases he applied the Nitric Acid freely, and produced a healthy sore which readily healed." In some cases, where the ulceration was very slow, and unaccompanied by much inflammation, the internal use of Arsenic has been found beneficial. " M. Dupuytren has lately found that it is a specific when externally applied, in conjunction with Calomel. His formula is the following powder:

R Hydrargyri submuriatis præcip. partes 199;
Oxidi Arsenici albi, partem 1:
                    Tere optime.

" If any crust cover the surface, let it first be removed by a poultice or other means; then sprinkle the sore with the above powder, by means of a little puff. The sore puts on a healthy character and heals under this management. If the powder do not adhere, it may be mixed with Gum Arabic in powder, augmenting the quantity of the Arsenic." The circumstance that Arsenic cures Lupus has, probably, given rise to the opinion, that Cancer has been cured by that mineral. In three or four less severe cases of lupous tubercles in the face, which had made no progress towards ulceration, I have seen the solution of Muriate of Barytes, taken internally, materially amend the complaint.

Books which may be consulted on Lupus.

PATRIX, l'Art d'appliquer le Caustique Arsenical, 8vo. 1817.
PLUMBE on Diseases of the Skin, 8vo. 1827.
RAYER, Traité des Maladies de la Peau, 8vo. 1826.

———

GENUS VIII.   ELEPHANTIASIS.

Syn. Ἔλεφας, ἐλεφαντία, ἐλεφαντίασις, σατυρίασις, λεοντίασις, ἡλάκλειον πάθος (*G.*): Elephantiasis (*Sag. Cull.*): Elephantiasis Indica (*Sauv.*): Elephanta Arabum (*Vog.*): Elephantiasis Arabica (*Good*): Lepra Elephantiaca seu Arabica. (*Auct.*) Mal rouge-lèpre des jointures (*F.*): Koostum (*Tam.*) Ruggit pittee (*Duk.*): Pedda-rogum (*Tel.*): Vhénghum, Koosthum (*Sans.*): Dzudham (*Arab.*): Khorah (*Hind.*): Der Elefantenaussatz, der Aussatz, die Feldsucht (*German*): Radesyge, Syedalsahed (*Norwegian*): *Black Leprosy.*

As the Elephantiasis is almost unknown in this country, and I have only seen four instances of the disease, I must speak of it principally as it is described in books; and should have omitted the subject altogether, had it not appeared to me that some comment on the mistakes of translators and their followers, as well as on the history of the disease in general, might contribute to put the matter in a clearer light than that in which it now stands.

The Elephantiasis (Plate LXVIII. of BATEMAN) (as described by the Greeks *) is principally characterised by the appearance of shining tubercles,

* The terms ἐλέφας and ἐλεφαντίασις were applied to this tubercular disease by Aretæus, and the succeeding Greek writers, partly, perhaps, on account of some resemblance of the diseased skin to that of the elephant; but principally from the formidable severity and duration of the disease. " For it is disgusting to the sight," says Aretæus, " and in all respects terrible, like the beast of similar name." (De Diuturn. Morb. lib. ii. cap. 13.) And Aëtius observes, " Elephantiasis quidem à magnitudine et diuturnitate nomen accepit." (tetrabibl. iv. serm. i. cap. 120.) So also the poet : —

> " Est lepræ species, elephantiasisque vocatur,
> Quæ cunctis morbis major sic esse videtur
> Ut major cunctis elephas animantibus exstat."
> Macer de Herbar. Virtut.

The same disease was described by the Arabians, under the appellation of Juzam or Judam, and is still designated by similar terms in Arabia and Persia, viz. Dsjuddam, and Madsjuddam, according to Niebuhr. (Description de l'Arabie, tom. iii. p. 119.) The translators, however, of the works of the Arabian physicians into Latin, committed an extraordinary blunder, in rendering this appellation by the Greek term Lepra; by which they misled their brethren (who henceforth called Elephantiasis the Arabian Leprosy), and contributed to introduce much confusion both into medical and popular language in the use of the term. The Arabians have not employed the word Lepra; but have designated the varieties of scaly and tubercular diseases by appellations in their own language, as distinct and definite as those of the Greeks. (See Avicenna, lib. iv. fen. 3. tract. 3.—Alsaharavius, tract. 31.—Haly Abbas, Theoricè, lib. viii. cap. 15, and Pract. cap. 14. — Avenzoar, lib. ii.)

of different sizes, of a dusky red or livid colour,
on the face, ears, and extremities; together with a
thickened and rugous state of the skin, a diminu-
tion or total loss of its sensibility, and a falling off
of all the hair, except that of the scalp.

The disease " is said seldom to appear in youth;
but the only case of it which the editor ever saw,
was that of a boy of fourteen years of age, a native of
Jamaica, in whom the disease developed itself two
months after he arrived in this country." It is
described as very slow in its progress, sometimes
continuing for several years, without materially
deranging the functions of the patient. During
this continuance, however, great deformity is gradually produced. The alæ of the nose become
swelled and scabrous, and the nostrils dilate; the
lips are tumid; the external ears, particularly the
lobes, are enlarged and thickened, and beset with
tubercles; the skin of the forehead and cheeks
grows thick and tumid, and forms large and prominent rugæ, especially over the eyes: the hair of
the eyebrows, the beard, the pubes, axillæ, &c.
falls off; the voice becomes hoarse and obscure;
and the sensibility of the parts affected is obtuse,
or totally abolished, so that pinching or puncturing
them gives no uneasiness.* This disfiguration of
the countenance suggested the idea of the fea-

---

* From an interesting account of the Elephantiasis by Mr. Robinson,
a resident in India, it appears that this insensibility occurs only in the
Baras or *Leuce;* his description of which will be found in a subsequent
page.

tures of a satyr or a wild beast; whence the disease was by some called *Satyriasis**, and by others *Leontiasis*.†

As the malady proceeds, the tubercles begin to crack, and at length to ulcerate: ulcerations also appear in the throat, and in the nose, which sometimes destroy the palate and the cartilaginous septum; the nose falls; and the breath is intolerably offensive: the thickened and tuberculated skin of the extremities becomes divided by fissures, and ulcerates, or is corroded under dry sordid scabs, so that the fingers and toes gangrene, and separate, joint after joint. ‡

---

* The term *Satyriasis*, or *Satyriasmos*, was also deemed applicable to the disease, on account of the excessive libidinous disposition said to be connected with it. See Aretæus, loc. cit., and Aëtius, tetrab. iv. serm. i. cap. 120. But in all the cases which I have seen, they produced the contrary condition, destroying both the power and the appetite. Mr. Robinson, however, says that its first effect is an increase of the venereal passion, which becomes lost during its progress.

† The two Greek writers, just quoted, attribute this name to the laxity and wrinkles of the skin of the forehead, which resembles the prominent and flexible front of the *lion*. But the Arabian writers ascribe it to a different source. Haly Abbas says the countenance was called *leonine*, because the white of the eyes becomes livid, and the eyes of a round figure; and Avicenna observes that the epithet was applied to the disease, because it renders the countenance terrible to look at, and somewhat of the form of a lion's visage. loc. cit. These appellations prove that the allusions were entirely metaphorical, and did not refer to any resemblance in the skin of patients to the hide of these beasts.— M. Alibert has figured two varieties of Elephantiasis; viz. in plate 52., under the title of "Lepre tuberculeuse," where it is incipient on the eyebrows; and, in plate 34., affecting the nose and lips, where it is called "Lepre leontine." His "Lèpre elephantiasis," plate 33., is the Barbadoes leg.

‡ Alsaharavius thus states the symptoms of the *juzam*, when fully formed:—"The colour of the skin is changed, the voice is lost, the

Aretæus and the ancients in general consider Elephantiasis as an universal *cancer* of the body, and speak of it with terror: they depict its hideous and loathsome character, its contagious qualities, and its unyielding and fatal tendency, in strong metaphorical language, which, indeed, tends to throw some doubt on the fidelity of their description. The very appropriation of the name is poetical; and Aretæus has absurdly enough prefixed to his description of the disease an account of the elephant, in order to point out the analogy between the formidable power of the beast and of the disease. It is probable, that his terrors led him to adopt the popular opinion respecting the

hairs have entirely disappeared; the whole surface of the body is ulcerated, discharging a putrid sanies, with extreme fœtor; the extremities begin to fall off, and the eyes weep profusely." Lib. Practice, tract. 31. cap. 1.

"The accuracy of this description is confirmed by Dr. Kinnis's very minute detail of the symptoms of the disease, as it appears in the Isle of France.† He describes the tubercles as differing in form, being flat, oval, and irregular: larger on the forehead and bridge of the nose, but smaller and more confluent on the cheeks, 'which,' he remarks, 'sometimes hang down from the bones, stretching and depressing the corners of the mouth.' He further says, 'the lips, when affected, were penetrated by hard, whitish bodies, like recently-formed cicatrices.' The tumours are not confined to the external surface, but, according to Dr. Kinnis, are observed in the mouth, on the palate, uvula, fauces, and tonsils, of a yellowish-red or a red colour, smooth, shining, and about the size of a split pea: yet so little inconvenience was experienced by the affected from these tubercles in the mouth, that 'one or two were not even aware of their existence previous to examination.' It is a curious fact, that the palms of the hands and the soles of the feet were seldom tuberculated in those cases which Dr. Kinnis examined. He found the pulse generally weak, 'and above a hundred in a minute.'" T.

† Edinburgh Med. and Surg. Journ. vol. xxii. pp. 286—294.

malady, without the correction of personal observation: for, although his account has been copied by subsequent writers *, and the same popular opinions have been constantly entertained, there is much reason to believe that some of the prominent features of his portrait are incorrectly drawn.

Notwithstanding the care with which the separation and seclusion of lepers have been enforced, in compliance with the ancient opinion, there is great reason to believe that Elephantiasis is *not contagious.*† M. Vidal long ago controverted that opinion, having never observed an instance of its communication from a leprous man to his wife, or *vice versâ* ‡, although cohabiting for a long series of years. Dr. T. Heberden daily observed many examples of the same fact in Madeira, and affirms

* It is impossible to read the description of this disease (as said to occur at Barbadoes) by the learned Dr. Hillary, without a conviction that that respectable physician had in his mind the history detailed by the eloquent Greek (Aretæus), and not the phænomena of the disease, as he had himself seen it. See his Obs. on the Air and Dis. of the Island of Barbadoes, p. 322, 2d edit.

† Turner quotes from several ancient authors to prove its contagious nature.—Treatise on Diseases of the Skin, 4th edit. pp. 14, 15. T.

‡ See his Recherches et Obs. sur la Lèpre de Martigues, in the Mém. de la Soc. Roy. de Méd. tom. i. p. 169. — Dr. Joannis, a physician at Aix, who investigated the disease in the lazar-house at Martigues, in 1755, also asserts the rarity of its communication between married persons. See Lond. Med. Obs. and Inquiries, vol. i. p. 204.—Indeed, several able physicians, two centuries before, though bending under the authority of ancient opinion, yet acknowledged their astonishment at the daily commerce of lazars with the healthy, without any communication of the disease. See Fernel, de Morb. Occult. lib. i. cap. 12.: Forest. Obs. Chirurg. lib. iv. obs. 7.: also the works of Fabricius, Plater, &c. Fernel, indeed, admits that he never saw an instance which proved the existence of contagion.

that " he never heard of any one who contracted the distemper by contact of a leper." Dr. Adams has given his testimony to the same truth, remarking that none of the nurses in the lazar-house at Funchall have shown any symptoms of the disease ; and that individual lazars have remained for years at home, without infecting any part of their family.* " Dr. Whitlaw Ainslie, who saw many cases of the disease in India, is decidedly of this opinion ; but he regards it as hereditary. Its non-contagious nature is also confirmed by Dr. Kinnis."

. With respect to the *libido inexplebilis,* which is said to be one of the characteristics of Elephantiasis, the evidence is not so satisfactory. Its existence, however, is affirmed by most of the modern writers, with the exception of Dr. Adams " and Dr. Kinnis." MM. Vidal and Joannis mention it among the symptoms of the disease at Martigues.† Dr. Bancroft, senior, states its occurrence in the Elephantiasis of South America ‡ : and Prof. Niebuhr asserts, that it appears in the Dsjuddam of Bagdat.§ But Dr. Adams observed, on the contrary,

---

* See his Obs. on Morbid Poisons, 2d edit chap. 18.

† M. Vidal particularises the case of Arnaud, a sailor, who had been afflicted with the tubercular Elephantiasis six months, when he died of putrid fever. " Il n'avoit cessé, presque jusqu'à sa mort, de ressentir les ardeurs d'un assez violent Satyriasis."

‡ " Lepers are notorious for their salacity and longevity." Nat. Hist. of Guiana, p. 385.

§ " Loc. cit. The story related by Niebuhr, of a lazar gratifying this propensity by infecting a woman by means of linen sent out of the lazar-house, and thus obtaining her admission, appears, however, to be entitled to little credit.

in the lazars of Madeira, an actual wasting of the generative organs in the men, who had been seized with the malady subsequent to the age of puberty, and a want of the usual evolution of them, in those who had been attacked previous to that period. * Is the Elephantiasis in Madeira now less virulent than that of former times? has it undergone some change in its character? or is the ancient account of the disease incorrect? " Elephantiasis is very prevalent in the island of Java; and a Dutch physician, on whose authority this is stated, observed that it attacked women more rarely than men."

It is generally affirmed, that the Elephantiasis was extensively prevalent in Europe, in the middle ages, especially subsequent to the crusades; and it is certain, that every country abounded with hospitals, established for the exclusive relief of that disease, from the tenth to the sixteenth century †; and that an order of knighthood, dedicated to an imaginary St. Lazarus, was instituted, the members of which had the care of lepers, and the

* Dr. Kinnis saw no instance of this in the Isle of France, " the testicles in males, and the breasts in females, being constantly of their natural size." T.

† The number of these establishments, however, has been greatly misrepresented, in consequence of an error of quotation from Matt. Paris, which has been echoed by several authors. That historian has been made to assert, that, in the thirteenth century, there were 19,000 lazarettoes in Christendom; whereas he only states that the Knights Hospitalers were then in possession of so many *manors*. " Habent Hospitalarii novemdecim millia maneriorum in Christianitate," are his words. See his Histor. Angl. ad ann. 1244; also Du Cange, Gloss. voc. Lazari; Mezeray, Hist. de France.

control of the lazarettoes, assigned to them, and ultimately accumulated immense wealth. From these facts, however, nothing satisfactory is to be collected, respecting the actual prevalence of Elephantiasis at those periods. For although it is obvious, from the nature of the examination instituted by the physicians of those lazarettoes, that the tubercular disease was the object of their enquiry, yet it is also evident, that, in consequence of the general application of the term, *leprosy*, to the Elephantiasis, to the leprosy of the Jews *, to the proper scaly Lepra, and even to other cutaneous affections, which have no affinity with either of the diseases just mentioned, almost every person, afflicted with any severe eruption or ulceration of the skin, was deemed *leprous*, and was received into the lazarettoes. This fact, indeed, is acknowledged by many of the physicians to these hospitals, in the sixteenth century and subsequently.

---

* This appears to have been the *Leuce* of the Greeks, the white *Baras* of the Arabians, and the third species of *Vitiligo* of Celsus. (See Hippocrat, Περι Παθων. Avicen. loc. cit. — Cels. de Med. lib. v. cap. 28.) The two characteristic symptoms of the Hebrew leprosy, which are pointed out in the Mosaic account, are the *whiteness of the hair* of the parts affected, and the *depression* of the skin. " And if the *hair* of the plague is *turned white*, and the plague in sight be *deeper* than the skin of his flesh, it is a plague of leprosy," &c. (Leviticus, chap. xiii.) Thus also Avicenna: " There is this difference between the white Alguada (*Alphos*) and the white Baras; the hairs grow upon the skin affected with the former, and they are of a black or brown colour: but those which grow in the Baras are *always white*, and at the same time the skin is *more depressed* or *sunk* than the rest of the surface of the body." (loc. cit.) And Celsus: " λευκη habet quiddam simile alpho; sed magis albida est, et altius descendit; in eaque *albi pili* sunt, et lanugini similes."

Greg. Horst, who was one of the appointed ex-
aminers at Ulm, towards the close of that century,
and who has given a minute detail of his investiga-
tions, admits that, " where the tubercles of the
face, the thick lips, acuminated ears, flattened
nose, round eyes (the essential symptoms of Elephantiasis) are absent; yet if the patients are
affected only with a dry and foul Scabies, with
pustular eruptions, fissures, and branny exfoliations,
which constitute the *Psora* of the Greeks, — or
even with great itching, emaciation, ulceration, and
exfoliations of thicker scales, which are the *Lepra*
of the Greeks, — nevertheless they are sent to the
lazarettoes, if they are poor, for the means of sub-
sistence. Hence it happens," he adds, " that,
here and elsewhere, *very few instances of real Ele-*
phantiasis are found in the lazarettoes, while *many*
are there, affected only with an obstinate Psora or
Lepra Græcorum."* Forestus, who held a similar
office at Alcmaer and Delft, in the same century,
affirms that a very small proportion of the persons
who wandered about the Low Countries, as lepers
and beggars, were true lepers; but were merely affected with Scabies, or some external defœdation of
the skin. " Nay," he says, " not one in ten of them
is truly a leper, or afflicted with the legitimate Elephantiasis."† Riedlin makes a similar observation
respecting the patients admitted into the leper-

* See his Obs. Med. lib. vii. obs. xviii. epist. J. H. Hopfnero.
† See his Obs. Chirurg. lib. iv. obs. vii. schol.

hospital at Vienna. *Indeed, there is little doubt, that every species of cachectic disease, accompanied with ulceration, gangrene, or any superficial derangement, was deemed *leprous;* and hence that, in the dark ages, when the desolation of repeated wars, and the imperfect state of agriculture, subjected Europe to almost constant scarcity of food, the numerous modifications of Scurvy and Ignis sacer, which were epidemic during periods of famine, and endemic wherever there was a local dearth, were in all probability classed among the varieties of leprosy; more especially as the last stage of the Ignis sacer was marked by the occurrence of ulceration and gangrene of the extremities, by which the parts were mutilated, or entirely separated. † " With regard to the causes of this disease, independent of its hereditary taint, nothing satisfactory has been suggested. The Vytians of Lower India," says Dr. Ainslie, "reckon eighteen varieties of India, all of which they conceive to be produced by one or other of the following causes : 1. Drinking milk after eating fish to excess; 2. eating fla-

---

* " Sicuti vero non *nisi rarissimè* inveniuntur, quibus Leprosi nomen meritò et reverà attribui posset, uti quidem leprosi à plerisque auctoribus describuntur; sed *plerumque* hisce domibus illi includuntur, qui Scabie siccâ, fædâ, et diu jam instante, laborant," &c. D. V. Riedlin, Lineæ Med. vol. iii. Ann. 1697. Mens. Maio.

† It would be foreign to my purpose to enter into any detail here respecting the history and symptoms of the Ignis sacer, which was correctly ascribed by Galen (de Succor. Bonit. et Vitio, cap. 1. — De Natur. Humor. lib. ii. cap. 3. &c.) to the use of unsuitable food. It has been well described by Lucretius, lib. vi. In more recent times, it has been erroneously supposed to originate from various deleterious substances taken with the food, and not from actual deficiency of nutriment. See above, pp. 134, 135.

tulent food; 3. eating to excess the grain of the Dolichos *lablab*; 4. drinking cold water after having perspired much; 5. eating to excess the seed of the Sesamum *Orientale;* 6. checking vomiting so as to allow undigested matter to get into the bowels; 7. sensual indulgence in the daytime; 8. habitual costiveness; 9. the bites of a cat, and of certain snakes, a certain lizard, and certain wasps; 10. worms. Such are the absurd causes to which the natives of a country, in which the disease prevails, ascribe Elephantiasis. Dr. Ainslie says it is more common on the coast than in the interior; and he supposes that this may arise from the natives eating a bad kind of fish; or too much salt fish, of which they are very fond. He adds, that he never knew a native of Great Britain or Ireland to have the disease; but had seen a Swede, two Danes, and a German labouring under it."

Under the head of Elephantiasis, Dr. Winterbottom appears to have described the *Leuce,* and not the Elephantiasis of the Greeks; the *Baras,* and not the *Juzam* of the Arabians. The principal symptoms which he witnessed were the *pale* colour of the skin (in black subjects) and its loss of sensibility, which are distinctly stated as the leading symptoms of Leuce, by Celsus, and by the other Roman and Greek physicians, as well as of Baras by the Arabians.* Some of the Greeks and Arabians,

* See Celsus de Medicina, lib. v. cap. 28. — Aëtius, tetrab. iv. serm. i. cap. 123. — Paul. Æginet. lib. iv. cap. 5. — Actuarius, Meth. Med. lib. ii. cap. 11.

indeed, seem to consider the Leuce, or Baras, as possessing an affinity with Elephantiasis, and sometimes terminating in it *; and, if they be not modifications of the same disease, it is probable that some of the symptoms of the one (Leuce), such as the insensibility, and change of the colour and strength of the hair, may have been transferred in description to the other. † The numerous large tubercles of the nose, forehead, and ears, which are deemed characteristic of Elephantiasis, did not appear in the disease seen by Dr. Winterbottom. The swellings or tuberosities of the joints of the hands and feet, which terminate in ulcerations, that occasion the fingers and toes to drop off, appear also to belong to the two diseases in common, and afford another proof of their affinity. Nevertheless, as we have nowhere any account of the regular succession of the tubercular state (Elephantiasis or Juzam) to that of mere discoloration and insensibility (Leuce or Baras), we are not warranted in drawing the conclusion, that they are but de-

---

* Avicenna applies the term *Baras,* with the epithet *black,* to the rugged and scaly state of the skin in Elephantiasis: (lib. iv. fen. 3. tract. 3. cap. i. — and fen. 7. tract. 2. cap. 9.) and Alsaharavius expressly states, that when the disease arises from putrid phlegm, it commences with Baras, or with white Bohak (Alphos of the Greeks), and becomes Juzam in its advanced stage. Lib. Pract. tract. 31. cap. 1. See also Dr. Thomas Heberden's account of Elephantiasis in the Island of Madeira. (Med. Trans. of the Coll. of Physicians, vol. i. p. 27.)

Plenck describes it under the name Lepra der Aussatz. Vide Doct. de Morb. Cutan. p. 67. .

† This conjecture has been confirmed by Mr. Robinson, in the paper above alluded to.

grees or stages of the same disease. * Accurate histories of the Elephantiasis, Leuce, and other modifications of the formidable cutaneous diseases, that occur in hot climates, and especially where agriculture and the arts of civilisation are imperfectly advanced, must be deemed still among the *desiderata* of the pathologist.

While the fifth edition of this work is in the press (Dec. 1818), I have had the satisfaction of perusing a valuable paper, written by Mr. Robinson, a medical practitioner in India, which confirms the accuracy of my description of the tubercular Elephantiasis, and supplies the desideratum above noticed, by furnishing a clear and distinct history of the Baras, or white leprosy, as well as the notice of a remedy adequate to its cure.

This paper will probably appear in the 10th vol. of the Transactions of the Med. and Chirurg. Society of London; but I am permitted to extract the following description:—"One or two circumscribed patches appear upon the skin, (generally the feet or hands, but sometimes the trunk or face,)

---

* It is curious, that the Foolas, on the coast of Africa, employ the Arabian terms, but, if Dr. Winterbottom was correctly informed, in an inverted sense. They divide the disease into three species, or rather degrees: 1. the *damadyang*, or mildest leuce, when the skin is merely discoloured and insensible in patches; 2. the *didyam*, (sometimes written sghidam, dsjuddam, and juzam,) when the joints of the fingers and toes are ulcerated and drop off, the lips are tumid, and the alæ nasi swell and ulcerate; and 3. the *barras*, when these symptoms are increased, and, from ulcerations in the throat and nose, the voice becomes hoarse and guttural. See his Account of the Native Africans in Sierra Leone, vol. ii. chap. 4.

rather lighter coloured than the neighbouring skin,
neither raised nor depressed, shining and wrinkled,
the furrows not coinciding with the lines of the
contiguous sound cuticle.   The skin thus circumscribed is so entirely insensible, that you may with
hot irons burn to the muscle, before the patient
feels any pain.*   These patches spread slowly until
the skin of the whole of the legs, arms, and gradually often the whole body, becomes alike devoid
of sense: wherever it is so affected, there is no
perspiration; no itching, no pain, and very seldom
any swelling.   Until this singular apathy has occupied the greater part of the skin, it may rather be
considered a blemish than a disease : nevertheless
it is most important to mark well these appearances,
for they are the invariable commencement of one
of the most gigantic and incurable diseases that
have succeeded the fall of man; and it is in this
state chiefly (though not exclusively) that we are
most able to be the means of cure.   The next
symptoms (which occur in some patients at two
months, but in others not till after five or six years,)
are the first which denote internal disease or derangement of any functions.   The pulse becomes
very slow (from 50 to 60), not small but heavy,
' as if moving through mud;' the bowels are very
costive, the toes and fingers numbed, as with frost,

* In the cases of real tubercular Elephantiasis, described by Dr. Kinnis, " the parts affected with the disease were benumbed, or, as the patients sometimes expressed it, ' asleep,' but they had never entirely lost
their sensibility." — Edin. Journ, l. c.   T.

glazed and rather swelled, and nearly inflexible.
The mind is at this time sluggish and slow in apprehension, and the patient appears always half
asleep. The soles of the feet and the palms of the
hands then crack into fissures, dry, and hard as the
parched soil of the country; and the extremities
of the toes and fingers under the nails are incrusted
with a furfuraceous substance, and the nails are
gradually lifted up, until absorption and ulceration
occur. Still there is little or no pain; the legs and
fore-arms swell, and the skin is every where cracked
and rough. Contemporary with the last symptoms,
or very soon afterwards, ulcers appear at the inside
of the joints of the toes and fingers, directly under
the last joint of the metatarsal or metacarpal bones,
or they corrode the thick sole under the joint of
the os calcis, or os cuboides. There is no previous
tumour, suppuration, or pain, but apparently a simple absorption of the integuments, which slough
off in successive layers of half an inch in diameter.
A sanious discharge comes on; the muscle, pale
and flabby, is in turn destroyed; and the joint being penetrated as by an auger, the extremity drops,
and at length falls a victim to this cruel, tardy, but
certain poison. The wounds then heal, and other
joints are attacked in succession, whilst every re-
volving year bears with it a trophy of this slow
march of death. Thus are the limbs deprived one
by one of their extremities, till at last they become
altogether useless. Even now death comes not to
the relief of, nor is it desired by, the patient, who,

'dying by inches,' and a spectacle of horror to all
besides, still cherishes fondly the spark of life remaining, and eats voraciously all he can procure:
he will often crawl about with little but his trunk
remaining, until old age comes on, and at last he
is carried off by diarrhœa or dysentery, which the
enfeebled constitution has no stamina to resist.
Throughout the progress of this creeping but inveterate complaint, the health is not much disturbed, the food is eaten with appetite, and properly
though slowly digested. A sleepy inertness over-
powers every faculty, and seems to benumb, almost
annihilate, every passion as well of the soul as of
the body, leaving only sufficient sense and activity
to crawl through the routine of existence."

Mr. Robinson adds, that he has never seen this
disease attack the larger joints, destroy the nose,
nor affect any of the bones, except those of the
hands and feet; and that the tuberculated Elephantiasis, though it sometimes supervenes, is by no
means connected with, caused by, or necessarily
subsequent to it.

Mr. Robinson affirms that the cure of this disease may be generally accomplished in the early
stage, by the use of a plant which grows abundantly
in India, and which appears to possess remedial
qualities which entitle it to an introduction into
the Pharmacopœias of Europe, namely, the *asclepias
gigantea*, especially in combination with alterative
doses of mercury and antimony, and with topical
stimulants.

By the surgeons of the present day the appellation of Elephantiasis is appropriated to a disease, altogether different from the malady originally so called by the Greeks; namely, to an énormously tumid condition of the leg*, arising from a repeated effusion and collection of a lymphatic and gelatinous matter in the cellular membrane under the skin, in consequence of inflammation of the lymphatic glands and vessels. The skin itself is much thickened in the protracted stages of this extension, and its vessels become much enlarged; its surface grows dark, rough, and sometimes scaly. †
This condition of the surface, together with the huge mis-shapen figure of the limb, bearing some resemblance to the leg of an elephant, suggested the application of the term. ‡ As the effusion first takes place after a febrile paroxysm, in which the inguinal glands of the side about to be affected are

---

* *Syn.*—Elephantiasis (*Auct. var.*): Bucnemia (*Good*): Anay kaal (*Tam.*): Huttie kā pāwny (*Duk.*): Yeanugay kāloo (*Tel.*): Ghéjapádhá vāyoo (*Sans.*): Daíl fil (*Arab.*): Drusenkrankheit (*German*): Yara-skin (*Polynes Isles*): Barbadoes leg (*Hillary*): Cochin leg.

† See Alibert's plate of "Lepra elephantiasis," No. 35., where this is well represented.

‡ The appellation of *elephant*, or *elephant-disease*, was, in fact, applied to this affection by the Arabians, confessedly from this resemblance: (see Haly Abbas, Theor. lib. viii. cap. 18.;—Avenzoar, lib. ii. cap. 26.;—Alsaharavius, Pract. tractat. xxviii. cap. 11, &c.) hence the translators were puzzled, and misinterpreted *Juzam* by the Greek term, *Lepra*. The translator of Haly Abbas was alone correct in rendering the Arabic names: having given the proper classical appellation of *Elephantiasis* to the tubercular Juzam, he translates this name (denoting the *elephant-leg* by the term *Elephas*. (loc. cit.; — also Theoricè, lib. viii. cap. 15.; and Practicè, cap. 4.) For, as this disease had not been noticed by the Greek physicians, even by those of the Eastern empire, there was no classical term by which it could be rendered.

inflamed, and the limb is subsequently augmented in bulk by a repetition of these attacks, Dr. Hendy termed the malady "the glandular disease of Barbadoes," in which island it is endemial.* In England it is often called "the Barbadoes leg."† Except when these paroxysms occur, the functions and constitution of the patients are not materially injured, and they often live many years, incommoded only by carrying about "such a troublesome load of leg."‡

In this country the disease is only seen in its inveterate stage, after repeated attacks of the fever and effusion have completely altered the organisation of the integuments of the limb, and rendered it altogether incurable. In this state, the swelling is hard and firm, does not pit on pressure, and is entirely free from pain. The skin is thickened and much hardened; its blood-vessels are enlarged, particularly the external veins, and the lymphatics distended; and the cellular substance is flaccid, and sometimes thickened, and its cells much loaded

* See his inaugural dissertation, and subsequent treatise on the subject, London, 1784; also Rollo's "Remarks on the Disease lately described by Dr. Hendy," &c. 1785.

† The disease is not exclusively confined to the leg; it sometimes appears in the arms, and even on the ears, breasts, scrotum, &c. Hillary on the Diseases of Barbadoes, p. 315.; — Hendy, part i. sect. 2.

‡ See Hillary on the Climate and Dis. of Barbadoes. It is affirmed by Dr. Clarke, however, and by Dr. Winterbottom, that the agility of the patients, who are affected with this unseemly deformity, at Cochin, and on the Gold Coast, is not impaired by it. (See Clark's Obs. on the Dis. in Long Voyages to Hot Climates; Winterbottom, loc. cit. p. 113.) Dr. Hendy observes that, in consequence of the gradual augmentation of the bulk, patients are not in general sensible of the weight, except when they are debilitated by indisposition.

with a gelatinous fluid. The muscles, tendons, ligaments, and bones, are generally in a sound state. — In this advanced stage, the disease is altogether irremediable; and indeed little success seems to have attended the practice employed in the earlier stages, which has been chiefly directed to alleviate the febrile paroxysms by laxatives and diaphoretics, and subsequently to strengthen the system by Cinchona. Local bleeding has never been employed; for there are no leeches in Barbadoes, according to Dr. Hendy; but after the fever and inflammation have subsided, he strongly recommends the binding of the limb in a tight bandage, as the means of exciting absorption, and of reducing the swelling.*

* While this sheet was in the hands of the compositor, I was favoured by Mr. J. Mason Good, a gentleman distinguished by his knowlege of the oriental languages, with some observations relative to the original Arabic appellations of these diseases, which, while they confirm the views which I had entertained in general, throw additional light on the subject.

"The Leprosy of the Arabs," he says, "appears to have been called by themselves immemorially, and is still called, *juzam* and *juzamlyk*, though vulgarly and more generally *judam* and *judamlyk*, from an Arabic root, which imports erosion, truncation, excision. The term *juzam* has passed from Arabia into India, and is the common name for the same disease, among the Cabirajas, or Hindu physicians, who also occasionally denominate it *Fisádi khún*, from its being supposed to infect the entire mass of blood, but more generally *khora*."

I learn also from this communication, that the original Arabic term, which was used to denote the *tumid leg*, above mentioned, was *dal fil*, which is literally *elephant disease*; and further, that "*dal fil* is the common name for the *swelled leg* in the present day among the Arabians who sometimes contract it to *fil* alone, literally *elephas*."

But although the Arabians in general distinguish the *Juzam* from other diseases; yet I have observed, that they sometimes mentioned the *baras* (*leuce*) as having an affinity with it, calling some forms of the Juzam *black baras*. Mr. Good remarks, that "*juzam* itself has occa-

In conclusion, then, it will be seen that the
terms Elephantiasis and Lepra have been thus confounded. The word Lepra (which should be confined to a *scaly* disease) has been erroneously applied to the proper Elephantiasis (a *tubercular*
disease). Elephantiasis again, which is so distinctly described by the Greek writers, has been
transferred, by the Latin translators of the Arabian
writers, to the local affection of the leg, (the *elephas* of these writers, the *Barbadoes* leg, and the
glandular disease of Dr. Hendy,) and is commonly
used in that acceptation by practitioners at present.
But it has been also misapplied to the white disease of the skin, called by the Greeks, Romans, and
Arabians, Leuce, Vitiligo, and Baras (or Beras)
respectively; and thence, by an easy step, it has
been again transferred, by some unlearned persons,
even to the scaly Lepra; while the term Lepra has

---

sionally been employed in the same loose manner; and has been made
to import leucè or vitiligo, as well as proper or black judam; though in
the former case it is commonly distinguished by the epithet *merd*, i. e.
pilis carens, as *merd-juzam*, *bald juzam*. The proper and more usual
name for this last disease, is *beras* or *aberas*, sometimes written *alberas*,
though less correctly, as this last is *beras*, with a mere prefix of the definite article."

Mr. Good adds, " that one of the most celebrated remedies for this
disease (*juzam*) employed by the Cabirajas, or Hindu physicians, is
arsenic (*Shuce.* in India *sanc' hya*) mixed in pills with black pepper," six
parts of the latter being added to one of the former: the pills are ordered to be of the size of small pulse, and one of them is to be swallowed morning and evening, with some betel leaf.

Since the publication of the former editions, I have had an opportunity of seeing two cases of Elephantiasis, which have been under treatment in London during the greater part of the present year (1814);
and in both, the arsenic had been fully tried, and proved to be entirely
void of any remedial power.

been often indiscriminately applied to all these affections. I trust, the foregoing statements may contribute to elucidate this matter. " With regard to the remedial treatment of Elephantiasis, our experience in this country affords us little assistance.

" Among the multifarious remedies proposed and employed by the ancients, one of the most likely to prove useful was Decoction of Elm Bark in the proportion of ℥iv of the bark to ℔iij, boiled down one half. After bleeding and purging, Willis recommended a Mixture in which the sharp-pointed Dock, Rumex *acutus* (*Oxylapathum*) was the most active ingredient. * This plant was also used along with Bryony, Scabious Mallow, and Chamomile flowers in the formation of a bath; and it also entered a liniment. In India the chief reliance is placed on a powder (termed *mudai*) prepared from the root of the Esclepias *Gigantea* †, a plant described by Dr. Ainslie in the Mat. Med. of Hindostan. This author, in a letter to the Editor, says, "I found, when the disease was taken early, that mercurials, judiciously administered in small doses, were almost the only remedy that did good. I thought that in two or three cases, treated in this way, I entirely removed it. Nothing can be done without the frequent use of the tepid bath, so that the skin may be kept in the cleanest state possible."

* Willis de Impetigine sive Lepra Græc. Sect. 3. c. 7. T.
† Edin. Med. & Chir. Trans. vol. i. p. 414. T.

Books that may be consulted on Elephantiasis.

ADAMS, DR. On Morbid Poisons, 8vo. 1807.

ASIATIC Researches, vol. ii.

ALARET, (Hist. de l'Eléphant. des Arabes, 1800.

EDINBURGH Med. and Surg. Journ. vol. iii. p.18.—vi. p.161. Oct. 1824.

JACKSON's Account of Marocco, 8vo. 1810.

LONDON Med. & Chir. Trans. Vol. x.

RAYER, Traité des Malad. de la Peau, 8vo. 1826.

RAYMOND, Hist. des Eléphantiasis, 1767.

RECHERCHES ASIATIQUES, 4to. 1805.

RUETTE, Essai sur l'Eléphantiasis, 8vo. 1802.

GENUS IX. FRAMBŒSIA.

YAWS.

Syn. Frambœsia (*Auct. Var*):

Synon. Lepra fungifera (*Cartheuserus*): Anthracia rubula (*Good*): Pian (*Native American*): der Schwammförmige Aussatz (*German*): *Yaws.*

Def. IMPERFECTLY SUPPURATING TUMOURS, GRADUALLY INCREASING FROM SPECKS TO THE SIZE OF A RASPBERRY; WITH A FUNGOUS CORE: ONE TUMOUR GENERALLY GROWING LARGER THAN THE OTHERS. FEVER SLIGHT BUT CONTAGIOUS: OCCURRING ONCE ONLY DURING LIFE.

The nature of this disease, which is indigenous in Africa, and has been thence conveyed to the West Indies and America, has been imperfectly investigated by European practitioners; and as it is perhaps never seen in England, a very brief account of it here will be sufficient.*

* Yaws, *sibbens,* raged in Scotland in the 17th century; and even at this period it is occasionally met with in the Shetland Islands. T.

M. Alibert has figured two diseases as examples of Frambœsia, under the titles of "Pian ruboide," and "P. fungoide," which were seen

The eruption of the Yaws sometimes commences without any precursory symptoms of ill health; but it is generally preceded by a slight febrile state, with languor, debility, and pains of the joints, resembling those of rheumatism.* The whole skin at this period seems as if dusted with flour. After several days, minute protuberances † appear on various parts of the skin, at first smaller than the head of a pin, but gradually enlarging, in some cases to the diameter of a sixpence, and in others even to a

---

at the hospital St. Louis at Paris; but they are obviously not Yaws. The first of them appears to be a neglected Porrigo, or a Sycosis, of the scalp (plate 35.); and the other a species of wen (plate 36.)

Dr. James Thomson objects to the disease being classed with the Tubercula. The eruption is at first papular, then pustular, and ultimately fungoid.—Edin. Med. and Surg. Journ. vol. xv. p. 322. T.

* The earlier writers on this disease assert, that the general health is not impaired by this eruption during the first stages. But on the authority of Dr. Winterbottom, and of Dr. Dancer, I have stated that a *febricula* is the ordinary precursor of the Yaws. Dr. Winterbottom indeed, observes that the successive eruptions which occur are also usually preceded by slight febrile paroxysms, sometimes by rigors. See his account of the Nat. Africans of Sierra Leone, vol. ii. chap. 8.; — and Dancer's Medical Assistant.

† It is not easy to discover the precise character of this eruption, from the varying language of authors. An anonymous writer, who gave the first explicit account of the disease (see Edin. Med. Essays, vol. v. part ii. art. 76.), says they are at first "level or smooth with the skin," but soon "become protuberant *like pimples*." Dr. Hillary, who has copied much from this writer, describes them as "*pimples*," though smooth and level with the skin, but soon becoming "protuberant *pustules*." (On the Dis. of Barbadoes, p. 359.) And Dr. Winterbottom, who has given, on the whole, the most perspicuous description of the disease, calls them "*pustules*" from their first appearance. Again, as to the contents of these eruptions, the anonymous author and Dr. Hillary say that *no pus*, nor any quantity of ichor, is found in them, but speak of a little *ichor* as drying upon the surface; while Dr. Winterbottom says, they are "filled with an opake whitish fluid," and when they burst, "a thick viscid matter is discharged."

greater extent: they are most numerous, and of the largest size, in the face, groins, axillæ, and about the anus and pudenda. But the crop is not completed at once; new eruptions appear in different places, while some of the earlier ones dry off. When the cuticle is broken, a foul crust is formed on the surface, from under which, on the larger protuberances, red fungous excrescences often spring up, which attain different magnitudes, from that of a small raspberry to that of a large mulberry, which fruit they somewhat resemble from their granulated surfaces. * " The period in which these shoot is very uncertain; varying from one month to three months." When the eruption is most copious, these tubercles are of the smallest size: and when less diffuse, they are largest. " In debilitated habits they bleed on the slightest touch." Their duration and progress are various in different constitutions, and at different periods of life. Children suffer less severely than adults, and are more speedily freed from the disease: in them, according to Dr. Winterbottom, the duration of the Yaws is from six to nine months; while, in adults, it is seldom cured in less than a year, and sometimes continues during two or three. " The fungous tubercles attain their acme, according to Dr. Thomson, and the anonymous writer already quoted, more

---

* Hence both the popular appellation of *Yaw,* which in some African dialect signifies a *raspberry,* and the nosological title, *Frambœsia,* from the French *Framboise,* which denotes the same fruit. See Sauvages, Nosol. Meth. class. x. ord. iv. gen. 23.

rapidly in the well-fed negroes than in those who are ill-fed and thin; and they likewise acquire a larger size in the former than in the latter." They are not possessed of much sensibility, and are not the seat of any pain, except when they appear upon the soles of the feet, where they are confined and compressed by the hard and thickened cuticle: in that situation they render the act of walking extremely painful, or altogether impracticable. They never suppurate kindly, Dr. Winterbottom says, but gradually discharge a sordid glutinous fluid, which forms an ugly scab round the edges of the excrescence, and covers the upper part of it, when much elevated, with white sloughs. When they appear on any part of the body covered with hair, this gradually changes in its colour from black to white, independently of the white incrustation from the discharge. "It frequently falls off, and never grows again." They leave no depression of the skin.*

* The anonymous writer in the Edin. Med. Essays, and after him Dr. Hillary and others, have deemed the Frambœsia to be the Hebrew leprosy, described by Moses. (Leviticus, chap. xiii.) In some respects, and especially in the appearance of what is called "raw flesh," in the leprous spots, together with *whiteness of the hair*, the description of the leprosy of the Jews is applicable to the Yaws. But the leprosy is described by the great legislator as beginning in several ways, or appearing under several varieties of form, in only one of which this rising of "raw flesh" is mentioned: and the two circumstances, which all these varieties exhibited in common, were a depression of the skin, and whiteness of the hair. Now this change in the colour of the hair is common to the Frambœsia, and to the Leuce, as stated; and it is conjoined, in the latter, with cutaneous depression. It seems pretty obvious, indeed, that the term leprosy was used, in the Scriptures, to denote several diseases of the skin, against which the law of exclusion was enforced, and others, to which it did not apply. An instance of the latter occurs in Gehazi, whom we find still in the employment of Elisha, and even con-

The period, during which the eruption is in progress, varies from a few weeks to eight months. "When no more pustules are thrown out," Dr. Winterbottom observes, "and when those already upon the skin no longer increase in size, the disease is supposed to have reached its acme. About this time it happens, on some part of the body or other, that one of the pustules becomes much larger than the rest, equalling or surpassing the size of a half-crown piece : it assumes the appearance of an ulcer, and, instead of being elevated above the skin like others, it is considerably depressed ; the surface is foul and sloughy, and pours out an ill-conditioned ichor, which spreads very much, by corroding the surrounding sound skin : this is what is called the *master* or *mother-yaw ;*" *Mama-pian,* by the negroes. When arrived at its acme, however, the eruption continues a considerable time without undergoing much alteration, often without very materially injuring the functions; and it seldom proves dangerous, except from the mischievous interference of ill-directed art.*

The Frambœsia is propagated solely by the con-

---

versing with the king, after the leprosy had been inflicted upon him, " and his seed for ever." (2 Kings, chap. v. & vi. & chap. viii. ver. 4.)

Dr. Hibbert (Edin. Journ. of Med. Science, vol. i. p. 287.) has satisfactorily proved, that the *great Gore, Pox,* or *Morbus Gallicus* of the 15th century, was Frambœsia. The name Sibbens, by which it is known in Scotland, is a corruption of the Gaelic word Sivvens, wild rash. T.

* " All this time the patient is in good health, does not lose his appetite, and seems to have no other uneasiness but what the nastiness of the sores occasions," &c. Edin. Med. Essays, vol. v. p. 789. The fact is stated by Hillary in the same words, p. 343.

tagion of the matter, discharged from the eruption, when it is applied to the wounded or broken skin of another person, who has not previously undergone the disease. * "It may be communicated by using the same spoon, by kissing, and by coition when its seat is in the genital organs, in which case it is often mistaken for syphilis." Like the febrile eruptions, the Frambœsia affects the same person only once during life; but, unlike them, it is not propagated by effluvia. In Africa it is usually undergone during childhood. The period, which elapses between the reception of the contagion and the commencement of the disease, is nowhere mentioned: but in the case of a Dane, whom Dr. Adams saw at Madeira, the patient had been ten months absent from the West Indies before he felt any indisposition. †

With respect to the treatment of Frambœsia, nothing very satisfactory is to be collected from the writings of the practitioners to whom we are indebted for the history of the disease. The native Africans, according to Dr. Winterbottom, "never ttempt to cure it, until it has nearly reached its height, when the fungi have acquired their full size, and no more pustules appear." And the

* The complaint is sometimes inoculated by flies, in those hot countries where the skin both of the diseased and the healthy remains uncovered. Hence, Dr. Bancroft says, "none ever receive it whose skins are whole; for which reason the whites are rarely infected; but the backs of the negroes being often raw by whipping, and suffered to remain naked, they scarcely ever escape it." Nat. Hist. of Guiana, p. 385. See also Winterbottom, pp. 141—143.

† See Memoirs of the Med. Soc. of London.

practitioners in the West Indies soon learned, by
experience, that active evacuations retard the natural progress of the disease; and that mercurials,
although they suspended it, and cleared the skin
of the eruption, yet left the patient still susceptible of, or rather still impregnated with the virus,
which speedily evinced its presence, by a reappear-
ance of the symptoms more severe and tedious
than before.   In truth, the disease, it would seem,
like the pustular and exanthematous fevers of our
own climate, will only leave the constitution, after
it has completed the various stages of its course,
and removed the susceptibility of the individual to
future infection; and no medicine, yet discovered,
has had any influence in superseding this action,
or in accelerating its progress.   Unless, therefore,
any urgent symptoms should require alleviation
(which seldom, if ever, happens), it is advisable to
dispense with the administration of medicine, and
to be content with restricting the patient to a moderate and temperate regimen, during the first
stage of the malady. *   When the eruptions begin
to dry, or as soon as they cease to multiply and
enlarge, the disease appears to require the same
management as other slow and superficial ulcerations, accompanied with a cachectic state of the

---

* The anonymous writer in the Edin. Essays recommends the following bolus every night until the yaws are at their height.
    ℞ Florum Sulphuris Ðj
       Camphoræ gr. v.
       Theriacæ Andromachi ʒj
       Syrupi Croci q. s. ft. bolus, q. q. nocte horâ somni sumendus, T.

system; viz. a light, but nutritious diet, a dry and wholesome air, warm clothing, moderate exercise, and a course of tonic medicine, especially of Sarsaparilla, or Cinchona, with the mineral acids, or with Antimonials and small doses of Mercury, according to the circumstances of the individual habit. The effects of Mercury, however, exhibited so as to excite salivation, * as the early West Indian practitioners recommend, seem to be of a very questionable nature, especially when it is unaccompanied by the vegetable decoctions; and it is certain that patients have, in some cases, soon recovered under the use of the latter, when the mercurials were omitted.† The native Africans employ decoctions of the bark of two or three trees, which are gently purgative, as well as tonic, and likewise wash the sores with them, after carefully removing the crusts. ‡

* This treatment is often followed by a train of harassing symptoms, called by the negroes the *bone-ach*. "The unhappy sufferer is tormented with deep-seated pains in the bones, especially round the joints, which are occasionally aggravated to a violent degree; the periosteum becomes thickened, inflamed, and painful, and nodes are formed on the bones. When these symptoms have continued for some time, the bones are affected with caries, and even become soft and lose their form."

† See Dr. Winterbottom's "Account," &c. vol. ii. pp. 158, 59; and Schilling, De Frambœsia, quoted by him.

‡ In a very short but able account of this disease, which I lately saw in MS., the mercurial treatment was said not only to be unsuccessful, but to aggravate the affection of the skin; and much advantage was ascribed to strong decoctions of the woods of Vervain, wild Senna, &c. when the scabs began to fall off; and to the frequent ablution of the diseased parts with warm water, and to the use of lime-water as a drink previously. These decoctions were also found to relieve "the small eruption, bone-ach, and joint-evil often consequent on the bad treatment, or mere palliation," by Mercury.

The *master-yaw* sometimes remains large and troublesome, after the rest of the eruption has altogether disappeared. It requires to be treated with gentle escharotics, and soon assumes a healing appearance under these applications. Paring off the cuticle, and the stronger caustics are requisite for the cure of the *crab-yaws*, or tedious excrescences, which occur on the soles of the feet.

Order VIII.

MACULÆ.

THIS Order comprises those discolorations of the skin which are permanent, and most of which are the result of an alteration of the natural texture of the part. It comprehends, therefore, several varieties of connate and acquired disfigurations of the skin, some of which are not capable of being removed, and most of them are removable only by surgical means. The various maculæ, that have been described in medical and surgical writings, are included under the terms EPHELIS, NÆVUS, SPILUS, and moles, with other appellations applied to the more anomalous appearances.

GENUS I. EPHELIS.

Syn. Ephelis à sole (*Sauv.*): Nigredo à sole (*Sennert*): Epichrosis Ephelis (*Good*): Sommers-prose; die Leberflecke (*German*): Hâle (*F.*): *Sun Burn.*

Def. THE CUTICLE SPOTTED WITH DARK FREC-KLES, CONFLUENT OF CORYMBOSE ; DISAPPEARING IN THE WINTER.

The term EPHELIS denotes not only the *freckles,* or little yellow *lentigines,* which appear on persons

of fair skin, and the larger brown patches, which
likewise arise from exposure to the direct rays of
the sun, as the name imports ; but also those large
dusky patches, which are very similar in appearance, but occur on other parts of the surface, which
are constantly covered.* (Plate LXIX. of BATEMAN.)
Lory and some other writers have endeavoured
to make distinctions between Lentigines and Ephelides; but there does not appear to be any essential difference between them, and all the ancient
writers have properly treated of them together.†

The larger Ephelides, especially those which
occur on the sides, abdomen, and other covered
parts, sometimes differ little from the Pityriasis
versicolor, or actually degenerate into it; the cuticle becoming rough with minute furfuraceous
scales. The brief description of the Ephelis given
by Celsus is, indeed, equally applicable to both.
" Nihil est nisi asperitas quædam, et durities, mali

---

* " Nomen inditum απο τs ηλιs, non quod à sole tantum vitia illa in
cute contrahuntur, sed quod à reliquis inducta causis, similem asperita-
tem et colorem habeant." Gorræi Defin. ad voc. εφηλιν.—This acceptation of the term is sanctioned by the authority of Hippocrates, who
gives the same appellation to the spots which sometimes occur in pregnant women, and to those occasioned by the solar rays. " Quæ utero
gerunt in facie maculam habent, quam εφηλιν vocant."—Lib. Περι αφορων.
Also Περι γυναικειων, lib. ii. Sauvages has improperly classed with Ephelis
the mottled and dusky red hue of the shins of those who expose their
legs constantly to strong fires in the winter; and also the livid patches
of scurvy which arise from extravasation of blood under the cuticle.
Nosol. Meth. class. i. gen. iii. spec. 4. & 6.—See also Plenck de Morb.
Cut. class. i. spec. 2.; and Plater has, by an extraordinary mistake, called
the pustules of Scabies Ephelides. De Superfic. Corp. Dolore, cap. 17.

† See Oribas. de Loc. Affect. Cur. lib. iv. cap. 52., and Synops. viii.
35.—Aëtius, tetr. ii. serm. iv. cap. 11.—Actuar. Meth. Med. iv. cap. 13.

coloris." *   I have occasionally known the dingy
hue of these maculæ, as well as of the patches
of Pityriasis, give rise to a suspicion of syphilitic
infection.   But independently of the history of the
previous symptoms, the paucity of these patches,
their want of elevation or depression, their perma-
nency, and their final evanescence, without any
tendency to ulceration, or even to inflammation,
will enable those, whom a habit of inspecting such
appearances has not sufficiently instructed, to discriminate them.

Celsus apologizes, as has been already observed,
for prescribing the treatment of Ephelides and
freckles, and such trifling discolorations of the
skin ; and the same apology must still be urged:
" eripi tamen fœminis cura cultus sui non potest."
The uniform practice both of ancient and modern
authors has been to apply some gentle astringent
and discutient lotion or liniment to the parts affected. † From the time of Hippocrates, bitter almonds
have been recommended as possessed of such
discutient properties. ‡ They have probably no
virtues, " except those of a sedative nature," which

---

* De Medicina, lib. vi. cap. 5. — M. Alibert has thought the common
freckle and the larger Ephelis worthy of two beautiful engravings ; the
former, in plate 26, is called " Ephelide lentiforme ;" and the latter, in
plate 27, " Ephelide hepatique."

† In the remedies adapted to all these superficial and cuticular discolorations, according to Oribasius, " mediocri adstrictione et abster-
sione opus est." Synops. lib. viii. cap. 33. The same observation is
stated from Crito, by Aëtius, tetr. ii. serm. iv. cap. 11. See also Actuarius, Meth. Med. lib. iv. cap. 13.

‡ Hippoc. Περι γυναικειων, lib. ii. Oribasius says, " Amygdalæ amaræ
sunt facultatis perspicuè attenuantis, ut ephelin expurgent." De Virtute
Simplic. lib. ii. cap. i.

are not possessed by the ptisan, decoctions of Tares, and some other mucilaginous and detergent applications, recommended by the same authors. Some gentle restringent or stimulant is commonly advised, however, by these writers. Celsus employed resin, with a third part of fossil salt, and a little honey;—and Actuarius combined vinegar, honey, and bitter almonds, for the same purpose. * Wine was likewise recommended as a vehicle for these and other substances. " Geoffroy praises a combination of bullock's gall, and solution of Potassa (Oleum tartari per deliquium et aqua.)" † Solutions of White Vitriol and precipitated Sulphur have also been used.

The principle of these applications was correct but it may be pursued in a more simple and effectual manner by lotions of Alcohol, in its pure state or diluted with some distilled water, " or with the addition of a few drops of Hydrocyanic acid," if the skin be irritable;—by dabbing the spots two or three times a day with the diluted mineral acids, in the proportion of about a drachm of the strong Sulphuric Acid to a pint of water, or the same quantity of Muriatic Acid to half a pint; by using, in a similar manner, the Liquor Potassæ diluted with about twenty times its quantity of water; " or, a solution of Perchloride of Mercury (*Corrosive Sub-*

* Celsus, loc. cit.—Actuarius, loc. cit.—Dr. Withering recommend an infusion of horseradish in milk, as a cosmetic. See his Botan. Arrang. of Brit. Plants. Of these cosmetic lotions, however, we may say with Celsus, " pene ineptiæ sunt."

† Mém. de l'Acad. des Sciences.

limate), in the emulsion of bitter almonds, in the proportion of one grain of the salt and six fluid ounces of the emulsion."

GENUS II. NÆVUS, &c.

Syn. Maculæ Maternæ; Nævi, Spili (*Auct. var.*): Metrocelis (*Good*): Khal (*Arab.*): Bak (*Turc.*): Envie; Tache congénitale (*F.*): die Muttermahle (*German*): *Mother Spots.*

Def. CONGENITAL SPOTS AND DISCOLORATIONS OF THE SKIN.

The various congenital excrescences and discolorations of the skin, to which the appellations of Nævus, Spilus, moles, &c. have been applied, may be conveniently treated of together. They exhibit many peculiarities of form, magnitude, colour, and structure, and are seen on almost every part of the surface of the body in different instances. Some of them are merely superficial, or stain-like spots, and appear to consist of a partial thickening of the rete mucosum, sometimes of a yellow, or yellowish-brown, sometimes of a bluish, livid, or nearly black colour. To these the term Spilus* has been more particularly appropri-

---

* Σπιλος, *macula.* This discoloration seems to be included by Sauvages under his first species, Nævus *sigillum*, and by Plenck, under N. *lenticularis*, spec. i. of his Arrangement. See Sauvages, Nos. Meth. class. 1. gen. 4.; Plenck, Doctrina de Morb. Cutan. p. 37.

ated. Others again exhibit various degrees of thickening, elevation, and altered structure of the skin itself*, and consist of clusters of enlarged and contorted veins, freely anastomosing, and forming little sacs of blood. These are sometimes spread more or less extensively over the surface, occasionally covering even the whole of an extremity, or one-half of the trunk of the body; and sometimes they are elevated into prominences of various form and magnitude. Occasionally these marks are nearly of the usual colour of the skin; but most commonly they are of a purplish red colour, of varying degrees of intensity, such as the presence of a considerable collection of blood-vessels, situated near the surface, and covered with a thin cuticle, naturally occasions.

The origin, which was anciently assigned to these marks by physicians, and to which they are still ascribed by the vulgar (*viz.* the influence of the imagination of the mother upon the child in utero), has occasioned their varieties to be compared with the different objects of desire or aversion, which were supposed to operate on the passions of the mother: whence the following Nævi have been described. The flat and purple stains were considered as the representative of claret, or of port wine (Plate LXXI. Fig. 1. of BATEMAN)†; and

---

* Sauvages comprehends all these excrescences under Nævus *maternus*, spec. 2.; and Plenck under his four remaining species, N. *flammeus, tuberculosus, cavernosus,* and *malignus.*

† Nævus flammeus (*Plenck*): Fevermahl (*German*).

sometimes of a slice of bacon, or other flesh. Sometimes the stains are regularly formed, like a leaf,
with a very red border, and lines, like veins, across
from a central rib, forming the Nævus *foliaceus*
(Plate LXX. of BATEMAN); and sometimes a small
red centre with branching lines, like legs, has suggested the idea of a spider, or N. *araneus* * (Plate
LXXI. Fig. 2. of BATEMAN). But those Nævi
which are prominent have most commonly been
compared to different species of fruit, especially
to cherries, currants, and grapes, when the surface
is smooth and polished; or to mulberries, raspberries, and strawberries, when the surface is granulated: whence the Nævus *cerasus* (Plate LXXI.
Fig. 1. of BATEMAN), *ribes, morus, rubus, fragarius,*
&c. † (Plate LXXII. of BATEMAN).

Some of these excrescences are raised upon a
neck or pedicle; while some are sessile upon a
broad base. Some of them again, although vivid
for some time after birth, gradually fade and disappear: some remain stationary through life, but
commonly vary in intensity of colour at different
seasons and under circumstances easily explained;
and others begin to grow and extend, sometimes
immediately after birth, and sometimes from incidental causes at a subsequent period, and from small
beginnings become large and formidable bloody
tumours, readily bursting, and pouring out impe-

* See the Plate of Bateman, fig. 8. *x*.
† See Bierling Adversaria Curios. obs. ix. — Valentin. Prax. Med.
Infallib. cap. 1. — Strobelberger de Curand. pueril. Affect. cap. 17. —
Septaliûs de Nævis.

tuous and alarming hæmorrhages, which, if they do not prove suddenly fatal, materially injure the health by the frequent depletion of the system.*
Sometimes, however, after having increased to a certain degree, they cease to enlarge, and thenceforth continue stationary, or gradually diminish, till scarcely any vestige remains. †

In some instances, however, these preternatural enlargements and anastomoses, which constitute the Nævi, are not merely cutaneous.   A similar mor-

---

* A most striking case of this kind came under the notice of the Editor about ten years since. The little patient was born without any apparent mark upon the body, nor did any appear for eight days after birth, when a small point, resembling a red minute tubercle, appeared on the forehead, and gradually increased to the size of a crown-piece, when it was showed to the Editor. This spot was surrounded by many small points, at different distances from the main spot; and these gradually enlarging ran into one another, forming larger spots; which again in turn coalesced with others, until they finally were added, as their diameters increased, to the main spot. (ATLAS, pl. xxv.) The extent which the whole occupied, and the eye being also involved in the disease, prevented extirpation from being proposed or attempted; and the only curative measure resorted to was an effort to obliterate the Nævus, by exciting ulceration in various parts of it. This partially succeeded; but, before the plan had advanced beyond the second sore, the child was attacked with Hydrocephalus and died. A post mortem examination explained satisfactorily the nature of the disease. The arterial system was natural, but the venous was so thin in the coats of the vessels, that there was not sufficient power to return the blood, which of course accumulated in the veins; and those in the vicinity gradually assumed the same diseased state. The most remarkable part of the case, and on account of which it is mentioned in this place, was the extension of the disease to the bones of the cranium. The Editor is not aware of any case of a similar kind being on record: the scull-cap is in the Museum of Anatomy of Dr. Alexander Monro, of Edinburgh, to whom the Editor presented it; and an accurate engraving of it will be found in the Atlas of Plates attached to this edition of the Synopsis. T.

† See Mr. Abernethy's Surgical Works, vol. ii. p. 224. et seq.

bid structure may take place in other parts: it sometimes occupies the whole substance of the cheek, according to Mr. Abernethy, and has occurred in the orbit of the eye; and Mr. John Bell affirms, that it affects indifferently all parts of the body, even the viscera. *

The origin of these connate deformities is equally inexplicable with that of other anomalous and monstrous productions of nature; but it would be insulting the understanding of the reader to waste one word in refutation of the vulgar hypothesis, which ascribes them to the mental emotions of the mother; an hypothesis totally irreconcilable with the established principles of physiology, and with the demonstrable nature of the connection between the fœtus and the parent, as well as with all sober observation.

It is important, however, to know, that very slight causes of irritation, such as a trifling bruise, or a tight hat, will sometimes excite a mere stain-like speck, or a minute livid tubercle, into that diseased action, which occasions its growth. This growth is carried on by a kind of inflammatory action of the surrounding arteries; and the vary-

* The ordinary Nævi appear to consist of *venous* anastomoses only: but some of them, even when congenital, are of that species of morbid structure which Mr. John Bell has denominated " aneurism by anastomosis," and which, he says, is made up of " a congeries of small and active arteries, absorbing veins, and intermediate cells," somewhat analogous to the structure of the placenta, or of the gills of a turkey-cock. See his Principles of Surgery, vol. i. discourse xi.; also Mr. Abernethy's Surg. Works, loc. cit.

ing intensity of colour arises from the different
degrees of activity in the circulation. Thus these
marks are of a more vivid red in the spring and
summer, not in sympathy with the ripening fruit,
but from the more copious determination of blood
to the skin, in consequence of the increase of the atmospheric temperature. The same increased determination to the surface is also produced tempo-
rarily, and, with it, a temporary augmentation of
the florid colour of the Nævi, by other causes of
excitement to the circulation; as by active exercise,
by heated rooms, or the warmth of the bed, by
drinking strong liquors, or high feeding, by emotions of the mind, and, in women, by the erethism
of menstruation.

These considerations will serve to suggest the
proper means of treating the Nævi and Spili, where
any treatment is advisable. When they are merely
superficial, without elevation, which would render
them liable to accidental rupture, and without any
tendency to enlarge and spread, there appears to
be no good reason for interfering with them. The
applications mentioned by the older writers were
doubtless as futile as they were disgusting; such as
saliva, the meconium of infants, the lochial blood
of women, the hand of a corpse, &c.: and the
severe resource of the knife, even if the deformity
of a scar were much less than that of the original
mark, is scarcely to be recommended.

But when the Nævi evince a tendency to enlarge,
or are very prominent excrescences, and either

troublesome from their situation *, or liable to be ruptured, some active treatment will then be required. Either their growth must be repressed by sedative applications, or the whole morbid congeries of vessels must be extirpated by the knife. " The latter is the only certain plan of cure. It has been recommended to inclose them with a ligature under the skin ; and thus cutting off their supply of blood, destroy their growth; and where they are sufficiently early attended to, no plan is better : but if more advanced, there is no security but in the complete extirpation, by dissection, of the diseased part."

All strong stimulants externally must be avoided, as they are liable to produce severe inflammation, and even constitutional disorder.

The consideration of the mode in which these vascular excrescences grow, by a degree of inflammatory action in the surrounding vessels, suggested to Mr. Abernethy the propriety of maintaining a constant sedative influence upon those vessels, by the steady application of cold, by means of folded linen kept constantly wet. This practice has succeeded, in several instances, in repressing the growth of these unnatural structures, which have afterwards shrunk, and disappeared, or ceased to be objects of any importance. — Pressure may, in some instances, be combined with this sedative

---

* A *cherry-nævus* on the lip, for instance, has prevented the act of sucking.

application, and contribute to diminish the dilatation of the vessels. " I have seen Nævi under parts of the dress, which exerted a constant pressure upon them, completely obliterated by this means ; " but in the majority of cases, pressure is the source of great irritation to these maculæ, and cannot be employed. — The temporary enlargement of these prominent Nævi by every species of general excitement, would teach us to enjoin moderation in diet, exercise, &c. during the attempts to subdue them.

The mode of extirpation is within the province of the surgeon ; and the proper choice of the mode, under the different circumstances, is directed in surgical books. From the days of Fabricius Hildanus[*], the propriety of radically removing every part of the diseased tissue of vessels has been inculcated : " and where there is any doubt of this having been effected, the bottom of the wound should be rubbed with Nitrate of Silver, or some other escharotic ; " but Mr. John Bell has most satisfactorily stated the grounds of that precept, by explaining the structure of these excrescences, as well as the source of the failure and danger, when they are only cut into or opened by caustic. I shall, therefore, refer the reader to his " Discourse," already quoted.

The varieties of Spilus, or mere thickening and discoloration of the rete mucosum, are sometimes removable by stimulant and restringent applications.

---

[*] Fab. Hild. Oper. cent. v. obs. 46.

A combination of lime and soap is extolled by several writers: and lotions of strong spirit, with the Liquor Potassæ, as recommended for the treatment of the Ephelides and of Pityriasis, certainly sometimes remove these maculæ.

With respect to those brown maculæ, commonly called *Moles*, I have little to observe: for no advantage is obtained by any kind of treatment. It is scarcely safe, indeed, to interfere with them: for when suppuration is induced in them, it is always tedious, and painful, the matter emitting at the commencement an extremely fetid odour. When moles are irritated by accident, or rudely treated, so as to produce excoriation, they are liable, it is said, to become gangrenous, and thus to produce sudden fatality.

Moles are not always congenital. I lately saw an instance in a lady of remarkably fair and delicate skin, where a numerous crop of small moles appeared, in slow succession, upon the arms and neck. Congenital moles, indeed, are not always stationary; but they sometimes enlarge, gradually, for a time, and afterwards disappear.

INDEX.

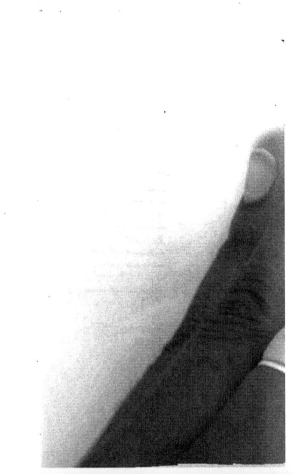

INDEX.

H H

INDEX.

INDEX.

THE END.

LONDON:
Printed by A. & R. Spottiswoode,
New-Street-Square.

Lightning Source UK Ltd.
Milton Keynes UK
UKOW05f2332200716

278899UK00011B/478/P